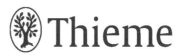

Optical Coherence Tomography in Glaucoma

Jullia A. Rosdahl, MD, PhD
Associate Professor of Ophthalmology
Department of Ophthalmology
Duke University School of Medicine
Durham, North Carolina, USA

214 illustrations

Thieme
New York • Stuttgart • Delhi • Rio de Janeiro

Library of Congress Cataloging-in-Publication Data is available from the publisher.

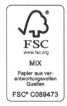

© 2022 Thieme. All rights reserved.

Thieme Medical Publishers, Inc.
333 Seventh Avenue, 18th Floor,
New York, NY 10001, USA
www.thieme.com
+1 800 782 3488, customerservice@thieme.com

Cover design: © Thieme
Cover images source: © Ryan McNabb
Typesetting by DiTech Process Solutions, India

Printed in Germany by Beltz Grafische Betriebe

5 4 3 2 1

ISBN: 978-1-68420-247-8

Also available as an e-book:
eISBN 978-1-68420-248-5

To my husband Joe and my children Brian and Katie.

To the medical students, residents, fellows, colleagues, and patients who inspire, delight, and teach me every day.

Jullia A. Rosdahl, MD, PhD

Contents

11.   Special Considerations: High Refractive Errors 152

Ki Ho Park and Yong Woo Kim

12.   Future Directions: Optical Coherence Tomography Angiography for Glaucoma 165

Darrell WuDunn

Preface

Every time I look at an optical coherence tomography (OCT) image, I am struck by the detail and I marvel at our ability to see neuronal layers in vivo and in such a way that it can impact people's vision, and really their lives. What a tool we have, and what a privilege to assemble a book on OCT for glaucoma with experts and leaders in glaucoma care.

I remember the first time I saw an OCT image, as a resident at the Massachusetts Eye and Ear Infirmary in Boston; it was a time-domain image, quite hazy by today's spectral domain standards, and Dr Simmons Lessell was sharing his amazement at the technology. Dr Teresa C. Chen, one of the contributors to this book, was doing seminal work on OCT and other computerized imaging modalities; she was my clinical mentor when I was a resident. Boston, Massachusetts, as described by Dr Joel S. Schuman, is really the birthplace of OCT, and I love his chapter describing its inception and history. My personal appreciation for OCT truly developed during my glaucoma fellowship at the Duke Eye Center; the Duke Glaucoma Service is filled to the brim with outstanding teachers, but Dr Sanjay Asrani was and continues to be our OCT champion.

The importance and power of OCT in glaucoma care is really a global endeavor, with almost 10,000 citations on PubMed for "OCT Glaucoma" at the writing of this book. Our goal with this book is to provide a practical guide, especially for trainees and doctors new to glaucoma, but with pearls, examples, and novel topics such that even those who are more experienced would deepen their knowledge. With this in mind, I reached out to colleagues who had the expertise and skill, people I knew personally such as Drs Teresa C. Chen and Felipe A. Medeiros, and people I knew only by reputation such as Dr Ki Ho Park; thankfully for all of us, all of the contributors kindly agreed. It has been such a privilege and delight to include their work in this book, including the cover image from Ryan McNabb, PhD, and Anthony Kuo, MD, at the Duke Eye Center. I have learned so much by bringing this book to you, and I hope that you find it most useful in caring for your patients.

Jullia A. Rosdahl, MD, PhD

Acknowledgments

We wish to acknowledge all who have made this book possible, from the editorial team at Thieme, who provided the opportunity to create this book and have so kindly shepherded the process, to those teachers and clinicians and colleagues who have taught us what we know about optical coherence tomography. Most importantly, though, we are grateful to our patients, who allow us into their lives and eyes and who are the reason we wrote this book and the reason our readers are reading it, in the hopes of making those lives and eyes better.

Jullia A. Rosdahl, MD, PhD

Contributors

Ahmad A. Aref, MD, MBA
Associate Professor and Vice-Chair for Clinical
  Affairs
University of Illinois at Chicago College of
  Medicine
Illinois Eye & Ear Infirmary
Chicago, Illinois, USA

Teresa C. Chen, MD
Associate Professor and Senior Scientist
Massachusetts Eye and Ear Infirmary
Harvard Medical School
Boston, Massachusetts, USA

Ian Conner, MD, PhD
Assistant Professor
Department of Ophthalmology
University of Pittsburgh School of Medicine
Pittsburgh, Pennsylvania, USA

Elizabeth Ann Zane Cretara, MD
Assistant Professor of Ophthalmology
University of New Mexico
Albuquerque, New Mexico, USA

Rachel A. Downes, MD
Department of Ophthalmology
New York University (NYU) Grossman School of
  Medicine
New York, New York, USA

Mays A. El-Dairi, MD
Associate Professor
Department of Ophthalmology
Duke University School of Medicine
Durham, North Carolina, USA

Sharon F. Freedman, MD
Professor
Departments of Ophthalmology and Pediatrics
Duke University School of Medicine
Durham, North Carolina, USA

Lawrence S. Geyman, MD
University of Illinois at Chicago College of
  Medicine
Illinois Eye & Ear Infirmary
Chicago, Illinois, USA

Tanya S. Glaser, MD
Assistant Professor
Department of Ophthalmology
Duke University School of Medicine
Durham, North Carolina, USA

Divakar Gupta, MD, MMCi
Assistant Professor
Department of Ophthalmology
Duke University School of Medicine
Durham, North Carolina, USA

Ying Han, MD, PhD
Professor of Ophthalmology
Department of Ophthalmology
University of California at San Francisco
San Francisco, California, USA

Michael P. Kelly, FOPS
Department of Ophthalmology
Duke University School of Medicine
Durham, North Carolina, USA

Yong Woo Kim, MD, PhD
Assistant Professor
Department of Ophthalmology
Seoul National University Hospital (SNUH)
Seoul, South Korea

Catherine M. Marando, MD
Massachusetts Eye and Ear Infirmary
Harvard Medical School
Boston, Massachusetts, USA

Felipe A. Medeiros, MD, PhD
Joseph AC Wadsworth Distinguished Professor
of Ophthalmology
Professor of Electrical and Computer
Engineering
Duke University School of Medicine
Durham, North Carolina, USA

Julius Oatts, MD, MHS
Assistant Professor
Department of Ophthalmology
University of California at San Francisco
San Francisco, California, USA

Elli Park, MD
Boston University School of Medicine
Boston, Massachusetts, USA

Ki Ho Park, MD, PhD
Professor and Chair
Department of Ophthalmology
Seoul National University Hospital (SNUH)
Seoul, South Korea

Jullia A. Rosdahl, MD, PhD
Associate Professor of Ophthalmology
Department of Ophthalmology
Duke University School of Medicine
Durham, North Carolina, USA

Joel S. Schuman, MD, FACS
Elaine Langone Professor & Vice Chair for
Ophthalmology Research
NYU Langone Health, NYU Grossman School of
Medicine
New York, New York, USA

Hana L. Takusagawa, MD
Affiliate Associate Professor of Ophthalmology
Oregon Health & Science University, and
Eugene VA Health Care Center
Eugene, Oregon, USA

Atalie Carina Thompson, MD, MPH
Assistant Professor
Department of Ophthalmology
Wake Forest School of Medicine
Winston-Salem, North Carolina, USA

Andrew Williams, MD
Assistant Professor
Department of Ophthalmology
University of Pittsburgh School of Medicine
Pittsburgh, Pennsylvania, USA

Darrell WuDunn, MD, PhD
Professor and Chair
Department of Ophthalmology
University of Florida College of Medicine –
Jacksonville
Jacksonville, Florida, USA

1 Introduction: Practical Guide, OCT for Glaucoma

Jullia A. Rosdahl

Summary

This is an introduction with a reader's guide for our book on optical coherence tomography (OCT) for glaucoma. OCT is an invaluable tool for the diagnosis and management of glaucoma. This textbook provides a practical guide for the use of OCT in the clinical care of glaucoma patients: Including background on the development of OCT; in-depth descriptions of OCT of the optic nerve and retina in glaucoma patients, with chapters dedicated to illustrative case examples, artifacts, structure–function correlations, comparison of common devices, and anterior segment OCT; special considerations for OCT for childhood glaucomas and patients with high refractive errors; and future directions, namely, OCT angiography, swept-source OCT, and artificial intelligence. This introductory chapter also includes suggestions on how to use this guide depending on the reader's background and interests.

Keywords: optical coherence tomography, glaucoma, readers guide, optic nerve, retina, retinal nerve fiber layer

1.1 Introduction

Glaucoma is a group of eye diseases characterized by the loss of neural tissue at the optic nerve head, with "cupping" first visualized in the 1800s with Dr Helmholtz' ophthalmoscope, and the associated loss of peripheral vision. Over the last several decades, advances in computerized imaging have enabled doctors to visualize and quantify the optic nerve tissue to an astounding degree. In the 2000s, optical coherence tomography (OCT) became an integral part of the care of glaucoma patients, from screening glaucoma suspects, to the diagnosis of glaucoma, and for following patients with glaucoma to assess for progression of the disease.

The purpose of this guide is to serve as both a reference for understanding how OCT is used for the diagnosis and treatment of glaucoma, as well as a practical guide for "everyday" use to help doctors use this technology with greater skill and confidence.

1.2 Overview of the Guide

Summaries of each chapter provide an overview of the guide.

1.2.1 Development of OCT

OCT is a now a fixture in eye clinics around the world but only came to exist less than 30 years ago. Following decades of research on how evolving laser technologies could have clinical applications, in 1991 the first OCT captured an image of the eye. The history of OCT research and development is discussed by summarizing the science, sharing insights on the economic risks and successes, and highlighting clinical impacts.[1]

1.2.2 OCT of the Optic Nerve

Assessing the optic nerve is critical in the evaluation of glaucoma patients. Computerized imaging technologies such as OCT provide quantitative measurements of optic nerve head parameters, including the retinal nerve fiber layer (RNFL). A systematic approach to OCT interpretation is discussed, including attention to potential limitations and artifacts.[2]

1.2.3 OCT of the Macula

Retinal imaging of the macula, with attention to the retinal ganglion cell layer, inner plexiform layer, and nerve fiber layer, can supplement the information obtained with the peripapillary RNFL. Applications of macular imaging for glaucoma, advantages and disadvantages, and pitfalls to avoid are discussed.[3]

1.2.4 Illustrative Case Examples

Case examples illustrate the use of OCT in glaucoma diagnosis and management. Cases spanning the spectrum of glaucoma severity are discussed, from glaucoma suspect, early to advanced glaucoma, as well as examples of glaucomatous progression. Characteristic findings from other chapters (3, 4, 6, and 7 in particular) are reinforced.[4]

1.2.5 Structure–Function Relationship

The relationship between structure and function of the optic nerve is the basis of our pathophysiological understanding of glaucoma. This chapter describes structure–function mapping, the temporal relationship between structural damage and functional defects, and how structural changes are linked to functional changes in glaucoma.[5]

1.2.6 Comparison of Common Devices

OCT devices produced by several manufacturers are available for clinical use. Differences in imaging specifications, analysis techniques, normative databases, and diagnostic capabilities are discussed for the Cirrus 6000 (Carl Zeiss Meditec AG, Jena, Germany), Spectralis (Heidelberg Engineering GmbH, Heidelberg, Germany), Avanti RTVue XR (Optovue, Inc., Fremont, CA, USA), and 3D OCT (Topcon Corporation, Tokyo, Japan).[6]

1.2.7 Artifacts and Masqueraders

All OCT machines have artifacts. Critical assessment for artifacts and attention to ocular pathology unrelated to glaucoma are discussed, with relevant clinical examples of "red" and "green" "OCT diseases" and future directions.[7]

1.2.8 Anterior Segment OCT in Glaucoma

OCT of the anterior segment provides noninvasive, high-resolution, cross-sectional images of the anterior segment structures. This technology can provide a useful supplement for the diagnosis and management of glaucomas, particularly primary angle closure disease.[8]

1.2.9 Special Considerations: OCT in Childhood Glaucoma

OCT is an important tool for the management of childhood glaucoma, especially since children with glaucoma may not be able to perform visual field testing. Special considerations for the use of OCT in children are discussed, including how to acquire OCT images and suggestions for interpreting OCT images from pediatric eyes.[9]

1.2.10 Special Considerations: High Refractive Errors

Special care should be taken when interpreting OCT scans in eyes with high refractive errors, given the rising prevalence of myopia and that myopia is a risk factor for glaucoma. Causes of OCT scan errors are discussed as well as newer parameters to improve the accuracy of glaucoma diagnosis in myopic eyes.[10]

1.2.11 Future Directions: OCT Angiography for Glaucoma

OCT angiography is an emerging technology giving detailed images of the microvasculature of the optic nerve and retina. Although its role in the diagnosis and management of glaucoma is still unclear, growing evidence shows good correlation between OCT angiography of the optic nerve and surrounding structures, and tissue loss and visual field loss from glaucoma.[11]

1.2.12 Future Directions: Swept-Source OCT for Glaucoma

Swept-source OCT is an emerging technology using a tunable, longer wave of light than spectral domain OCT, allowing for high resolution with improved range of depth and increased scan speed. How this new technology fits in the framework of clinical glaucoma care is not yet clear, but current research is investigating the role of swept-source OCT in imaging the optic nerve and macula, as well as the anterior segment and choroid, for glaucoma.[12]

1.2.13 Future Directions: Artificial Intelligence Applications

Artificial intelligence refers to the development of computer programs to automate tasks to mimic human behavior. Deep learning is a type of artificial intelligence and uses a neural network to learn from a training dataset; these algorithms can process complex data such as ophthalmic images. Although research is still needed to study the performance of deep learning algorithms in real-world settings, these algorithms can be trained to distinguish between eyes with glaucoma and control eyes on OCT.[13]

1.3 How to Use the Guide

Depending on the background of the reader, this book can be approached in a variety of ways. Certainly, it can be read starting from Chapter 2 through Chapter 14, as a comprehensive summary of how OCT can be used for the care of glaucoma patients, which is recommended for trainees and doctors new to OCT. Readers with some general knowledge and experience with OCT may find individual chapters to be more useful; and starting with Chapter 5 to review the Illustrative Cases may help to reveal knowledge gaps to be filled by the reading specific chapters. Readers with an already significant background in OCT will likely find the chapters on Anterior Segment OCT (Chapter 9), special considerations (Chapters 10 and 11), and future directions (Chapters 12, 13, and 14) most useful. Anyone with an interest in the history of medicine will find Chapter 2 to have unique insights into the development of this technology.

1.4 Conclusion

This book is designed to be a practical guide, summarizing the clinical utility of the OCT technology, covering the basics and more advanced analyses, common clinical scenarios as well as more rare situations such as pediatric cases and high refractive errors, and aspects of OCT that are on the cutting edge such as OCT angiography, swept-source OCT, and artificial intelligence. We hope this guide helps the reader to use OCT with greater skill and confidence to care for their patients with glaucoma.

References

[1] Schuman JS. Spectral domain optical coherence tomography for glaucoma (an AOS thesis). Trans Am Ophthalmol Soc. 2008; 106:426–458

[2] Gracitelli CPB, Abe RY, Tatham AJ, et al. Association between progressive retinal nerve fiber layer loss and longitudinal change in quality of life in glaucoma. JAMA Ophthalmol. 2015; 133(4):384–390

[3] Tan O, Chopra V, Lu AT, et al. Detection of macular ganglion cell loss in glaucoma by Fourier-domain optical coherence tomography. Ophthalmology. 2009; 116(12):2305–14.e1, 2

[4] American Academy of Ophthalmology Preferred Practice Patterns. Primary Open Angle Glaucoma PPP, November 2015. https://www.aao.org/preferred-practice-pattern/primary-open-angle-glaucoma-ppp-2015

[5] Medeiros FA, Zangwill LM, Bowd C, Mansouri K, Weinreb RN. The structure and function relationship in glaucoma: implications for detection of progression and measurement of rates of change. Invest Ophthalmol Vis Sci. 2012; 53 (11):6939–6946

[6] Aref AA, Rosdahl JA. Optical coherence tomography in glaucoma diagnosis. 2019 Focal Points Collection. Volume XXXVII, Number 11. American Academy of Ophthalmology; November 2019

[7] Chen TC, Hoguet A, Junk AK, et al. Spectral-domain OCT: helping the clinician diagnose glaucoma: a report by the American Academy of Ophthalmology. Ophthalmology. 2018; 125(11):1817–1827

[8] Leung CK, Weinreb RN. Anterior chamber angle imaging with optical coherence tomography. Eye (Lond). 2011; 25(3):261–267

[9] Hess DB, Asrani SG, Bhide MG, Enyedi LB, Stinnett SS, Freedman SF. Macular and retinal nerve fiber layer analysis of normal and glaucomatous eyes in children using optical coherence tomography. Am J Ophthalmol. 2005; 139(3):509–517

[10] Kim YW, Park KH. Diagnostic accuracy of three-dimensional neuroretinal rim thickness for differentiation of myopic glaucoma from myopia. Invest Ophthalmol Vis Sci. 2018; 59 (8):3655–3666

[11] Miguel AIM, Silva AB, Azevedo LF. Diagnostic performance of optical coherence tomography angiography in glaucoma: a systematic review and meta-analysis. Br J Ophthalmol. 2019; 103(11):1677–1684

[12] Takusagawa HL, Hoguet A, Junk AK, Nouri-Mahdavi K, Radhakrishnan S, Chen TC. Swept-source OCT for evaluating the lamina cribrosa: a report by the American Academy of Ophthalmology. Ophthalmology. 2019; 126(9):1315–1323

[13] Thompson AC, Jammal AA, Berchuck SI, Mariottoni EB, Medeiros FA. Assessment of a segmentation-free deep learning algorithm for diagnosing glaucoma from optical coherence tomography scans. JAMA Ophthalmol. 2020; 138 (4):333–339

2 Development of Optical Coherence Tomography

Joel S. Schuman and Rachel A. Downes

Summary

Optical coherence tomography (OCT), now a fixture in eye clinics around the world, was developed less 30 years ago. Following decades of research on potential clinical applications for evolving laser technologies, a prototype instrument captured the first OCT images in 1991. A mere 5 years later, a global medical device company launched the first commercial OCT instrument. OCT has since flourished, producing a strong return on investment for the governments and corporations that funded its creation and making an unmeasurable impact on patients' lives in not only ophthalmology but also in an array of other medical fields. OCT is the product of a resolute group of scientists, engineers, physicians, students, and businesspeople, and its story underscores the importance of persistence and collaboration. This chapter reviews the history of OCT research and development: briefly summarizing the relevant science, providing insight into the economic risks and ultimate successes of key players, and highlighting the profound impact on patient lives.

Keywords: OCT, optical coherence tomography, femtosecond laser, interferometry, Fourier transform, OCT-A, OCT-angiography

2.1 Introduction

Less than three decades have passed since the publication of the first optical coherence tomography (OCT) images of a retina.[1] In that time, OCT has evolved from a nascent technology with many skeptics to an integral component of eye care around the world. A 2011 publication estimated the global volume of OCT to be around 30 million ophthalmic images annually.[2] This figure was on par with the rate of magnetic resonance imaging (MRI) at the time.[2] Given that 9 years have passed since that analysis, and in light of the development of improved OCT technology and broadened applications of OCT in the interim, OCT volume is likely dramatically higher today. This chapter chronicles the development of OCT, providing context for its ascent and highlighting the individuals and ideas that made it possible (▶ Fig. 2.1).

2.2 Setting the Stage: Lasers Meet Medicine

2.2.1 Light in Flight

In 1971, Michael Duguay, then a researcher at AT&T Bell Laboratories, first proposed that the capture of echoes of light or "light in flight" could yield useful data about the composition of biological tissues.[3,4] With the use of a laser-activated Kerr shutter, he proposed a method of freezing the motion of light in order to noninvasively image tissues.[3,4] In the same year, Eric Ippen left Bell Labs for Massachusetts Institute of Technology (MIT; Cambridge, MA, USA) where doctoral student James Fujimoto soon joined him.[5] The pair and their collaborators began the hard work of developing a practical application for Duguay's theoretical proposal, and the work that would ultimately culminate in the invention of OCT began.[5]

By the 1980s, this group had their sights on skin and skin diseases as the first target for applying femtosecond laser technology to clinical medicine.[5] The researchers soon found that skin yielded a high degree of optical scattering in response to laser light and thus shifted their focus to the eye.[5] With transparent structures throughout its length —from cornea to lens to vitreous to retina—the eye proved to be the optimal test case for developing a practical medical application for capturing "light in flight."[5]

Ex vivo bovine and rabbit eyes were the subject of early work in this arena, and experiments on these animal models provided useful insights.[5] The earliest experiments utilized laser light with a wavelength of 625 nanometers (nm), resulting in scans with a sensitivity of −70 decibels (dB).[5] Later work would find that longer wavelengths were more effective in reducing attenuation from optical scattering, thus improving sensitivity.[5] For context, through this change among others, modern OCT machines have achieved three log units better sensitivity than those early scans.[5]

The original experiments sought to "see inside" of ophthalmic tissues through nonlinear cross-correlation, in which the instrument produced two beams of light: one directed at the tissue and one reference beam with a variable time delay.[5,6] By assessing the varying echo profiles and time delays of these beams (e.g., by analyzing and comparing

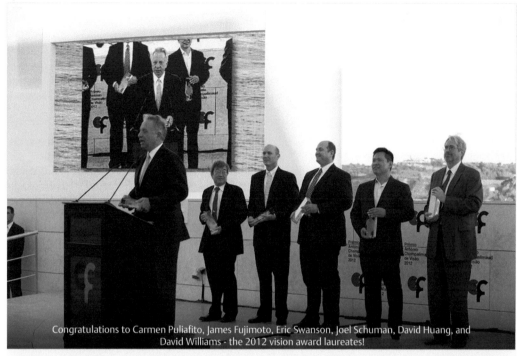

Congratulations to Carmen Puliafito, James Fujimoto, Eric Swanson, Joel Schuman, David Huang, and David Williams - the 2012 vision award laureates!

Fig. 2.1 Presentation of the António Champalimaud Vision Award in 2012 to James Fujimoto, David Huang, Carmen A. Puliafito, Joel S. Schuman, and Eric Swanson. Founded in 2005 in Lisbon, Portugal, the Champalimaud Foundation focuses on biomedical research and discovery with a central mission of improving the health and well-being of mankind. The Vision Award, first given in 2007, highlights contributions to the improvement and preservation of sight for people around the world. The Vision Award recognizes outstanding contributions to vision science in even-numbered years and exceptional work in alleviating visual problems, with a particular focus on developing nations, in odd-numbered years. In 2012, the inventors of optical coherence tomography (OCT) were honored in conjunction with David Williams, who was recognized for applying adaptive optics to the eye.

the backscattered and backreflected beams of light), the prototype devices produced inference patterns related to the structure of the tissue, culminating in the generation of an axial scan (A-scan).[5,6] As early as this initial work, there was a focus on applying the technology to assess pathological states.[5]

2.2.2 Interferometry

In the late 1980s, superluminescent diode interferometers replaced femtosecond lasers as the primary light source in OCT research.[5] Interferometry hastened the development of a feasible clinical product because it enabled the creation of instruments that were less expensive yet offered improved sensitivity.[5] Interferometry had its roots in the work of Sir Isaac Newton.[5,7] Its first real-world application was in the telecommunications industry, in which this technology improved the transmission of optical data.[5,7] Early OCT work

used Newton's classic technique of low-coherence or white-light interferometry.[7]

Interferometers worked by comparing an optical beam with a reference beam.[7] First, a laser source emitted a light, which a partially reflecting mirror called a beamsplitter divided into two perpendicular beams: one beam that would travel into the tissue of interest (e.g., the eye; this was the optical beam), and a reference beam.[7] A mirror at a known distance reflected the reference beam such that it traveled back to the beamsplitter at a known time delay (e.g., it served as a time reference).[7] At the beamsplitter, this reference beam interfered with the optical beam after it was backreflected and backscattered by the tissue.[7] Upon returning from the eye, the optical beam had multiple echoes resulting from the structural variations among the tissues within the eye.[7] In other words, intraocular structures had variable microscopic composition and were located at different distances from the light source such that each tissue type reflected and scattered the optical beam differently.[7] Thus, the variable echoes of light within the optical beam corresponded to microstructural nuances within the eye.[7] Ultimately, a detector compared the reflection and scattering of both beams, measuring the interference or correlation between them.[7] This method of time domain detection enabled ultrahigh-resolution time and distance measurements and eventually gave rise to the earliest commercial OCT instruments.[5,7]

Fercher and his collaborators at Medical University of Vienna (Vienna, Austria) published the first application of interferometry in medicine in 1988, measuring the axial length of *in vivo* human eyes; their results correlated with the acoustically measured axial lengths within 0.03 mm.[8] Despite its advantages in precision and speed, interferometry was not a practical medical tool.[5] Researchers and subjects struggled with its sensitivity to movement and vibration and the fact that bulk optics required very precise alignment in order to avoid signal loss.[5] In the US, John Apostolopoulous, then an undergraduate student at MIT, pioneered much of the early work in interferometry.[5] His experiments proposed a technique similar to nonlinear cross-correlation, but he substituted an inexpensive low-coherence diode laser for the femtosecond lasers used in the latter technique.[5] Apostolopoulous's experiments did not have sufficient sensitivity for generating scans of the eye, but he described a theoretical means for doing so in his unpublished 1989 bachelor's thesis.[5]

2.2.3 The Pivotal Role of Collaboration

The developers of OCT worked at an astonishingly fast pace to translate the "light in flight" principle to meaningful clinical impact. The diversity in background and level of training among those involved played a key role in facilitating this expeditious development. The team included a range of scientists from undergraduates like Apostolopoulous to senior principal investigators as well as the full spectrum of medical personnel from preresidency fellows to attending physicians.[5] In 1990, Eric Swanson, an engineer at MIT's Lincoln Laboratories, joined the mix.[5] In contrast to many academic enterprises, the emphasis of the work at Lincoln Labs is deeply pragmatic; there is a substantial focus on Department of Defense technology and advanced engineering with an emphasis on feasibility and implementation.[5] Swanson worked on intersatellite

optical communications and fiber optics networking.[5] Compared to the bulk optics previously used in interferometry, fiber optics mitigated alignment issues and enabled use in catheters or endoscopes.[5] The latter of these features enabled OCT development work in intravascular applications, including measurement of coronary artery plaques.[5] Swanson brought his content expertise and the Lincoln Labs implementation-oriented mindset to the OCT effort.[5] With the application of fiber optical elements and other contributions from Swanson, the feasibility of OCT improved dramatically: imaging speed became 100 times faster, the design became more compact (the prototype instrument that initially required a 1-square meter table could then sit on a platform just 19 inches wide), and the patient interface became more flexible.[5]

2.3 Optical Coherence Tomography: The Debut

2.3.1 OCT versus Ultrasound

Ultrasound (US) existed long before OCT, but both technologies hinged on strikingly similar principles. Whereas ultrasound generated images through the measurement of the time delay and intensity of backreflected and backscattered echoes of soundwaves, OCT sought to achieve the same with echoes of light waves.[7] Each technology had a set of advantages and drawbacks that made it most suitable for measurement of different biologic structures.[7] US required direct contact of the probe to the tissue it measured as well as the use of gel in order to couple the transmitter–receiver and the tissue, in order to transmit sound waves appropriately; OCT did not require physical coupling or the use of a coupling agent.[7] Although these features of US did not inhibit its application in imaging most structures of the body (e.g., intra-abdominal organs), they made it less attractive for imaging the fine structures of the eye.[7] US waves had a sufficiently low frequency to propagate to the deep structures of the body, but this came with the trade-off of poorer image resolution.[7] In contrast, the high frequency light waves emitted in OCT precluded penetration through most opaque biological tissues due to the high degree of scattering and absorption but could achieve much finer resolution.[7] This principle limited OCT's use to structures that were "optically accessible" (i.e., the optically clear components of the eye) and some structures in turbid media that could be accessed via catheters or endoscopes (e.g., coronary plaques).[7] Despite these drawbacks compared to US, OCT emerged as a superior technology for imaging of the eye's intricate microstructure, not only because an instrument that did not require contact with the eye was more tolerable for patients, but also because the use of shorter wavelength light permitted the collection of data that highlighted details as fine as the intricate layers of the retina with a much higher axial resolution than US.[7]

2.3.2 How OCT Works (▶ Fig. 2.2)

Starting from its earliest prototypes, OCT leveraged the intrinsic differences between tissues

within the eye to generate detailed images.[7] Various tissue-dependent phenomena occurred when the light beam from OCT instruments passed through the structures of the eye. For one, tissues could transmit light; that is, light could continue propagating into deeper tissue layers and structures, much like sound waves in US propagate from superficial skin, subcutaneous tissue, and fascia to the deep viscera.[7] Second, tissues could absorb light.[7] Tissues that absorbed light, such as those containing melanin or hemoglobin, effectively removed certain wavelengths from the beam.[7] This principle explained why the retinal pigment epithelium, a melanin-containing layer, appeared distinctly different in OCT images than

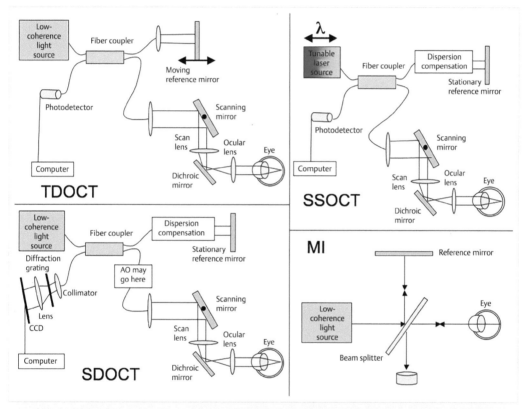

Fig. 2.2 Schematics of optical coherence tomography (OCT). Schematic diagrams are shown of time-domain OCT (TD-OCT), spectral domain OCT (SD-OCT), swept-source OCT (SS-OCT), and the original Michelson interferometer (MI) optical setup upon which OCT is based. A laser source emits a light which is divided into two perpendicular beams by a beamsplitter: one beam that travels into the eye (the optical beam) and the reference beam. A mirror at a known distance reflects the reference beam such that it travels back to the beamsplitter at a known time delay (a time reference). This reference beam interfers with the optical beam after it is backreflected and backscattered by the tissue. The returning optical beam has multiple echoes resulting from the structural variations among the tissues within the eye. The detector compares the reflection and scattering of both beams, measuring the interference or correlation between them. (*This figure is taken from an article entitled, "Spectral Domain Optical Coherence Tomography for Glaucoma (An AOS Thesis)" in the Trans Am Ophthalmol Soc 2008;106:426–458 and republished with permission of the American Ophthalmological Society.*)

2

microstructures that contained no or different pigments.[7] Third, tissues could reflect light back toward the receiver.[7] Reflection occurred at the borders of tissues or substances with different indices of refraction, such as at the air-corneal interface or vitreo-retinal interface.[7] Finally, tissues could scatter light; scattering occurred due to compositional variations within cells, often due to the presence of major intracellular components including nuclei and other organelles.[7] Because of this principle, OCT distinguished the layers of the retina that were composed of organelle-laden cell bodies from those that contained mostly axons; the composition of the latter included primarily cytoplasm and cell membranes with fewer organelles, thus resulting in a lesser degree of scattering when the incident beam met that layer.[7] Of note, when tissues scattered light, it propagated in multiple directions; the portion of that scattered light that propagated in the reverse direction of the incident beam was called backscattered light.[7] Since OCT instruments only detected light along the same axis as the incident beam, they only detected the backscattered portion of all scattered light.[7] Due to these principles, tissues with higher degrees of absorption appeared darker in OCT images, and those with a higher degree of scattering (and thus a more substantial amount of backscattered light) appeared brighter.[7]

These principles also explained why OCT was not optimal for imaging deep structures of the body.[7] Due to the strong absorption and scattering of light incident upon skin, the penetration of the beam was too shallow to reach deeper structures.[7] That is, when a tissue absorbed or scattered light too strongly, it effectively cast a shadow over deeper structures and tissues.[7] On the other hand, the primarily transparent structures of the eye transmitted most light and demonstrated a very low degree of reflection, absorption, and scattering.[7] OCT was developed with sufficient sensitivity to detect the very minor differences among layers that were all weakly absorptive, backreflective, and backscattering.[7]

Even in its earliest iterations, OCT produced images with microstructural precision on par with histological biopsies. Though the results appeared similar to histologic samples (and the results of early OCT scans were validated through histology), the mechanism of OCT was entirely different.[7] Whereas histology relied on external markers of cellular or subcellular components to differentiate structures, OCT leveraged intrinsic features.[7]

2.3.3 The First OCT Images

In the late 1980s, one of the authors of this chapter (Joel S. Schuman) became involved in the OCT development effort as a fellow at Massachusetts Eye and Ear Infirmary/Harvard Medical School.[9] He proposed measurements of the deeper structures of the eye (e.g., the retina and its intricate layers which, though all transparent, were optically distinct) via optical coherence domain reflectometry.[9] After the group's work validated the utility of optical coherence domain reflectometry for measuring structures throughout the eye via individual A-scans, another student working on the project, David Huang, then a Health Sciences Technology Student at Harvard Medical School and Massachusetts Institute of Technology, had the insight that the clear next step was transitioning from multiple A-scans to a two-dimensional B-scan analogous to B-mode ultrasound.[9] This transition marked the invention of OCT; the inventors named the technology optical coherence tomography and published the first OCT images in *Science*.[1,9]

The 1991 *Science* paper demonstrated features of postmortem, *in vitro* human retina with detailed depictions of the optic nerve head and nerve fiber layer.[1] The paper also featured images of a fibrocalcific plaque in a postmortem, *in vivo* human coronary artery specimen.[1] To generate the images, multiple A-scans were combined using a logarithmic false color or gray scale.[1] Following the generation of these images, the tissues underwent histologic evaluation, which recapitulated the structural findings and validated the technique.[1] This publication was not only scientifically interesting but also demonstrated promising clinical applications of OCT in the fields of ophthalmology and cardiology. Of note, a 1994 Japanese patent described a similar concept, though there was no corresponding publication in the literature to catalogue the work of that group.[10]

At this point, the multidisciplinary team of scientists, engineers, clinicians, and students who contributed to OCT's development saw the culmination of their efforts in the publication of the first OCT images. The contributions of this team, and Swanson's engineering expertise, yielded a sound hardware platform for OCT.[9] However, the software was not yet adequate for imaging *in vivo* specimens.[9]

2.3.4 Providing Clinical Value

The resolution of the first axial images from ophthalmic OCT was approximately 10 to 20 μm, a figure that bested standard B-mode US by 10 to 20 times or more.[11] Compared to preceding technologies like US, this impressive resolution was a major component of OCT's competitive advantage.[5] By providing fine detail about the microstructure of a patient's eye, OCT could inform treatment decisions in diseases where subtle changes were clinically meaningful, such as macular degeneration, glaucoma, and diabetic retinopathy.[5] Throughout the mid-1990s, Schuman and Puliafito led a prodigious collection of data at New England Eye Center in order to clinically validate and provide normative data for OCT.[5] With the support of NIH funding (Fujimoto and Schuman, PIs), the group collected OCT images for more than 5,000 patients, with a particular focus on glaucoma and diseases of the retina.[5] In 1995, Puliafito et al published the first OCT atlas, which provided a framework for clinicians to interpret OCT for an array of retinal pathologies.[12]

OCT boasted a range of possible clinical applications, from screening, diagnosing, and staging ophthalmic diseases to monitoring their progression, treatment response, and recurrence.[9] OCT's potential reach extended to both general and subspecialty eye clinics, as it provided insights into the full breadth of eye disease, including pathology of the cornea, anterior chamber, vitreous, retina, and optic nerve.[9] For instance, following its invention and subsequent commercialization, OCT became integral in the management of glaucoma, as it detected early changes in retinal nerve fiber layer (RNFL) thickness that were imperceptible on standard examination yet were clinically meaningful in that they defined glaucoma damage and portended future disease progression.[9] By providing a means to identify these changes, OCT helped ophthalmologists make earlier and more objective medical and surgical treatment decisions.[9] The aforementioned collection of normative data, which included data on global and regional RNFL thickness, enabled eye care providers to put their patients' OCT images into a broader context to understand disease staging and progression.[9]

2.4 Commercialization

2.4.1 From the Bench to the Bedside: The Need for Speed

At the time of the 1991 *Science* issue that featured the first OCT images, the prototype OCT required several minutes' time to generate the 100 A-scans that were used to generate the corresponding B-scan.[1,5] Although this was sufficiently fast for

imaging the types of *in vitro* tissues that the paper featured, the scan time was too slow for real patients to be able to remain completely still, not blink, and tolerate the procedure.[1,5] OCT could not be a realistic clinical product until it became much faster.

Algorithm development was a vital piece of the transformation of OCT from a scientifically interesting concept to a commercially viable product.[5] Michael Hee, another Health Sciences Technology student at Harvard Medical School and Massachusetts Institute of Technology, was an essential contributor to OCT software development.[5,9] Hee and collaborators developed numerous indication-specific scanning and processing protocols including radial scanning to assess macular edema, circumpapillary scanning to evaluate glaucoma, and automated algorithms that quickly extracted key, clinically relevant data (e.g., topographic thickness maps in macular edema and global and regional RNFL thickness measurements in glaucoma).[5,9] Hee's 1997 graduate thesis, "Optical Coherence Tomography of the Eye," remains a useful OCT reference to this day, and the algorithms on which he worked as a graduate student were incorporated into commercial OCT systems for decades.[5,9]

2.4.2 The First Commercial OCT

In 1992, Fujimoto, Puliafito, and Swanson founded the first OCT company, dubbed Advanced Ophthalmic Devices (AOD).[13] The founders of AOD and their collaborators recognized that OCT would need to overcome substantial regulatory hurdles and skepticism in the ophthalmology community in order to garner meaningful clinical adoption.[5,13] Although the initial commercial enterprise for OCT was a startup, larger industry players soon developed an appetite for the novel technology. In 1994, medical device giant Humphrey Zeiss (Zeiss; now Carl Zeiss Meditech, Inc; Dublin, CA) acquired AOD and licensed the original OCT patent from MIT.[5] John Moore, the then president of Zeiss, took a risk by committing significant capital and human resources to the OCT project.[5] He designated Jay Wei, an engineer, as the lead for commercial development, and Wei collaborated closely with the original inventors on the development of Zeiss's first commercial OCT instrument, OCT 1000.[5]

In 1996, Zeiss launched OCT 1000, the first FDA-approved OCT instrument, a mere 5 years after the publication of those first OCT images in *Science*.[5,9] Clinical adoption of this new technology was sluggish, with only 180 units sold in the first 3 years.[5]

In 2000, Zeiss launched its second-generation instrument, OCT 2000, which included improved ergonomics over its initial offering.[5] These upgrades failed to move the needle in terms of sales, and in 2001, the company sold just 400 units.[5] Disappointing sales figures and waning corporate interest in the technology (Moore left Zeiss by this point, and the new executive team was less enthusiastic about OCT) threatened to halt further commercialization of OCT.[5] Zeiss seriously entertained the idea of scrapping OCT altogether, and the original inventors had to campaign against this.[5]

In 2002, Zeiss launched Stratus OCT, and this third-generation instrument finally produced the long-awaited sales figures the original team envisioned.[5,9] Stratus boasted similar image resolution to its predecessors but markedly faster speed and increased scan density, ultimately yielding superior image quality.[5,9] Beyond these advantages, Stratus addressed concerns from clinicians and technicians about the size and complexity of the earlier OCT machines.[9] The original risk of investing in OCT finally paid off, as the insights that Zeiss gained by analyzing the technical, clinical, and marketing weaknesses of OCT 1000 and OCT 2000 ultimately enabled the company to produce a revolutionary ophthalmic imaging device.[5]

Beyond the strength of the Stratus OCT product, the Stratus launch benefitted from an evolving pharmaceutical landscape in ophthalmology. As expensive antivascular endothelial growth factor (anti-VEGF) therapies entered the market, payors and clinicians had an incentive to ensure appropriate and judicious use.[5] OCT offered a uniquely precise, quick, quantitative, objective, and noninvasive method of detecting treatment response, suggesting whether further injections were likely to be fruitful for individual patients.[5] In this new environment of high-cost drugs, Zeiss enhanced the value proposition of OCT by positioning it as a tool for facilitating appropriate resource allocation.[5]

OCT soon became an international success: by 2004, an estimated 10 million OCT images had been captured worldwide; by 2006, this figure doubled and commercial OCT sales climbed to more than cumulative 6,000 units; by 2008, greater than 10,000 commercial OCT instruments were in use around the world.[5,13] OCT had slowly but steadily become the standard for ophthalmic imaging.[5]

2.4.3 OCT Instrument Design

Although each new OCT instrument featured novel design elements, several themes have carried through the different generations and manufacturers.[7] First, each instrument had a method of ensuring alignment of the incident light beam with the target tissue.[7] For some, this was as simple as a real-time video of the patient's pupil; some included a video camera to view the fundus in real time; some models featured an integrated scanning laser ophthalmoscope; and several included a motorized chin rest to enable fine adjustments in patient position without the need to reposition the table or instrument.[7] For finer adjustments, OCT instruments usually incorporated mechanisms for adjusting the patient's fixation; this was typically a moveable computer-generated fixation target within the patient's field of view.[7] In terms of scanning, most machines were optimized for a specific working distance from the eye, and the OCT beam pivoted about the pupil to capture the full area of interest.[7] OCT instruments were created with patient safety in mind, and thorough research has validated their safety.[7] Furthermore, the duration and intensity of light exposure to the retina have been governed by international standards.[7]

2.5 The Fourier Switch

The early generations of OCT utilized time-delay (TD-OCT) technology.[5] That is, the instruments measured the time delay of the reflected signal and used these data to generate a cross-sectional image.[5] Fourier-domain technology, which ultimately gave rise to spectral domain OCT (SD-OCT) and swept-source OCT (SS-OCT), offered a means for generating higher quality images in a shorter time.[5] Whereas TD-OCT measured each light echo sequentially, Fourier-domain OCT measured them simultaneously.[7] In Fourier-domain OCT, A-scans were analyzed via a Fourier transform of detected frequencies, enabling rapid collection of A-scans and volumetric data; the faster OCT instruments that came from this technology provided a clinical product that was easier for patients, technicians, and clinicians.[5,14]

2.5.1 Spectral Domain OCT

Work in SD-OCT began as early as the 1991, with key publications emerging in the mid-1990s.[5,9] In 2001, Wojtkowski et al published the first study that showcased SD-OCT in a clinical context.[15] The paper described SD-OCT as a means of using wavelength rather than light time-of-flight to determine the location of a reflection of light.[15]

SD-OCT exhibited 50- to 100-fold higher sensitivity than TD-OCT.[7] SD-OCT facilitated collection of volumetric data via three-dimensional "cubes" that contained comprehensive structural information.[16] These three-dimensional datasets enabled generation of layer-specific retinal maps, including clinically relevant subanalyses such as RNFL thickness maps for assessment of glaucoma stage and progression.[7] SD-OCT also made the generation of *en face* views possible through the summation of axial scans; *en face* views allowed the viewer to better appreciate the extent of retinal pathologies and identify specific B-scans to evaluate further, much like spot films and coronal views in computed tomography (CT) scans can assist viewers in selecting specific transverse cuts that warrant further assessment.[7,16] By using known anatomic features as benchmarks (e.g., the retinal pigment epithelium), SD-OCT generated *en face* images at various levels.[7] Once SD-OCT provided three-dimensional data, surgical planning based on OCT became more feasible.[9]

In 2006, Optovue, Inc. (Fremont, CA) launched the first SD-OCT instrument in the US market, becoming the first commercial Fourier-domain OCT offering.[9] Optovue, a company that Jay Wei founded following his departure from Zeiss in 2003, was Zeiss's first major OCT competitor.[9] Optovue launched its device, named RTVue, at the 2006 annual meeting of the American Academy of Ophthalmology.[9] In the following year, Zeiss launched a competing SD-OCT instrument, Cirrus HD-OCT.[9] Both companies enjoyed success following the launch of these SD-OCT instruments, with each achieving sales exceeding 1,000 units before the end of 2008.[9]

In an unusual twist in medical device development, there was no clear patent ownership of SD-OCT technology.[9] As such, a substantial number of competitors entered the SD-OCT field in the mid-2000s.[9] This included a range of both large and small companies such as Bioptigen (Research Triangle Park, NC), Heidelberg Engineering (Heidelberg, Germany), Ophthalmic Technologies Inc. (Toronto, Ontario), Optopol Technology (Zawiercie, Poland), Reichert Ophthalmic Instruments (Depew, NY), and Topcon Medical Systems Inc. (Paramus, NJ).[9] Although the competition in the SD-OCT sector forced companies to innovate thoughtfully and quickly, challenges with pricing and reimbursement ultimately precluded smaller players from maintaining successful SD-OCT businesses.[5,9]

Consumers quickly recognized the value of SD-OCT in terms of image quality, speed, and ease of use (▶ Fig. 2.3 and ▶ Fig. 2.4). Since the launch of SD-OCT, the majority of the OCT market growth has been in this and other advanced OCT technology sectors, and TD-OCT instruments have become effectively obsolete.[9]

2.5.2 Swept-Source OCT

SS-OCT offered even greater image quality and more than 100-times faster imaging speed than SD-OCT, yet it struggled to find a successful commercial niche.[5] SS-OCT, which incorporated fiber optics and photonics components developed in the 1980s, emerged in the early 2000s as a method of marking interference and time delays with a frequency-swept laser.[5] In other words, the laser produces a "sweep" of frequency ranges, and the various time delays in the light that is backreflected/backscattered from the tissue are labeled with different frequencies.[7] Compared to SD-OCT, SS-OCT enabled imaging with longer wavelengths of incident light, facilitating deeper penetration of the incident light (and thus providing an optimized technology to precisely image the deeper structures of the eye including the choroid and ONH) and mitigating attenuation from certain ocular opacities (e.g., cataracts).[5,7] In addition, SS-OCT used a photodetector in place of the line scan camera and spectrometer in SD-OCT; photodectectors minimized optical transmission losses, yielding higher sensitivity.[7]

Despite its advantages, the commercial growth of SS-OCT instruments was sluggish due to their high price points in the absence of a clear way to recoup cost.[5] That is, there was not an obvious means for clinics and health systems to obtain high enough reimbursement for SS-OCT relative to SD-OCT to offset the greater capital investment of purchasing a SS-OCT instrument, particularly if they had recently purchased an SD-OCT device.[5] Exacerbating this cost issue, customers became wary of investing in every generation of OCT out of concern that the instruments will become obsolete before they see sufficient return on their investment.[5] Interestingly, in areas of medicine outside of ophthalmology, including cardiology, gastroenterology, and dermatology, commercial SS-OCT devices have done better than SD-OCT.[5] Notwithstanding these challenges, some OCT experts have surmised that in time, SS-OCT devices may evolve into a lower-cost, smaller-footprint alternative to SD-OCT through the incorporation of photonic integrated circuit technology.[5]

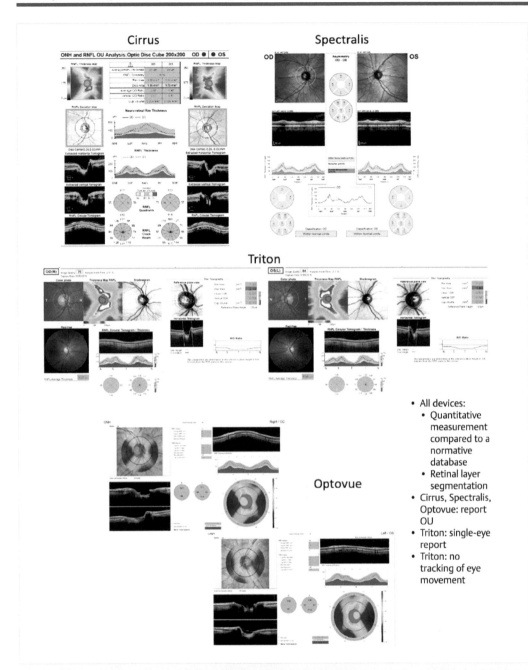

Fig. 2.3 Optical coherence tomography (OCT) reports on Cirrus, Spectralis, Triton, and Optovue instruments depicting the optic nerve heads of a healthy subject. The reports vary in format and some details each highlights. The essential take-aways through a number of common formats that enable the clinician to understand in which optic nerve head (ONH) regions and by how much the retinal nerve fiber layer (RNFL) thickness of the patient varies from healthy subjects in the normative dataset. As expected, in the case of this healthy subject, RNFL thickness is within the healthy range from the normative data in all ONH regions. All machines also segment retinal layers to enable layer-specific thickness measurement. Of the instruments included in this figure, all but the Triton enable tracking of eye movement to minimize motion artifact.

2

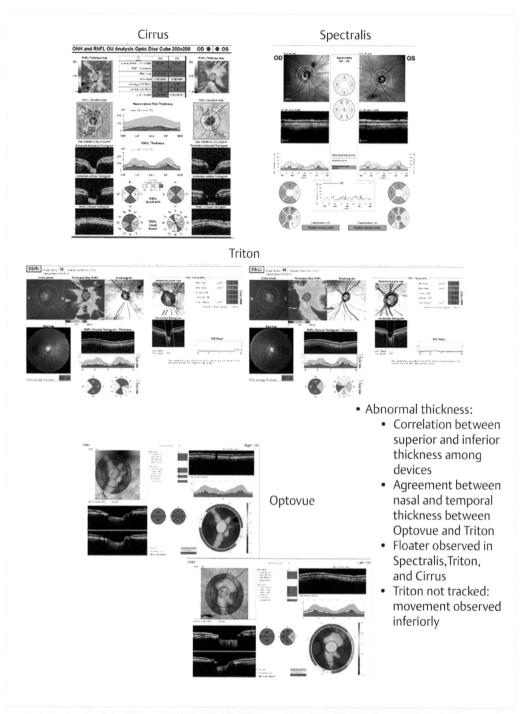

Cirrus

Spectralis

Triton

Optovue

- Abnormal thickness:
  - Correlation between superior and inferior thickness among devices
  - Agreement between nasal and temporal thickness between Optovue and Triton
  - Floater observed in Spectralis, Triton, and Cirrus
  - Triton not tracked: movement observed inferiorly

Fig. 2.4 Optical coherence tomography (OCT) reports on Cirrus, Spectralis, Triton, and Optovue instruments depicting the optic nerve heads of a subject with glaucoma. In contrast to the reports in ▶ Fig. 2.3, these reports demonstrate markedly diminished retinal nerve fiber layer (RNFL) thickness with notable inter-eye and inter-region differences in the degree of RNFL thickness loss. Among Optovue and Triton, there is correlation between inferior and superior thicknesses. The Spectralis, Triton, and Cirrus instruments document a vitreous floater. The Triton instrument image shows movement artifact inferiorly.

2.6 OCT-Angiography

The next phase of OCT development focused on precise imaging of vasculature through OCT-angiography (OCT-A). OCT-A appealed to academic researchers and industry interests alike because many prevalent eye diseases involve the ophthalmic vasculature (e.g., choroidal neovascularization in age-related macular degeneration [AMD]; capillary dropout in diabetic retinopathy).[17] In 2006, work on OCT-A began through parallel efforts in the US at Oregon Health Sciences University (OHSU; Portland, OR) and in Japan.[17] OCT-A required faster processing speeds and software algorithms than were available in any antecedent OCT generations, so progress was minimal over the first few years of development.[17] As such, the research team at OHSU, led by David Huang and Ricky Wong, focused their efforts on the creation of novel angiography algorithms.[17] The product of this work was an algorithm called split-spectrum amplitude decorrelate angiography (SSADA), which yielded 11-times the number of images compared to prior generations without an increase in scan time; through this achievement, SSADA effectively made OCT-A a commercial possibility.[17]

By 2014, Optovue launched the first commercial OCT-A instrument, AngioVue, in the international market.[17] Optovue struggled to launch the product in the US due to regulatory obstacles.[17] The company eventually succeeded, and AngioVue entered the US market in 2016.[17] In addition to collecting extensive data at record-high speeds, AngioVue featured a registration and tracking system that protected image quality when eye movements occurred.[17] In 2015, Zeiss beat Optovue in the US market with the FDA approval and launch of AngioPlex OCT-A, its OCT-A offering. In September 2018, Heidelberg obtained FDA approval for an OCT-A module that could be applied to its Spectralis machine, bringing a third OCT-A product to the US market.[17]

2.7 Impact

2.7.1 Financial

Academic institutions, medical device companies, and, via government funding, tax payers all made substantial financial contributions toward the development of OCT. Of the many corporations that launched commercial OCT instruments, nearly half had affiliations with government-funded research institutions.[5] A prior analysis sought to quantify government spending, and it estimated

that the US government invested around $100 million from 1995 to 2015 and that, globally, governments invested approximately $500 million from 2006 to 2016.[5,18] Without this generous funding, it is likely that the clinical adoption of OCT would have been significantly delayed or may have never succeeded; Swanson and Fujimoto, two important figures in the OCT development story, have surmised that the substantial government funding for OCT accelerated its development by as much as a decade.[5] Ample funding from government and industry enabled the scientists, engineers, physicians, and students who developed OCT to be creative and perseverant in their quest to produce an impactful clinical tool.[5]

OCT has provided a healthy return on investment (ROI) to its investors.[5] 2016 estimates stated that OCT had brought in a cumulative revenue of around $5 billion since the launch of OCT 1000 and an annual revenue of around $1 billion in that year alone.[5] To assess the government-specific ROI from OCT, Fujimoto and Swanson extrapolated a 2009 PricewaterhouseCoopers analysis in an effort to enumerate the sum of OCT-related employment and corporate taxes on local, state, and federal levels.[5,19] They estimated that globally, governments have recouped approximately $500 million in direct OCT tax revenue.[5] As this is not inclusive of taxes collected throughout the supply chain or for ancillary services, such as installation and maintenance, the actual sum is likely to be even higher.[5] Based on this analysis, it is expected that global governments have recouped their initial investment on OCT and stand to gain from its future successes. In addition to these direct returns, OCT has guided more judicious use of anti-VEGF therapy, providing additional financial benefit to governments, insurers, and patients.[5]

The financial impact of OCT reached beyond providing ROI to its investors; OCT has also been a significant source of job creation.[5,20] In 2016, Swanson collected historical employment data from 70 companies that sell OCT components or instruments.[20] He accumulated data on a range of positions including scientists, engineers, salespeople, marketing teams, administrative assistants, and executives.[20] In sum, he found that these companies provided 20,000 person-years of high-quality employment.[20] This estimate was likely a conservative one, as Swanson's analysis did not include positions at academic institutions, ranging from students with work-study jobs to full-time faculty, nor did it include the companies that participate in the OCT supply chain.[20]

2.7.2 Scientific and Clinical

Within ophthalmology, OCT has had an immeasurable impact on patient morbidity and quality of life. It has enabled near-specialist level of care in general ophthalmology clinics, promoted personalized medical and surgical treatment decisions, and facilitated timely referral to specialists when necessary. Among ophthalmologists, there has always been a strong appetite for new and improved applications of current and future generations of OCT. For instance, intraoperative OCT emerged as an area of interest for many academic ophthalmologists and industry interests.[14] Some researchers have proposed projecting OCT images over a surgical site. Others have suggested continuously capturing OCT images before, during, and after fine retinal procedures such as epiretinal membrane peel or removal of the inner limiting membrane.[14]

OCT has impacted patients beyond those with ophthalmic diseases. In cardiology, intravascular OCT adoption increased to around 100,000 procedures annually by the mid-2010s.[7] Given the prevalence of cardiovascular disease in developed nations, where it is the leading cause of death in adults, the potential impact of OCT in this area could have widespread implications for reducing morbidity and mortality for cardiac patients around the world.[7] Cancer is the second-leading cause of death among adults in the developed world, and OCT has proven fruitful in the diagnosis, monitoring, and research of many cancers, including those of the skin, gastrointestinal tract, breast, and female reproductive organs.[7] OCT research in oncology aimed to provide medical and surgical oncologists with a means of optimizing tissue selection and margin screening in real time.[7] In addition to these examples, pioneers in many other medical specialties began research in OCT over the past decade.[7]

This chapter not only showcased the fascinating story of OCT's invention and applications to date, but also sought to highlight the exciting developments yet to come. Although OCT's impact has been substantial, particularly in the field of ophthalmology, its use has been limited to just a fraction of its potential applications.

References

[1] Huang D, Swanson EA, Lin CP, et al. Optical coherence tomography. Science. 1991; 254(5035):1178–1181

[2] Swanson EA, Huang D. Ophthalmic OCT reaches $1 billion per year. Retin Physician. 2011; 45:58–59

[3] Duguay MA. Light photographed in flight. Am Sci. 1971; 59:551–556

[4] Duguay MA, Mattick AT. Ultrahigh speed photography of picosecond light pulses and echoes. Appl Opt. 1971; 10(9):2162–2170

[5] Fujimoto J, Swanson E. The development, commercialization, and impact of optical coherence tomography. Invest Ophthalmol Vis Sci. 2016; 57(9):OCT1–OCT13

[6] Fujimoto JG, De Silvestri S, Ippen EP, Puliafito CA, Margolis R, Oseroff A. Femtosecond optical ranging in biological systems. Opt Lett. 1986; 11(3):150–153

[7] Fujimoto JG, Moult EM, Swanson E, Potsaid B, Schuman JS, Duker JS. Optical coherence tomography: past, present, and future. In: Schuman JS, Puliafito CA, Fujimoto JG, Duker JS, eds. Everyday OCT: A Handbook for Clinicians and Technicians. Thorofare, NJ: SLACK Incorporated; 2017:101–120

[8] Fercher AF, Mengedoht K, Werner W. Eye-length measurement by interferometry with partially coherent light. Opt Lett. 1988; 13(3):186–188

[9] Schuman JS, Folio LS, Gabriele ML, Wollstein G. Optical coherence tomography (OCT) part II: its applications. In: Boyd B, ed. Modern Ophthalmology: The Highlights. Panama: Jaypee Highlights Medical Publishers, Inc.; 2011:317–330

[10] Tanno N, Ichimura T, Saeki A. inventors. Device for measuring the light wave of a reflected image. Japan Patent 6–35946. May 11, 1994

[11] Hee MR, Izatt JA, Swanson EA, et al. Optical coherence tomography of the human retina. Arch Ophthalmol. 1995; 113(3):325–332

[12] Puliafito CA, Hee MR, Schuman JS, Fujimoto JG. Optical Coherence Tomography of Ocular Diseases. Thorofare, NJ: SLACK, Incorporated; 1995

[13] Swanson E, Huang D. Ophthalmic optical coherence tomography market: past, present and future. Optical Coherence Tomography News. March 2009 http://www.octnews.org/articles/1027616/ophthalmic-optical-coherence-tomography-market-pas/

[14] Gabriele ML, Wollstein G, Ishikawa H, et al. Optical coherence tomography: history, current status, and laboratory work. Invest Ophthalmol Vis Sci. 2011; 52(5):2425–2436

[15] Wojtkowski M, Fercher AF, Leitgeb R. Phase-sensitive interferometry in optical coherence tomography. Proc SPIE, Light and Optics in Biomedicine. 2001;4515:250

[16] Wojtkowski M, Srinivasan V, Fujimoto JG, et al. Three-dimensional retinal imaging with high-speed ultrahigh-resolution optical coherence tomography. Ophthalmology. 2005; 112(10):1734–1746

[17] Ophthalmology Innovation Summit. "A History of OCT-A." Lecture by David Huang. 1 September 2016. https://www.youtube.com/watch?v=BwyVCVYT48A

[18] Eric A Swanson and James G Fujimoto. The ecosystem that powered the translation of OCT from fundamental research to clinical and commercial impact [Invited]. Biomed Opt Express. 2017; 8: 1638–1664

[19] Total Tax Contribution: How Much Do Large U.S. Companies Pay in Taxes? Survey with Business Rountable. Price Waterhouse Coopers; 2009. https://www.pwc.com/us/en/national-economic-statistics/assets/total_tax_contribution.pdf

[20] Swanson EA. Optical Coherence Tomography Industry Has Provided Well Over 20,000 Person-Years of Direct Employment. OCT News. 2016. http://www.octnews.org/articles/6323439/optical-coherence-tomography-industry-has-provided/

3 Optical Coherence Tomography of the Optic Nerve

Andrew Williams and Jullia A. Rosdahl

Summary

Assessment of the optic nerve is a critical component of glaucoma evaluation. Imaging technologies have evolved to provide quantitative measurements of optic nerve head parameters and to detect changes in measurements over time that may suggest glaucoma progression. Optical coherence tomography (OCT) in particular provides reproducible, reliable, and accurate measurements of optic nerve parameters, such as thickness of the retinal nerve fiber layer, and has become integral to clinical practice to guide physicians in glaucoma diagnosis and management. We describe in this chapter a systematic approach to OCT interpretation in clinical practice with attention to its limitations and potential artifacts.

Keywords: OCT, optic nerve, retinal nerve fiber layer, glaucoma, optic neuropathy, imaging, eye

3.1 Introduction

3.1.1 Glaucoma Imaging

Glaucoma is characterized by progressive loss of retinal ganglion cells that causes structural changes to the optic nerve and thinning of the retinal nerve fiber layer (RNFL) with subsequent corresponding visual field defects. Prompt recognition of early structural changes is critical to mitigate permanent vision loss from glaucoma. Visual field defects may not become apparent until 40% of retinal ganglion cells are lost, suggesting that perimetry alone may not capture early disease. Careful stereoscopic examination of the optic nerve remains a hallmark in detection and management of glaucoma, but subjective interpretation and two-dimensional documentation can limit the ability to identify subtle changes. Along the same lines, stereoscopic photographs of the optic nerve and monochromatic photographs of the RNFL are limited by only fair agreement in interpretation between glaucoma specialists and the lack of quantitative information.

Imaging modalities have been developed to aid ophthalmologists in optic disc assessment to monitor structural signs of glaucoma. Technologies such as the Heidelberg Retina Tomograph (HRT, Heidelberg Engineering, Heidelberg, Germany) emerged to provide quantitative information about the topography of the posterior fundus using confocal laser scanning microscopy (▶ Fig. 3.1). Similarly, the GDx scanning laser polarimeter estimated RNFL thickness by measuring its birefringence using polarized light (▶ Fig. 3.2). However, the detailed and precise imaging of the optic nerve possible with optical coherence tomography (OCT) is the most common computerized imaging of the optic nerve in current clinical practice. Commercially available OCT devices include Cirrus HD-OCT (Carl Zeiss Meditec, Dublin, CA), Spectralis (Heidelberg Engineering, Heidelberg, Germany), RTVue-100 (Optovue, Freemont, CA), 3D OCT-2000 (Topcon Medical Systems, Oakland, NJ), and RS-3000 Advance (Nikon, Tokyo, Japan). These different commercial devices utilize similar OCT acquisition principles but vary in scanning protocols and segmentation algorithms (discussed in depth in Chapter 7).

3.1.2 Optical Coherence Tomography

OCT noninvasively acquires a real-time image of the ophthalmic structures in optical cross section. Compared to previous models of time-domain OCT technology, spectral domain OCT (SD-OCT) produces higher resolution images by utilizing spectrally separated detectors and taking Fourier transform of broad spectral information (▶ Fig. 3.3). Using a near-infrared super-luminescent diode light, SD-OCT acquires 26,000 to 85,000 axial scans per second for an axial resolution of about 5 μm and transverse optical resolution of about 14 μm. Images are acquired either in raster scans (parallel frames), radial scans across the optic nerve, or as concentric circles to measure peripapillary RNFL thickness in a 3.46-mm scan circle centered on the optic nerve head (ONH). Software can now delineate Bruch's membrane opening (BMO) as standard reference for defining the region of the ONH, while previous device iterations required manual centration of the scan circle. Additionally, eye motion tracking recently has been incorporated to reduce noise and artifacts in acquired images. Software programs also contain a normative database of measurements from healthy subjects to aid interpretation of patient's measurements by comparing them to normal ranges.

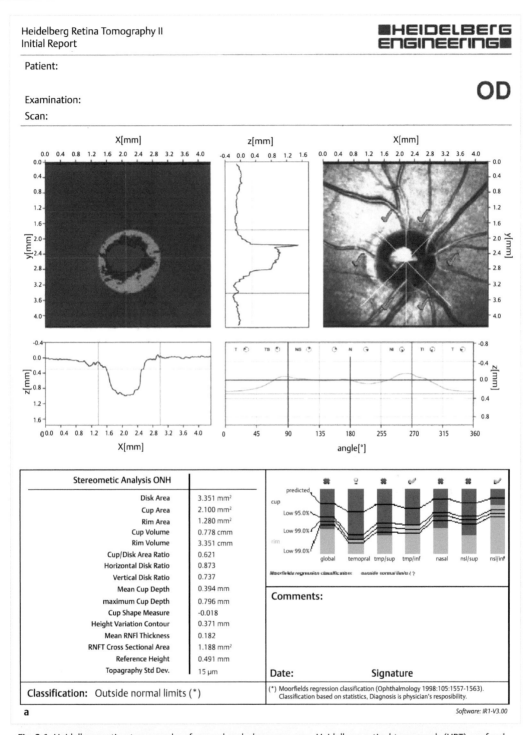

Fig. 3.1 Heidelberg retina tomographs of normal and glaucoma eyes. Heidelberg retinal tomograph (HRT) confocal images of the optic nerve are shown. **(a)** A healthy eye and

(Continued)

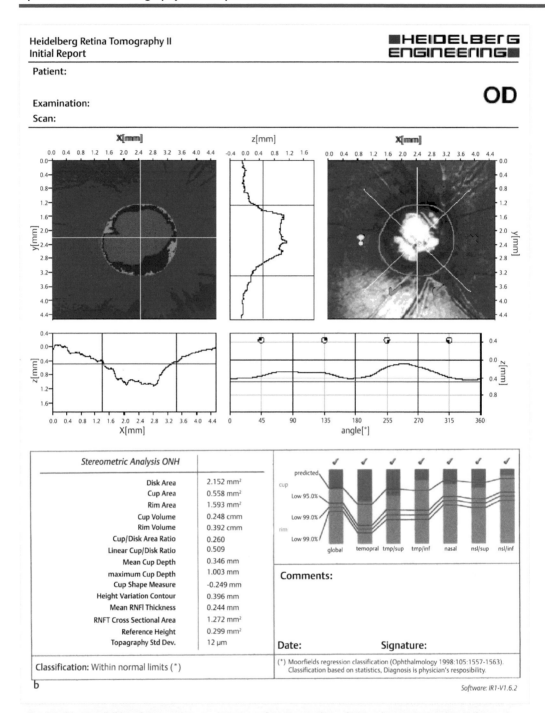

Heidelberg Retina Tomography II
Initial Report

■HEIDELBErG
EnGInEErInG■

Patient:

Examination:

Scan:

OD

Stereometric Analysis ONH	
Disk Area	2.152 mm²
Cup Area	0.558 mm²
Rim Area	1.593 mm²
Cup Volume	0.248 cmm
Rim Volume	0.392 cmm
Cup/Disk Area Ratio	0.260
Linear Cup/Disk Ratio	0.509
Mean Cup Depth	0.346 mm
maximum Cup Depth	1.003 mm
Cup Shape Measure	-0.249 mm
Height Variation Contour	0.396 mm
Mean RNFl Thickness	0.244 mm
RNFT Cross Sectional Area	1.272 mm²
Reference Height	0.299 mm²
Topagraphy Std Dev.	12 µm

Comments:

Date: Signature:

Classification: Within normal limits (*)

(*) Moorfields regression classification (Ophthalmology 1998:105:1557-1563).
Classification based on statistics, Diagnosis is physician's resposibility.

b

Software: IR1-V1.6.2

Fig. 3.1 *(Continued)* **(b)** a glaucomatous eye. (Courtesy of Dr Teresa Chen of Massachusetts Eye and Ear Infirmary.)

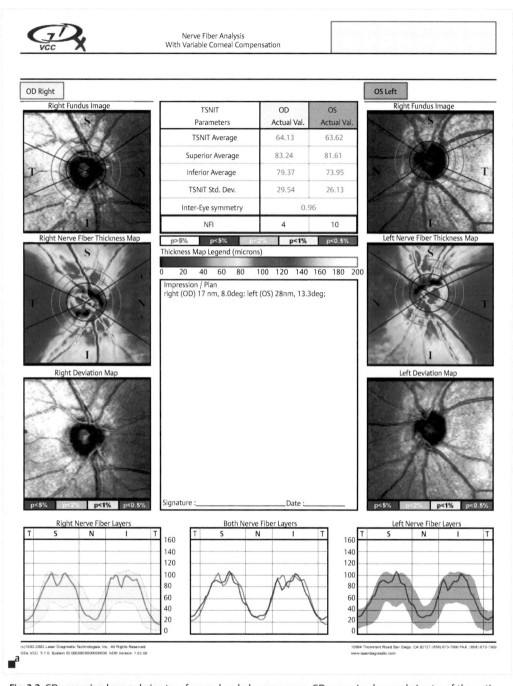

Fig. 3.2 GDx scanning laser polarimetry of normal and glaucoma eyes. GDx scanning laser polarimetry of the optic nerves are shown. (a) Healthy eyes and

(Continued)

Nerve Fiber Analysis
With Variable corneal Compensation

OD Right — Right Fundus Image — Right Nerve Fiber Thickness Map — Right Deviation Map — Right Nerve Fiber Layer

OS Left — Left Fundus Image — Left Nerve Fiber Thickness Map — Left Deviation Map — Left Nerve Fiber Layer

TSNIT Paremeters	OD Actual Val.	OS Actual Val.
TSNIT Average	32.23	25.79
Superior Average	44.81	32.00
Inferior Average	22.70	24.94
TSNIT Std. Dev.	11.53	8.45
Inter-Eye Summetry	0.50	
NFI	88	98

p>5% p<5% p<1% p<1% p<0.5%

Thickness Map Legend (microns)

0 20 40 60 80 100 120 140 160 180 200

Impression / Plan:
right (OD) 78nm, 13.8deg; left (OS) 82nm, 23.3deg;

Signature:_____ Date:_____

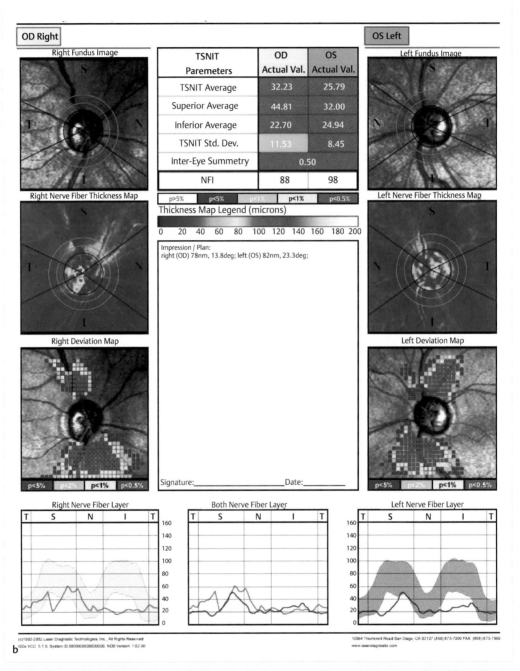

b

Fig. 3.2 *(Continued)* **(b)** glaucomatous eyes. (Courtesy of Dr Teresa Chen of Massachusetts Eye and Ear Infirmary.)

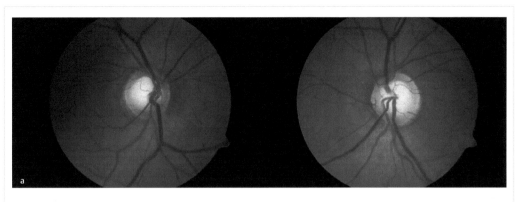

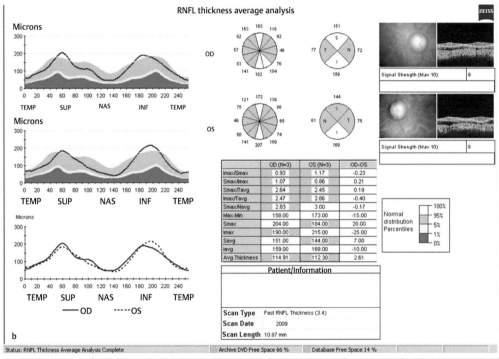

Fig. 3.3 Optical coherence tomography (OCT) imaging in a glaucoma suspect. These are optic nerve images of a 62-year-old man who was followed as a glaucoma suspect due to increased cup-to-disc ratio. **(a)** Optic nerve photos from approximately 10 years prior show physiologic cupping. **(b)** Time-domain OCT of the retinal nerve fiber layer (RNFL) showing normal thickness in both eyes.

(Continued)

3.2 OCT Output

3.2.1 Overview

Most commercial OCT platforms generate a printout to summarize quantitative and qualitative measurements of RNFL and ONH parameters. Depending on the software algorithm and technical capabilities of the device, these measurements include RNFL thickness, cup-to-disc ratio, neuroretinal rim area, and neuroretinal rim volume.

In addition, quality metrics are given to allow the interpreter to assess the validity of the data output. Patient identification and date of study are embedded in the report. Many printouts also include a

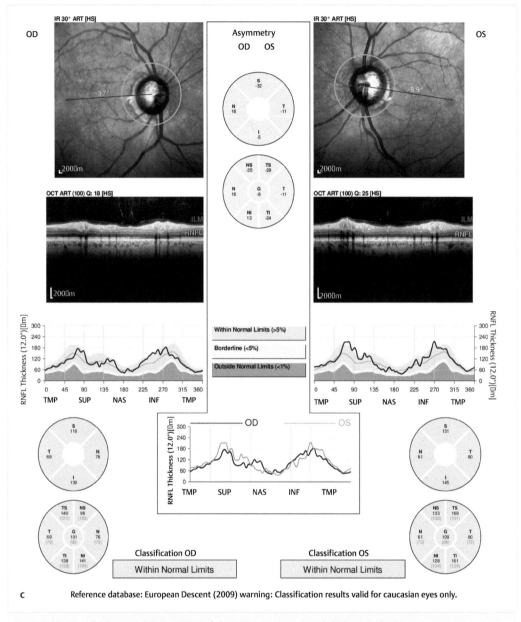

Fig. 3.3 *(Continued)* **(c)** Spectral domain OCT of the RNFL showing normal thickness in both eyes.

quality score or indication of signal strength, as lower quality images are more prone to artifactual measurements. Additionally, algorithmic delineation of the circumpapillary RNFL is demonstrated over acquired B-scan images in order for the user to assess accuracy of the RNFL tracing.

Retinal Nerve Fiber Layer Measurements (► Fig. 3.4 and ► Fig. 3.5)

Measurements of circumpapillary RNFL thickness feature prominently in the output and are given as a

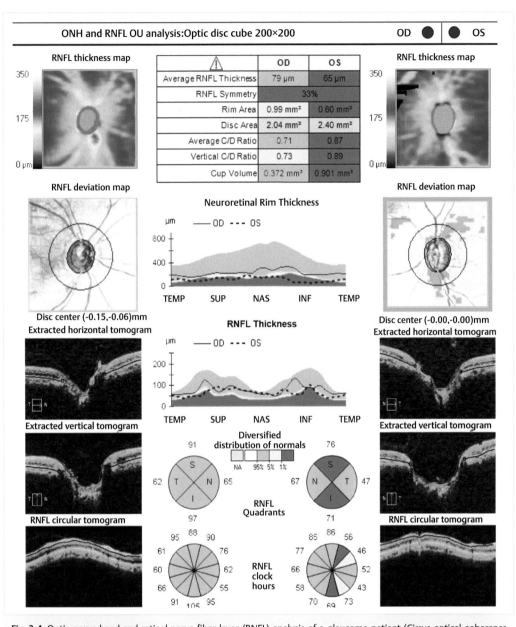

Fig. 3.4 Optic nerve head and retinal nerve fiber layer (RNFL) analysis of a glaucoma patient (Cirrus optical coherence tomography [OCT]). This is a Cirrus OCT report for a 70-year-old white woman with primary open-angle glaucoma that is moderate stage in the right eye and severe stage in the left. There is notable asymmetry in RNFL thickness between the two eyes. The superior and inferior thinning pattern on the left eye is also characteristic for glaucoma. There are superior and inferior arcuate defects on visual field testing of the left eye. The right eye demonstrates a superior nasal step consistent with moderate-stage disease, and progression analysis demonstrates thinning of the inferior RNFL quadrant over time (see ▶ Fig. 3.8). (Courtesy of Dr Ian Conner of the University of Pittsburgh.)

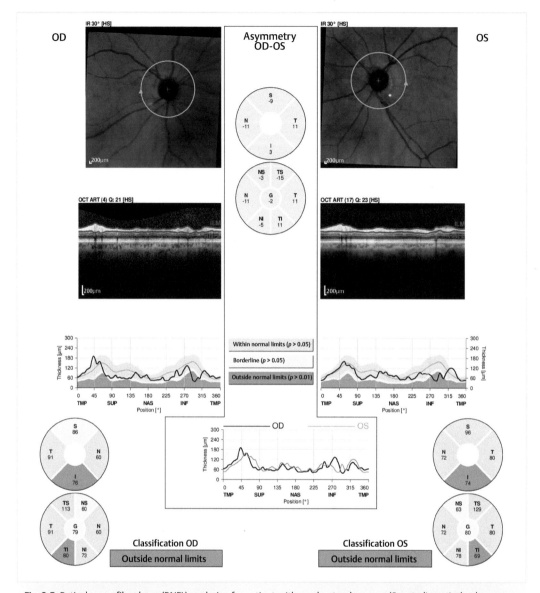

Fig. 3.5 Retinal nerve fiber layer (RNFL) analysis of a patient with moderate glaucoma (Spectralis optical coherence tomography [OCT]). This is a Spectralis OCT RNFL report of a 70-year-old woman with normal tension glaucoma. There is inferior thinning of the RNFL in both eyes. Her visual fields demonstrate early nasal defect superiorly in the right eye and dense superior nasal defect in the left eye.

global average, by quadrant, and by clock-hour for each eye. Summary measurements are presented in table form, including degree of RNFL symmetry, as asymmetry between eyes can be associated with glaucoma. Thickness maps illustrate RNFL measurements around the detected ONH, with warmer colors corresponding to thicker values in a classically butterfly-shaped distribution around the optic nerve. Deviations from normal thickness are also

illustrated in a deviation map to highlight potential areas of RNFL loss.

RNFL thickness is also graphed in a "TSNIT" plot, in which the circumferential RNFL thickness measurements are "unrolled" into linear form and presented from the temporal to inferior quadrants (the "Temporal-Superior-Nasal-Inferior-Temporal" plot). In normal eyes, this plot should demonstrate a characteristic double hump, with thickest RNFL measurements peaking at the inferior and superior regions.

Patient measurements are plotted over a normative measurement database, and interpretation of the probability of abnormal values is aided by color coding with red, yellow, green, and white shading. Red color highlights values in the lowest 1% of normative values and is considered outside normal limits. Yellow flags values from the 1st to 5th percentile and suggests borderline abnormality. Green indicates the middle 90% of normal, from 5th to 95th percentiles, and white flags values greater than the 95th percentile of normal subjects. Plots over normative values compare patient measurements with those from subjects of similar age, as age-related changes lead to RNFL thinning over time even in the absence of disease. Despite similar presentation and color coding of the TSNIT plot between devices, images cannot be directly compared from one OCT device to another because different manufacturers generate these plots from their own normative databases.

Optic Nerve Head Parameters

ONH analyses are generated by defining the boundary of the optic disc using the BMO. The area of the neuroretinal rim is measured as the minimum distance from the BMO to the internal limiting membrane (ILM), a parameter described at the BMO-MRW (Bruch's membrane opening minimum rim width). The Spectralis device acquires radial scans across the ONH to determine BMO-MRW and thus define the neuroretinal rim (▶ Fig. 3.6). For the Cirrus HD-OCT, ONH data is extracted from the 200 × 200 Optic Disc Cube scan using minimum area rather than distance to define the BMO-MRW, and normative measurement limits are corrected for optic disc tilt and size. Resulting metrics include cup-to-disc ratio, neuroretinal rim area, and neuroretinal rim volume. These ONH measurements complement RNFL data to detect glaucoma or progression, but themselves have less diagnostic accuracy. However, ONH parameters can suggest nonglaucomatous optic neuropathy if there is thin RNFL in the setting of normal neuroretinal rim and cup-to-disc ratio.

3.2.2 OCT Interpretation

As with perimetry, clinicians should interpret OCT output systematically in order to avoid overlooking information that could influence decision-making and to identify artifacts or anatomic variants that affect measurement values.[1] Although there is no standardized system for interpretation, several important components of the output summary should be regularly assessed for accuracy and reliability (▶ Fig. 3.7 and ▶ Table 3.1).

Table 3.1 Interpreting OCT output

Item	Description
1. Patient's name and age	Make sure age was entered correctly, as OCT measurements are compared to age-matched nomograms
2. Signal strength	On Cirrus OCT, values of 7 and above are preferred and values of 3 or below are quite poor For Spectralis OCT, a quality score of 15 or greater is preferred
3. Segmentation	Ensure B-scan tracings accurately outline the RNFL; rectangle-shaped areas of complete RNFL loss on thickness and deviation maps are likely segmentation artifact
4. Optic nerve tracing	Compare the delineation of the optic disc and optic cup to examination or photographs, as misidentified borders will skew measurements
5. TSNIT plot	Ensure that the superior and inferior RNFL peaks align with normative values and look for any area of complete loss, as values of RNFL thickness < 40 μm are likely artifactual
6. Asymmetry	Looks for discrepancy in average or quadrant RNFL thickness between eyes, as asymmetry can be suggestive of glaucoma
7. Thickness pattern	Does the RNFL thickness pattern makes sense for glaucoma? Do thin areas on OCT correspond to findings on clinical examination and perimetry?
8. Progression	Examine trends over time, including raw values, to assess disease progression
9. Refractive error and axial length	Be aware that myopic eyes are more prone to algorithm error due to increased axial length and optic disc tilt
10. Prior OCT scans	Make sure scan location is consistent across time points and be alert of artifacts from prior studies that could affect progression detection

Abbreviations: OCT, optical coherence tomography; RNFL, retinal nerve fiber layer; TSNIT, temporal-superior-nasal-interior-temporal.

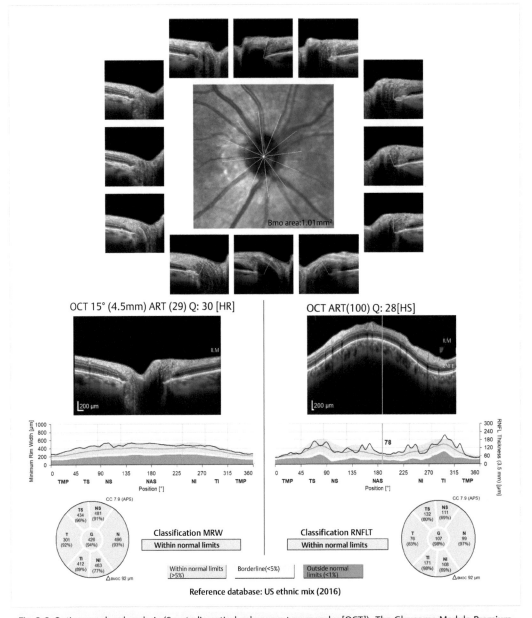

Fig. 3.6 Optic nerve head analysis (Spectralis optical coherence tomography [OCT]). The Glaucoma Module Premium Edition from Spectralis provides an analysis of the optic nerve head. This is an example from a patient who does not have glaucoma. The report includes analyses of minimum rim width (MRW) and retinal nerve fiber layer (RNFL) thickness at a diameter of 3.5 mm. MRW measurements at nine cross sections are displayed with arrows, colored green (normal), yellow (borderline), or red (outside normal limits). Temporal-superior-nasal-inferior-temporal (TSNIT) plots of the MRW and the RNFL thickness are shown. (Courtesy of Drs Felipe Medeiros, Eduardo Mariottoni, Alessandro Jammal, and Eric Cabezas at the Duke Eye Center.)

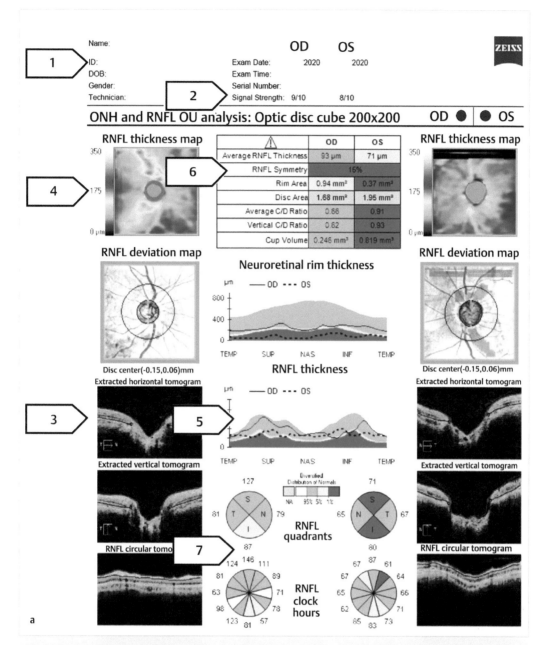

Fig. 3.7 Interpreting optical coherence tomography (OCT) of the optic nerve for glaucoma. Although there is no standard assessment for interpreting OCT measurements of the optic nerve, it is important to take a systematic and consistent approach in order to avoid misinterpretation of the data. An example of a systematic approach to interpreting Cirrus **(a)** and Spectralis

(Continued)

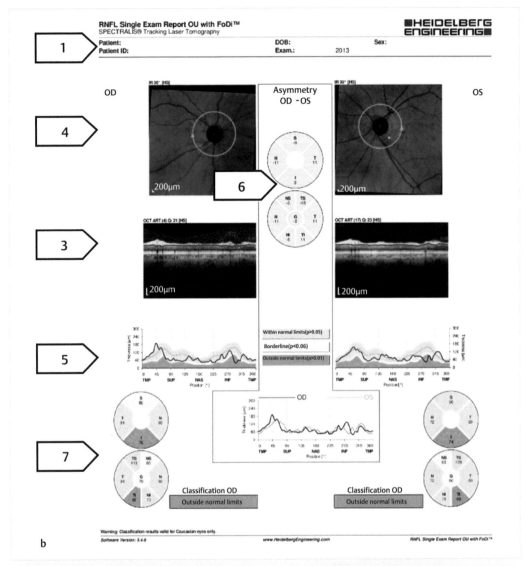

Fig. 3.7 *(Continued)* **(b)** OCT outputs is demonstrated. **Step 1:** Ensure the correct patient name and age. **Step 2:** Check the signal strength (Cirrus), as diminished signal can yield erroneous measurements. **Step 3:** Assess segmentation of the retinal nerve fiber layer (RNFL), as improper segmentation will result in incorrect measurements of RNFL thickness. **Step 4:** Compare the optic nerve tracing to fundus photographs or clinical examination. Accurate tracing can be affected by parapapillary atrophy or optic nerve tilt. Ensure proper centration. **Step 5:** Check the alignment of the temporal-superior-nasal-inferior-temporal (TSNIT) plots to be sure that the position of the superior and inferior peaks is generally aligned with those in the normative database. **Step 6:** Look for asymmetry in RNFL measurements between the two eyes. **Step 7:** Evaluate the pattern of RNFL thickness to assess whether it fits a pattern for glaucoma. In these examples from different patients, there is superior and inferior RNFL loss, which is consistent with a glaucoma diagnosis. Steps are described in more detail in ▶ Table 3.1.

Confirm Patient's Name and Age

Ensure that the output file is from the correct patient and confirm that age was put correctly, as measurements are made in reference to age-matched nomograms.

Check Signal Strength

Signal index can be diminished by nystagmus or media opacity, such as corneal scar, cataract, or vitreous opacity. OCT manufacturers have recommended threshold values of signal indices to guide interpretation of output reliability. For Cirrus HD-OCT, signal strength values of 7 or greater are preferred, and values of 3 or less have significantly diminished measurement reliability. For the Spectralis, the signal threshold is a quality score of 15 or greater out of a maximum of 45, and the recommended threshold for the RTVue-100 is a signal strength index of 39 of 100.

Evaluate for Segmentation Error

Examine the RNFL thickness and RNFL deviation maps for rectangular regions of complete RNFL loss, which are unlikely to reflect arcuate loss of RNFL thickness and likely represent segmentation error artifact. Evaluate the circumpapillary B-scan tracings to assess the accuracy of RNFL segmentation.

Check the Optic Nerve Tracing

Compare the delineation of the optic disc and optic cup to clinical examination or fundus photographs. Check that the scan is properly centered on the optic nerve. Tilted nerves and peripapillary atrophy are especially prone to algorithmic misidentification of optic nerve boundaries.

Evaluate the TSNIT Plot

Examine the RNFL thickness TSNIT plot to ensure that the superior and inferior peaks align with the normative data. Ocular torsion or long or short axial lengths may cause these peaks to be spaced further apart or closer together relative to normal data, leading to artifactually thin values in the superior and inferior quadrants. Additionally, any local area with thickness less than 40 µm likely represents segmentation artifact rather than true loss; even eyes with longstanding optic neuropathy have glial tissue and fibrotic changes to provide at least 40 µm of thickness in RNFL measurements.

Look for Asymmetry

Asymmetry in cup-to-disc ratio or RNFL thickness can be suggestive of glaucoma. Degree of asymmetry is reported as a percentage in some reports. Nonetheless, it is important to check the raw measurement values of RNFL thickness, especially by quadrant, as color-coded flags may not catch subtle abnormalities. A difference in average RNFL thickness greater than 9 µm between eyes could suggest glaucoma.

Assess Whether Abnormalities Fit a Glaucomatous Pattern

Do thin areas of RNFL measurement fit a glaucoma diagnosis? Classically, superior and inferior quadrants of the RNFL are the first to become thin, followed by the temporal quadrant. Atypical patterns may suggest artifact or an alternative diagnosis. Determine whether areas that are flagged as thin or progressively thinning correspond to clinical examination and perimetry.

Evaluate for Progression

Examine progression analysis output to investigate for changes in RNFL thickness over time that could suggest true disease progression. These data are often presented in both graphical and table formats. Normal age-related RNFL thinning occurs on a level of about −0.5 µm/year, while steeper loss suggests glaucomatous damage (often around −1 to −2 µm/year). Interpret regional progression in the clinical context of optic nerve examination and visual field data.

Check Refractive Error and Axial Length

Refractive error of the eye results in changes to relative magnification of peripapillary measurements, which are not taken into account in commercial algorithms. Myopic eyes are generally more prone to measurement error due to increased axial length and optic disc tilt. In pseudophakic patients, axial length may be more informative than refractive error to assess degree of myopic changes.

Compare to Prior Scans

Ensure scan location is consistent across timepoints. Take into account variation in signal strength and presence of artifact when interpreting progression, as algorithms for progression detection are vulnerable to errors made in image acquisition.

3.3 Utility of OCT in Glaucoma Management

3.3.1 Reproducibility

OCT scans of the optic nerve are highly reproducible, demonstrating consistent readings with repeated measurements. Test-retest evaluations in triplicate on glaucoma patients and controls have demonstrated excellent coefficient of variation measurements, in the order of 1 to 3%, indicating high reproducibility. Other studies have evaluated intersession variation by taking four separate measurements over a 1-month period, finding a 1 to 2% coefficient of variation, with the best reproducibility for cup-to-disc ratio and average RNFL thickness and the worst for nasal quadrant assessment. Based on these data, some researchers have estimated an inter-visit tolerance limit of about 4 μm, with values greater than 4 μm indicating a statistically significant change from baseline. However, this variation is likely to vary between commercial devices and reproducibility continues to improve with iterative technological improvements over time.

Incorporation of eye tracker technology has further reduced intersession measurement variation. Newer OCT devices can register follow-up scans automatically over previously scanned areas using anatomic retinal landmarks, increasing consistency between sessions and improving sensitivity to detect progression.

3.3.2 Reliability

Clinical decisions to initiate or to escalate glaucoma therapy often depend on RNFL thickness abnormality or loss on OCT, but clinicians must trust whether the images acquired for these measurements are reliable. Reliability metrics include signal strength and presence of artifact, such as image segmentation error.

Signal strength values correlate with RNFL measurement reliability, and low signal values suggest that output should be interpreted with caution. In one analysis of Cirrus OCT images, decreases in signal strength between 10 (perfect) and 3 yielded modest effect on measured RNFL, with an error of about 1 μm per 1-point decrease in signal strength. However, signal strength values less than 3 corresponded with a large error of 16 μm per 1-point decrease in signal strength, highlighting the importance of assessing OCT reliability when interpreting output.[9]

OCT measurements on patients with severe-stage glaucoma are more prone to decreased reliability due to diminished signal strength compared to images obtained from those with mild or moderate disease. Older age, black race, and long axial length are also associated with lower signal strength values. Additionally, the presence of artifact affects reliability independent of signal strength, although artifacts of one quadrant in RNFL thickness do not necessarily affect the values measured in other quadrants. Critical assessment of reliability is essential to interpret whether RNFL changes over time truly reflect progressive disease.

3.3.3 Progression Analysis

The high reproducibility of OCT imaging allows for comparisons of measurements over time to detect small glaucomatous changes to the ONH. Automated progression analysis algorithms trend measurements from registered images over time and calculate changes from baseline to latest study. For example, the Cirrus Guided Progression Analysis™ (▶ Fig. 3.8) provides event- and trend-based analysis of RNFL measurements and highlights changes that fall outside the limits of expected variability based on normative data. Tables of RNFL measurements are available in the printouts to summarize measurements over time with color coding to indicate whether thinning is outside expected values of measurement variability and age-related changes. Similar outputs are provided on other commercial OCT platforms (a Spectralis example is demonstrated in ▶ Fig. 3.9).

Although software guidance can alert the physician to areas of possible progression, there is no consensus on what quantity of change is truly significant. Test-retest standard deviation of SD-OCT measurements has been estimated to be as low as 1 μm. Accordingly, some authors argue that short-term RNFL changes of 4 or 5 μm should be suspicious of glaucomatous loss, but it is important to have multiple baseline measurements and confirmation of changes with subsequent scans in order to establish true change. Furthermore, sectoral measurements have less reproducibility than average RNFL values, and would therefore require greater change in thickness measurements for confidence in true progression, with estimates between 7 and 8 μm. Variability of image acquisition, such as subjective centration over the optic disc by the operator, decreases test-retest reliability of measurement values, as decentration as little as 0.1 mm results in approximately 2 μm variation of RNFL measurement. Even automated centration faces limitations. BMO provides a reliable landmark for ONH measurements, but the location of BMO may change over time due to intraocular pressure (IOP) fluctuations, connective tissue remodeling in the setting

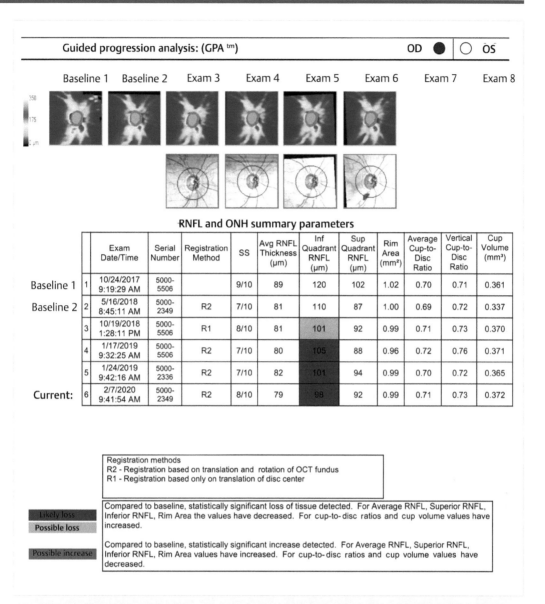

Fig. 3.8 Guided Progression Analysis (Cirrus optical coherence tomography [OCT]). The guided progression analysis on the Cirrus device trends retinal nerve fiber layer (RNFL) thickness values over time. RNFL thinning over time suggests glaucoma progression, and RNFL loss may not be evident on RNFL thickness measurements obtained at a single timepoint. This example is the guided progression analysis of the right eye from the same 70-year-old white woman whose RNFL analysis is provided in ► Fig. 3.4. Although the inferior RNFL thickness is greater than the fifth percentile for the patient's age, serial measurements over time indicate likely RNFL loss. The patient's visual field testing demonstrates a corresponding superior nasal step for the right eye, consistent with moderate-stage glaucoma. (Courtesy of Dr Ian Conner of the University of Pittsburgh.)

of glaucoma, or due to posterior migration with age. Further longitudinal studies are required to determine the stability of BMO position over time and how changes would affect reliability of ONH measurements.

Recent research has questioned the use of the "Rule of 5," or loss of 5 μm of average RNFL thickness between visits, to establish structural progression of glaucoma. This absolute cut-off lacked specificity for glaucoma progression due to measurement

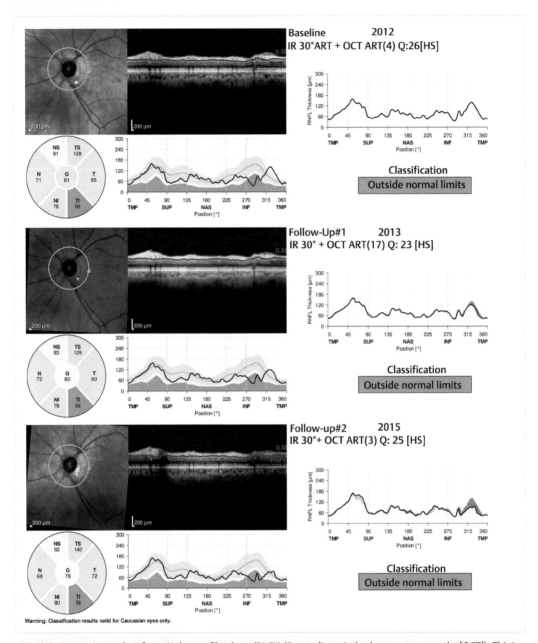

Fig. 3.9 Progression analysis for retinal nerve fiber layer (RNFL) (Spectralis optical coherence tomography [OCT]). This is a Spectralis OCT RNFL progression analysis report for a 70-year-old woman with normal tension glaucoma. There is an inferior notch at the baseline examination which corresponds with a superior nasal step on visual field testing. Over the following 3 years, there is progressive thinning of the RNFL inferiorly accompanied by a new arcuate defect on her visual field.

variability (with a quarter of glaucomatous eyes gaining 5 μm between visits over the 5-year period) and due to age-related loss, with a quarter of non-glaucomatous control eyes experiencing a 5 μm inter-visit loss during the course of the study.[8]

Although OCT measurements provide important quantitative information to aid in detection of structure changes, these data must be interpreted in the context of clinical evaluation and perimetry in order to detect true progression of disease.

3.3.4 Diagnostic Accuracy

OCT measurements provide valuable diagnostic information in glaucoma evaluation. In general, the average RNFL thickness and inferior quadrant RNFL thickness provide the best diagnostic accuracy for glaucoma, followed by RNFL thickness of the superior quadrant. Abnormalities in average RNFL thickness in glaucoma suspect eyes are highly specific for predicting visual field loss even several years later. Additionally, OCT measurements of ONH parameters can distinguish glaucomatous eyes from healthy eyes,[4] and RNFL measurements correspond to visual field testing in manifest glaucoma, with thinner readings correlating with areas of visual field defects.[5]

OCT parameters are meaningful structural measurements for patients with glaucoma. Faster rates of RNFL loss are associated with increased likelihood of visual field defects. Among glaucoma suspects with normal visual field testing at baseline, faster rate of RNFL thinning is strongly associated with development of manifest visual field loss. For every 1 µm/year faster rate of RNFL loss, there is an approximately twofold higher risk of visual field defect.[3] In the same vein, manifest glaucoma patients with RNFL thinning on trend-based progression analysis have a much higher chance of visual field progression compared to those with stable OCT measurements, with a hazard ratio of about 8.44 for visual field progression by Early Manifest Glaucoma Trial (EMGT) criteria.[10]

3.3.5 Correlation with Patient-Centered Outcomes

OCT measurements of RNFL correlate with meaningful patient-centered outcomes, including worsening quality of life scores and decreased driving simulation performance. Although blindness is the most feared outcome of glaucoma, evidence suggests that even mild disease results in decreased quality of life. Previous studies have used the National Eye Institute Visual Function Questionnaire (NEI VFQ-25) as a measure of vision-related quality of life in glaucoma patients and results generally correlate with degree of visual field loss, particularly in patients with advanced disease. Recent work has correlated progression of RNFL thinning by OCT with VFQ-25 scores, a relationship that remains significant even after adjustment for corresponding visual field loss.[2] Specifically, every 1 µm loss of binocular RNFL per year was associated with a loss of about 1 unit on the NEI VFQ-25 score, indicating that RNFL thinning corresponds with decreased visual function.

In the same vein, progressive RNFL loss has been found to correlate with decreased reaction time on driving simulations. Specifically, among glaucoma patients and controls, RNFL thickness was found to be inversely correlated with reaction times to low-contrast curve negotiation and to simulations of following a car moving at variable speeds.[6] OCT progression is strongly correlated with worsening visual function and correlates with quality of life and functional outcomes for glaucoma patients.[7]

3.4 Limitations and Pitfalls

3.4.1 Common Artifacts

Although OCT algorithms can label a patient output as normal or abnormal compared to controls, physicians must be able to recognize measurement artifacts in order to interpret these results accurately. The ability to recognize artifacts is critical, as they affect RNFL measurements in as much as a third of OCT scans from glaucoma patients.

Ocular pathology is a common confounder of measurement of RNFL thickness. Common culprits include focal media opacities, retinal disease, and myopia.

In contrast to global signal depression from cataract, focal medial opacities can lead to regional areas of decreased signal strength that could be misidentified as segmental RNFL thinning. These regional defects would also artifactually decrease the average RNFL thickness measurement. Common examples of focal media opacity include posterior vitreous detachment, prominent vitreoretinal interface opacity, vitreous hemorrhage, and asteroid hyalosis.

Retinal disease can also impact measurements of peripapillary RNFL thickness. Epiretinal membrane, traction from incomplete posterior vitreous detachment, and retinoschisis have been demonstrated to cause errors in both circumpapillary and macular analysis of RNFL thickness, and many of these artifacts are not readily apparent on the summary printout. Fortunately, macular B-scans and macular thickness maps often readily identify underlying confounding pathology and can alert the physician to interpret RNFL measurements with caution.

High myopia can also influence RNFL measurement values. Eyes with longer axial lengths tend to have thinner RNFL thickness, and ocular magnification influences measurements of ONH parameters. Additionally, myopic eyes tend to have temporally deviated RNFL bundles and vasculature that may not align with the normative data, as visualized on TSNIT plot. This misalignment can lead to artifactual flagging of superior and inferior quadrants as thin. Effects of refractive error are discussed in Chapter 11.

Lastly, multifocal intraocular lens implants can interfere with image acquisition. The varied focal points between concentric rings can lead to a wavy, horizontal artifacts in line-scanning images with gaps in the images wider in the center and narrower in the periphery.

Evaluation of acquired images is critical to identify measurement artifacts. Manual correction of segmentation errors can help to ensure accurate measurements are taken into account during clinical assessment.

Artifacts are discussed in depth in Chapter 8.

3.4.2 Pitfalls

Physicians interpret RNFL abnormalities in the context of ophthalmic history and physical examination. RNFL thinning is not specific for glaucoma, and it is essential to determine whether thin RNFL measurements could be due to nonglaucomatous optic neuropathy. Some signs suggestive of non-glaucomatous etiology include presence of an afferent pupillary defect, dyschromatopsia, optic disc pallor, and concomitant cranial nerve palsies, to name a few. In the presence of concerning neuro-ophthalmological signs, other causes of optic neuropathy should be considered, including compressive, inflammatory, infectious, and nutritional etiologies, before attributing RNFL loss to glaucoma.

RNFL thinning is also not specific for optic neuropathy, as retinal vein or artery occlusion, inherited retinal diseases, and transsynaptic neurodegeneration can also lead to loss of inner retinal layers. Evaluation of macular images and correlation with fundus examination can help to distinguish glaucoma from ischemic inner retinal processes.

Finally, thin RNFL measurements do not necessarily indicate RNFL loss. Congenital conditions can present with thin RNFL from birth, including optic nerve hypoplasia and superior segmental optic nerve hypoplasia. Complete history and examination coupled with perimetry is critical to establish a glaucoma diagnosis when OCT measurements are abnormal.

3.4.3 Green and Red Disease

Color coding of values as within or beyond normal ranges simplifies interpretation of results in a user-friendly printout. However, physicians must be aware that this color classification system is prone to false positives and false negatives.

Green Disease

There is a wide range of normal variation of ONH measurements in healthy eyes. As such, significant neuroretinal loss may occur for an individual while maintaining classification within the normal range (so-called "green disease"). Obtaining a baseline study is essential for monitoring structural progression over time, as significant thinning can occur even when individual values remain within the normal range.

Red Disease

Just as "green" measurements do not exclude glaucoma, "red" values are not diagnostic for glaucomatous disease. RNFL thickness measurements may read in the lowest 5th percentile due to image acquisition error, such as segmentation artifact from blinking or poor signal strength. Chorioretinal diseases in the macula can also lead to retinal thinning unrelated to RNFL loss from glaucoma. Erroneously flagged values also occur in myopic eyes, whose optical properties lead to minified structural measurements. Further complicating measurements in myopic eyes, peripapillary atrophy may be erroneously incorporated into optic nerve delineation and optic nerve tilt can disrupt *en face* measurement algorithms. Contour shift of the optic nerve can also disrupt the location of superior and inferior RNFL peaks in myopic eyes compared to the normative data, leading to "red disease" in regions where normative RNFL peaks are located.

3.4.4 Limitations

Information gleaned from OCT imaging has profoundly guided our management and understanding of glaucoma. Even so, OCT technology has its limitations. First, strict inclusion criteria for normative databases can limit applicability of normal ranges for clinical patient populations. Included subjects are predominantly adults of European ancestry without ocular comorbidities or high refractive error. Ongoing research aims to identify

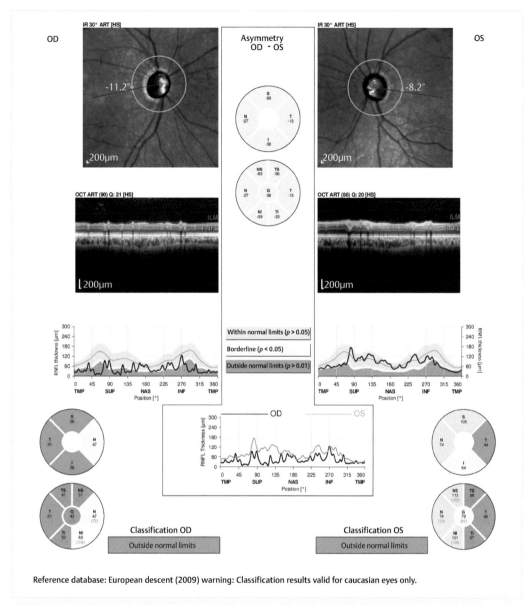

Fig. 3.10 Retinal nerve fiber layer (RNFL) analysis in a patient with severe glaucoma. This is a Spectralis optical coherence tomography (OCT) RNFL report for a 40-year-old man with juvenile open angle glaucoma. He has a history of eye pressures in the 40s and periods of nonadherence to treatment. There is profound thinning of the RNFL in the right eye, with inferior and temporal thinning in the left eye. Temporal thinning is not characteristic of glaucoma until later in the disease course. His visual field is profoundly depressed in the right eye and relatively intact in the left eye.

normative data for broader groups, including children and subjects of Indian ethnicity.

Second, a measurement floor of about 50 μm limits its utility of OCT of the optic nerve in advanced glaucoma (▶ Fig. 3.10). Measurement of retinal ganglion cell density at the macula may provide better sensitivity than peripapillary RNFL measurements in the setting of advanced disease, but central visual field assessment appears to have greater sensitivity in monitoring change in severe cases compared to available structural measurements. OCT of the macula for glaucoma patients is discussed in Chapter 4.

Third, as with many new technological developments in health care, cost of OCT devices can be a limitation for clinical uptake, particularly in developing countries. Fortunately, commercialization of the technology has allowed for widespread adoption of OCT and has made it increasingly accessible across many regions of the world.

Fourth, requirement of multiple baseline measurements and repeated measurements over time for progression analysis can cause a burden of frequent visits for glaucoma patients. However, the same is true for other parameters in glaucoma, such as IOP measurement and perimetry, and OCT measurements do not necessarily in themselves add to visit burden.

Fifth, presence of cataract and comorbid retinal disease can limit reliability and increase chances of artifact. Physicians must be cognizant of artifacts when interpreting OCT measurements. The authors hope that resources such as this textbook can help to inform clinicians in their approach and understanding of the use of OCT for their glaucoma patients.

3.5 Future Directions

OCT technology continues to evolve, and new developments provide exciting opportunities to advance structural assessment of optic nerve parameters in glaucoma. Incorporation of swept-source technology into SD-OCT (SS-OCT) allows for a longer wavelength and thus deeper penetration into ocular tissues. This swept-source technology allows for better visualization of choroid and sclera, heightening understanding of posterior segment diseases such as pachychoroid spectrum disorders. In the same vein, SS-OCT has also allowed for deeper imaging of the lamina cribrosa, allowing for measurements of glaucoma relevant parameters such as lamina cribrosa depth. SS-OCT is discussed in Chapter 13.

OCT angiography (OCT-A) allows for noninvasive assessment of superficial and deep vascular networks without intravenous dye by interpreting changes in images over time to derive blood flow. The role of OCT-A as a proxy for dye-based angiography is evolving in the treatment of retinal diseases. In glaucoma, OCT-A allows for noninvasive assessment of microvascular changes across different stages of disease. Beyond its use as a research tool, the utility of OCT-A in clinical management of glaucoma is yet to be determined. OCT-A for glaucoma is discussed in Chapter 12.

Another emerging imaging tool to incorporate into OCT is adaptive optics. Adaptive optics (AO) imaging controls for optical aberrations of the eye to enhance transverse resolution. Incorporation of AO into OCT images has allowed for high-resolution images of ONH structures, such as retinal nerve fiber bundles and lamina cribrosa pores and beams. Further research is needed to understand the role of these parameters in glaucoma management and how newer technologies can incorporate previous data acquired on current platforms.

3.6 Conclusions

The advent of SD-OCT has allowed for reliable, reproducible, and quantitative assessment of the optic nerve in detection and monitoring of glaucoma. These data provide critical information for assessment of glaucoma patients and allow for detection of structural progression. OCT-derived data on RNFL loss guide treatment escalations and follow-up intervals in clinical practice, and these measurements are used in close conjunction with perimetry and clinical examination. Moreover, advanced imaging of the optic nerve has brought with it an evolving concept of "pre-perimetric" glaucoma, in which loss of RNFL thickness is detected on OCT before the presence of a corresponding visual field defect. As technological capabilities advance, they continue to challenge and redefine our understanding and classification of glaucoma.

References

[1] Chen JJ, Kardon RH. Avoiding clinical misinterpretation and artifacts of optical coherence tomography analysis of the optic nerve, retinal nerve fiber layer, and ganglion cell layer. J Neuroophthalmol. 2016; 36(4):417–438

[2] Gracitelli CPB, Abe RY, Tatham AJ, et al. Association between progressive retinal nerve fiber layer loss and longitudinal change in quality of life in glaucoma. JAMA Ophthalmol. 2015; 133(4):384–390

[3] Miki A, Medeiros FA, Weinreb RN, et al. Rates of retinal nerve fiber layer thinning in glaucoma suspect eyes. Ophthalmology. 2014; 121(7):1350–1358

[4] Mwanza JC, Oakley JD, Budenz DL, Anderson DR, Cirrus Optical Coherence Tomography Normative Database Study Group. Ability of Cirrus HD-OCT optic nerve head parameters to discriminate normal from glaucomatous eyes. Ophthalmology. 2011; 118(2):241–8.e1

[5] Nilforushan N, Nassiri N, Moghimi S, et al. Structure-function relationships between spectral-domain OCT and standard achromatic perimetry. Invest Ophthalmol Vis Sci. 2012; 53 (6):2740–2748

[6] Tatham AJ, Boer ER, Rosen PN, et al. Glaucomatous retinal nerve fiber layer thickness loss is associated with slower reaction times under a divided attention task. Am J Ophthalmol. 2014; 158(5):1008–1017

[7] Tatham AJ, Medeiros FA. Detecting structural progression in glaucoma with optical coherence tomography. Ophthalmology. 2017; 124 12S:S57–S65

[8] Thompson AC, Jammal AA, Medeiros FA. Performance of the rule of 5 for detecting glaucoma progression between visits with OCT. Ophthalmol Glaucoma. 2019; 2(5):319–326

[9] Yohannan J, Cheng M, Da J, et al. Evidence-based criteria for determining peripapillary OCT reliability. Ophthalmology. 2020; 127(2):167–176

[10] Yu M, Lin C, Weinreb RN, Lai G, Chiu V, Leung CK. Risk of visual field progression in glaucoma patients with progressive retinal nerve fiber layer thinning: a 5-year prospective study. Ophthalmology. 2016; 123(6):1201–1210

3

4 Optical Coherence Tomography of the Macula

Divakar Gupta

Summary

Retinal imaging for glaucoma diagnosis and management has largely focused on quantifying characteristics of the optic nerve head (ONH), the peripapillary retinal nerve fiber layer (RNFL), and the retinal ganglion cell complex (GCC); this chapter focuses on optical coherence tomography (OCT) of the macula in glaucoma patients. These measurements are followed longitudinally to assess for changes due to glaucomatous progression. OCT measurements of the peripapillary RNFL and/or GCC may be affected by image acquisition techniques, image artifacts, and patient characteristics—all of which can limit the utility of peripapillary imaging or ONH imaging in glaucoma management. OCT imaging of macula retinal ganglion cells (RGCs) can supplement the information obtained with peripapillary imaging and may offer some advantages, including less variation in the RGC measurement and better image segmentation. Segmentation and interpretation of macular imaging may be influenced by artifacts that are different from those that affect peripapillary images. Further, certain populations of patients may have improved glaucoma surveillance using macular OCT scans such as patients with advanced glaucoma or myopia. Thus, macular imaging may complement the use of ONH or RNFL imaging and increase confidence of OCT findings. In this chapter, we discuss the applications, advantages and disadvantages, and potential pitfalls of OCT imaging of the macula for glaucoma diagnosis, management, and longitudinal follow-up.

Keywords: optical coherence tomography, macula, glaucoma, retinal nerve fiber layer imaging, retinal ganglion cell, glaucoma progression, imaging artifact

4.1 Retinal Imaging for Glaucoma

4.1.1 Glaucoma and Retinal Ganglion Cells

Ultimately, glaucoma is a collection of diseases that involve retinal ganglion cells (RGCs) dysfunction and/or loss. In patients with glaucoma, the structural changes of the optic nerve head (ONH) over time are due to RGC loss. Cell bodies of RGCs are found in the ganglion cell layer (GCL) of the retina, dendrites of RGCs are in the inner plexiform layer (IPL), and axons in the retinal nerve fiber layer (RNFL); RGC axons exit the eye through the optic nerve to synapse in the ipsilateral or contralateral lateral geniculate nucleus depending on where in the retina they originate. These three layers together (RNFL + GCL + IPL) are referred to as the ganglion cell complex (GCC).

However, glaucoma is not the only condition that affects the structure of the ONH or the peripapillary inner retina. Other findings include edema, pallor, and peripapillary abnormalities. ONH edema can occur in a variety of conditions; examples include elevated intracranial pressure, infection, inflammation, and acute ischemia. ONH edema leads to swelling of the RNFL, obliteration of the optic cup, and may be accompanied with retinal hemorrhages, cotton wool spots, or pallor. Optic disc pallor is another ONH finding that is not typical of glaucoma; this is more commonly seen in other optic neuropathies. ONH drusen may also change the contour of the optic nerve and mimic some of the visual field deficits seen in glaucoma and also affect peripapillary RNFL. Peripapillary atrophy around the optic nerve may be seen in variety of conditions including age-related macular degeneration, (pathologic) myopia, or in normal patients without other ocular comorbidities. Choroidal neovascular membranes can be seen juxtapapillary and may be a source of peripapillary RNFL thickening.

Similarly, GCC loss may also occur due to non-glaucomatous optic neuropathies or secondary to retrograde transneuronal degeneration, for example, after cerebrovascular accident or with an intracranial tumor (▶ Fig. 4.1). In glaucomatous optic neuropathy, however, there may be other clinical signs—optic nerve cupping, RNFL loss that respect the horizontal midline, optic disc hemorrhages, characteristic visual field changes on automated perimetry, etc.—that aid in the diagnosis of glaucoma.

Detecting structural changes in RGC layers is particularly important in glaucoma care as these changes may be the earliest clinical signs leading to a diagnosis of glaucoma. They may also be the first signs to confirm glaucomatous progression in

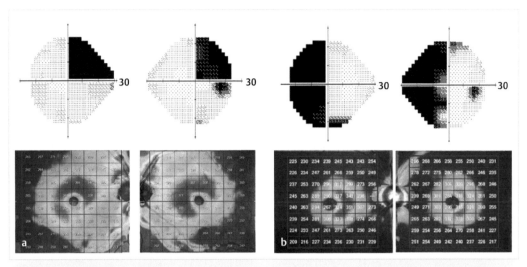

Fig. 4.1 Transsynaptic retrograde degeneration. Examples of corresponding macular optical coherence tomography (OCT) thickness loss in patients with cerebrovascular accidents. Both homonymous quadrantanopia **(a)** and hemianopia **(b)** show corresponding "homonymous" losses on macular OCT.

patients with known glaucomatous optic neuropathy. Significant structural changes (of up to 25–35% loss) can occur prior to visual field changes seen on automated perimetry.[1] Visual field defects may occur years after optic nerve or RNFL changes. Clinically, structural changes at the ONH or defects of the RNFL can be seen by slit lamp ophthalmoscopy or direct ophthalmoscopy or comparison of optic disc photography over time. These findings include vertical elongation of the optic cup, enlarged optic cup, optic rim notching, acquired optic pit, and wedge defects of the RNFL (which are more easily visualized using a green light or "red-free" light). Retina imaging is capable of detecting more subtle or smaller structural changes throughout the posterior pole which are challenging or impossible to see by clinical ophthalmoscopy alone.

Noninvasive imaging of the peripapillary and macula RGCs can be accomplished by a variety of techniques, including scanning laser ophthalmoscopy (SLO), scanning laser polarimetry, and optical coherence tomography (OCT). Retinal thickness analyzers have been used to measure total macular thickness. In this chapter, we will discuss the uses of spectral domain OCT (SD-OCT). SD-OCT is the most widely used commercially available device type for imaging retinal tissue. SD-OCT offers superior resolution and more efficient image acquisition relative to its predecessor time-domain OCT. SD-OCT is capable of imaging the macula, peripapillary region, and the ONH. There are many research and clinical applications of SD-OCT technology described in the literature for patients with glaucoma.

4.1.2 RGCs and the Macula

Although the peripapillary region has been the area that glaucoma specialists initially focused on when evaluating for glaucomatous disease, the macula has become an important structure to image for both the diagnosis and management of glaucoma. Unlike the peripapillary region, glaucomatous changes of the macula are not detected on ophthalmoscopy the way that some structural changes of the ONH/peripapillary RNFL can be seen on both OCT and ophthalmoscopy. The glaucomatous changes in the macula are more subtle and diffuse, less focal, than closer to the optic nerve, as the RNFL spans a greater area in the macula than it does around the optic nerve. The use of imaging of the macula in patients with glaucoma is of greater importance since the clinical signs of glaucoma disease are not able to be seen by fundus ophthalmoscopy.

In the macula RGCs are plentiful, with roughly 50% of RGCs localizing to the anatomic macula; the span of RGCs constitutes over 30% of total retinal thickness.[2] Cell bodies of RGCs are greater than one cell thick in the macula. This means that RGC death in the macula leads to significant and

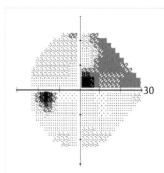

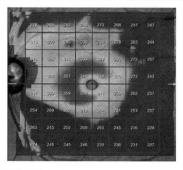

Fig. 4.2 Paracentral loss. Note the loss of annulus around the fovea inferotemporally in this patient's left eye. This corresponds to the superonasal paracentral and nasal step losses seen on automated perimetry.

measurable changes of the RNFL, GCC, and the total macular thickness on retinal imaging. This is an important advantage over peripapillary imaging, where changes in thickness over time are most sensitive to losses of RNFL (axons) and not RGC bodies.

Further, RGC loss in the macula intuitively correlates with visual field loss (on automated perimetry) than peripapillary RGC loss with visual field loss. The most common visual field testing locations are testing visual function in the macula surrounding the fovea (at the patient's fixation). Mapping RNFL loss around the peripapillary region to visual field losses involves following RGC axons from the optic nerve to their origination in the macula. Central defects seen on central visual field testing are more easily identified when looking at macular OCT imaging as opposed to peripapillary RNFL OCT images since the locations of these defects reside near the fovea (▶ Fig. 4.2).

Use of macular OCT marks a transition of how imaging for glaucoma is performed; initially, documenting and supplementing the clinical examination, to currently, providing structural information previously unattainable from clinical examination alone. ONH and peripapillary imaging was performed as the mainstay of glaucoma imaging and was primarily used to highlight areas of loss and supplement optic nerve ophthalmoscopy. Macular OCT can be used to complement peripapillary imaging and may offer internal validation of changes seen on peripapillary imaging. When an OCT finding is seen on macula or RNFL peripapillary imaging and is able to be correlated with the other OCT imaging location, the user can have more confidence that the finding is "real" and not the result of an artifact. Macular OCT may also allow for the possibility of detecting changes early, prior to visual field loss. The inner layers of the macula can show significant thinning prior to visual field deficits on perimetry.

There are some limitations to implementation. OCT scanning of the macula will add time to imaging acquisition protocols depending on the protocol and OCT machine manufacturer. Similar to RNFL protocols, macular imaging requires patient cooperation and fixation. Macula images may be susceptible to a variety of artifacts that can be related to patient characteristics, glaucomatous related changes, and other ocular comorbidities. In some cases, artifacts seen on the macula scan are not seen on the peripapillary scan and vice versa. Common artifacts seen on macula imaging are discussed later in this chapter.

4.2 OCT Image of the Macula

4.2.1 Devices and Segmentation

Currently, there are five major manufacturers of commercially available SD-OCT devices: (1) Cirrus from Carl Zeiss Meditec (Jena, Germany); (2) Spectralis from Heidelberg Engineering (Heidelberg, Germany); (3) 3D OCT-2000 from Topcon Medical Systems (Tokyo, Japan); (4) Avanti Widefield OCT from Optovue (Fremont, CA, USA); and (5) RS-3000 Advance 2 from Nidek (Gamagori, Japan). Three of these devices acquire raster scans of the macula in a square pattern (Spectralis, RS-300 Advance, 3D OCT-2000) and two acquire an ellipse or circle pattern of the macula (Cirrus, Avanti). The manufacturers report results as either total retinal thickness and/or a combination of RNFL, GCL, and IPL. There is no standard as to which size or shape is best for discriminating glaucomatous changes in the macula. Users should be aware of different shapes and sizes that are available for imaging the macula using SD-OCT.

To quantify RNFL, GCC, or total macular thickness measurements, automated segmentation software is used. Some manufacturers allow for the user to manually correct individual scan segmentation errors using their software. Segmented macula layers can discriminate glaucomatous and healthy control eyes.[3] Total macular thickness measurements are reproducible and segmented by OCT software. Total macular thickness may be more accurately segmented when compared with RNFL or GCC layers, due to the high reflectivity of the internal and external limiting membranes. However, total macular thickness measurement can be affected by nonglaucomatous pathologies, and may be influenced to a greater amount, compared to RNFL/GCC measurements, by pathologies that affect retinal thickness outside of the GCC. GCC segmentation may improve diagnostic ability of macular scans, and some studies have found improved diagnostic ability of macular GCC over total macular thickness.[4] GCC measurements are also highly repeatable by commercially available machines. The ratio between GCC and total macular thickness may also be an important measure in early glaucoma. Artifacts influence segmentation of the macula in ways that may differ from peripapillary RNFL scans; this depends on the source and location of the artifact and is discussed later in this chapter.

4.2.2 Correlation between Visual Field and Macular OCT

The function of the RGCs in the macula can be tested by automated perimetry—more so in center-weighted visual field tests, such as the Humphrey Visual Field (HVF) 10–2 pattern. This structure–function relationship is keenly important for the diagnosis of glaucoma. In the most common pattern of standard automated perimetry, the HVF 24–2 with a size III stimulus, nearly 230 ganglion cells are tested by a stimulus that excites a point near the fovea, and 10 ganglion cells are stimulated by a stimulus on an edge point.[5] The 24–2 pattern vastly under samples the center macula region; the center of the macula is the region with greatest range of RGC thickness. It is notable that estimates correlating structure and function have determined that a 52% loss of RGCs correlates with a 3 dB loss on the visual field.[5] This highlights the importance of using OCT for diagnosis of preperimetric disease glaucoma.

Pathologies of the RGCs in the macula inferior to the fovea will affect the superior visual field and pathologies of the superior macula will affect the inferior visual field. In normal eyes, perifoveal macular thickness is correlated with visual field

sensitivity on automated perimetry.[6] The mapping of macular structure to visual field is easier to visualize than the relationship between peripapillary RNFL and visual field. However, techniques to combine visual field and OCT data into combined probability maps will likely continue to help doctors understand the structure–function relationship in their patients with glaucoma.[7] These techniques will also be invaluable to patients to understand their condition and results of their visual field and retinal OCT testing.

Imaging around the optic disc does offer some advantages over imaging of the macula using OCT. Both acquisition locations, the RNFL and the macula, are known to correlate with glaucoma severity. Earlier studies found greater ability to distinguish glaucomatous and normal eyes using ONH or peripapillary OCT protocols compared to macular imaging in patients with glaucoma and normal tension glaucoma.[8,9] Visual field abnormalities also correlated better with peripapillary RNFL changes rather than macular OCT scan parameters.[10]

Changes in macula thickness do correlate with structural optic nerve changes, peripapillary RNFL thickness, and visual field. Performance of segmented macular volume and macular layers—macula nerve fiber layer (mNFL) or macular GCC—to distinguish healthy, glaucoma suspect, and glaucoma subjects (with different stages of disease) has been shown to be similar to peripapillary RNFL.[11] Macular scans can also be used to distinguish early from advanced glaucomatous disease. The relationship between visual field and OCT in different stages of glaucoma were similar whether they were evaluated by macular scans or peripapillary RNFL.[12] Macular thickness is also known to correlate with hemifield loss respecting the horizontal midline on visual field. This is similar to RNFL OCT changes and their relationship to visual field tests. Of note, the topographical relationship between OCT of the macula and visual field, and the comparison of probability maps of automated perimetry and OCT of the macula, are more direct and intuitive to the interpreter.

4.2.3 Complementing Peripapillary RNFL Scans with Macular OCT Scans

RGC death will lead to a decrease in RNFL thickness on retinal imaging. Thus changes in RGC macular thickness will also correlate with RNFL measurements on OCT (both macular and peripapillary) scans. This complementary nature of macular OCT to ONH or peripapillary OCT parameters is one of the greatest strengths of macular imaging.

Glaucomatous defects respect the horizontal midline (or the line that connects the fovea to the center of the ONH) and follow the RNFL bundles in an arcuate curvilinear path from macula RGC back to the optic nerve. Importantly, this pattern of loss can help differentiate glaucomatous changes from retina thickness measurement changes from other pathologies; examples include vascular occlusion, ischemic optic neuropathies, and macular degeneration. Macular scans are also easy and require minimal additional time to acquire in patients who are already having imaging around the optic nerve. Dilation is not required in most patients. The relationship between macula thickness and GCC also varies with disease stage.

Artifacts that affect the optic nerve and peripapillary are usually different from those that affect the macula. This allows the macula scans to complement the RNFL OCT, especially when peripapillary artifacts limit interpretation of peripapillary scans or when peripapillary OCT scans are uninterpretable, such as with myopic changes. Importantly, studies have found that RNFL analysis around the ONH can miss macular damage (seen on macular OCT, or 10–2 pattern visual field), which could represent early damage or progression of glaucoma; up to one out of three OCT reports from peripapillary RNFL can miss macular damage.[13] This highlights the importance of using macular scans, especially in patients who are not routinely undergoing a visual field testing dedicated to the central macula. Patients with low or normal tension glaucoma in particular may present with central defects. These defects can be easily missed or overlooked on traditional 24–2 strategy visual field testing and may not easily be seen on RNFL OCT reports. Other types of glaucoma may also have central visual field defects missed on traditional visual field testing strategies and may benefit from macular OCT scans.

Another consideration is that RNFL reports are typically presented as sectoral maps. This can lead to pathologic focal defects from glaucoma being "averaged" out in a sector or global indices. Sometimes this is coined "green" disease as reports show sectoral data in the color green to indicate that they are normal when analyzed using data from a normative database, when in fact there is focal RNFL loss that is pathologic. The macula SD-

OCT reports are typically not presented in this manner for scans done using a glaucoma protocol for image acquisition and analysis; they are presented without sectoral or global summary indices. This allows the end user to see glaucomatous patterns (such as arcuate or paracentral) of loss more easily. Careful analysis of the data in OCT raw scans is still needed to ensure these subtle (yet significant) changes are not overlooked.

4.2.4 Asymmetry Analysis

In the HVF test, one of the parameters reported is the glaucoma hemifield test, which compares sets of data points across the horizontal midline for asymmetry. In this same spirit, asymmetry reports of macular OCT data allow for comparison across the horizontal midline (intra-eye comparison) and also comparison between eyes (inter-eye comparison). In this case the comparison across the horizontal midline is done across the line that connects the fovea to the center of the ONH. Since glaucoma is a disease characterized by asymmetry (both between eyes and within an eye), these plots can highlight early or mild-to-moderate changes that may not be as easily seen on peripapillary RNFL sectoral maps. Quadrant analysis of macular asymmetry also correlates to functional declines in visual field sensitivity.[14]

Intra-eye comparison often tends to be more helpful than inter-eye comparison. Since glaucomatous changes respect the horizontal midline, early signs can be seen as asymmetry on these hemifield comparisons. They may appear in arcuate patterns in patients with glaucoma. These intra-eye comparisons are more helpful than comparing to a normative database.

4.3 Macular OCT and Glaucoma Management

4.3.1 Diagnosis and Progression

For the diagnosis of glaucoma, OCT of macula can be a useful tool. The doctor looks for the characteristic OCT patterns that correlate with the typical "visual field type" patterns seen in glaucoma, that is, assessing OCT scans of the macula for arcuate or paracentral RNFL/total macular thickness losses (relative to the other hemifield or to the other eye) or overall loss of RNFL volume. These losses will also respect the line that connects the fovea to the center of the optic nerve which is the anatomic equivalent to the horizontal midline on the visual field. In the same way that visual field deficits typically "point" toward the optic nerve, one may observe "grooves" or losses of the RNFL as a bundle can be followed back to the optic nerve. The contour of the overlying retinal vessels can be affected and are seen on three-dimensional reconstructions of images to follow the contour of these "grooves." These findings are similar to the RNFL wedge defects seen as loss of retinal sheen on retinal photos or on ophthalmoscopy.

Paracentral defects can be seen and can be one of the most helpful uses of the OCT macula map (▶ Fig. 4.2). The topographic map created in this central annulus of the macula shows deep paracentral defects in what is usually the thickest portion of the macula. Thus, it can be easier to detect a deficit that may otherwise be averaged out on the RNFL plot. Altitudinal RNFL defects of the macula can also be seen in more advanced glaucoma, but care should be taken to consider nonglaucomatous pathologies such as prior vascular occlusion or ischemic optic neuropathy. Similarly, in cases with patterns of loss that do not respect the fovea to optic nerve line (the RNFL raphe) or involve only the temporal edge of the macula map, nonglaucomatous pathologies should be considered.

Comparison of OCT maps over time can aid in the diagnosis of glaucomatous progression. Subtraction maps of OCT macula scans can highlight arcuate-shaped or paracentral defects that deepen over time, consistent with progression of disease. These defects can often be tracked back to the optic nerve. Also, corresponding defects can be seen on OCT peripapillary RNFL change plots or RNFL raw scans for confirmation. Macular scans have been shown to outperform peripapillary RNFL when it comes to detecting progression.[15] They may also hold an advantage in patients with advanced glaucoma, as the RNFL may have limited thickness to detect change, while the macula, and its greater population of RGCs, may be in a more dynamic range.

4.3.2 Barriers to Proper OCT Interpretation

There are many things that can influence the interpretation of OCT. There are limitations of the imaging acquisition, image processing, and software that the user should be aware of in order to avoid an improper interpretation. Importantly, in some cases these barriers can tell the doctor ordering the test that an OCT may not be a reliable way to follow this patient's disease or that caution should be used when interpreting the data.

Floor Effect

Special caution needs to be taken for a variety of situations that may lead to inaccurate interpretation of macular OCT maps. "Floor effect" is a phenomenon that many readers will be already aware of from their experience interpreting OCT RNFL scans. Since some macula protocols report GCL (or some other combination of the sublayers that make up GCC) there is the possibility that severe loss of RGCs in a region can lead OCT values that are near the "floor." This can be for a particular sublayer or even for total macular thickness. This "floor" is a thickness value that only shows the thickness of retinal support cells and/or retinal vasculature; the values of the RNFL, GCC, or total macular thickness are not reduced to zero even with complete neuronal loss. Even at the "floor" there are retinal support cells and vasculature present; thus, the RNFL (or the total macular thickness) is never a zero level of thickness. Yet at these low microns of thickness the OCT may not be dynamic enough to identify changes and therefore glaucomatous change will be more difficult to detect over time. Also, accurate automated segmentation is a greater challenge in more advanced RGC loss since the reflective borders between the nuclear layers and their neighboring layers are more difficult to discern.

Importantly, this is one of the instances when macula scans in glaucoma patients may impart an advantage over peripapillary imaging. Due to the density of RGCs in the macula, even when there are greater losses of RGCs, as seen in advanced or severe disease, there may be a greater ability (or dynamic range) to identify changes over time than at focal areas around the optic nerve. It has been shown in practice and research studies that patients with advanced glaucoma can still demonstrate glaucomatous progression on the macular OCT, even as it nears the "floor" or as the peripapillary RNFL is no longer reliably imaged.

Averaging out Phenomenon

Averaging out of pathology is a phenomenon that is commonly seen on the reports that the commercial platforms provide to the end user. In the peripapillary RNFL reports, a focal wedge defect in a hemisector or quadrant sector can be easily overlooked when it does not have an average thickness in the sector that is identified by the machine to be outside normal limits (which is usually done by comparing a patient's result to a normative database). Since early glaucomatous defects are commonly focal, doctors must be on the lookout for this "averaging out" from occurring.

Just as it is an issue with peripapillary RNFL interpretation, averaging out can still be a concern when looking at macular OCT results. In the classic "ETDRS" style OCT maps used to evaluate primary retinal pathologies, it would be easy to miss the focal defects that are seen in glaucoma. Also, glaucomatous defects in the macula may not fall proximal to the fovea and may be best seen in the more peripheral macula, often nasal to the macula. The manufacturers of the various OCT platforms have developed reports to highlight glaucomatous damage, but any report that shows results in average microns in a particular sector of an annulus is at risk for averaging out pathology. Caution should be exercised to ensure that the interpreter is not missing pathology (resulting in a false negative error), particularly in focal paracentral defects.

One advantage of the macular OCT over the peripapillary OCT reports is that the macular data are not compared to a normative database. In that way, we are identifying changes in macular thickness by looking at progression or comparing across hemi-fields or between eyes.

Contact Lens Effects

Patients who are imaged with and without their contact lenses can also have OCT scans that appear different. Contact lenses in patients with high refractive error can cause optical aberration and changes in the size of the acquired image. This is particularly important when comparing follow-up scans (in a patient who intermittently wears contact lenses) or comparing a patient to a normative database, or when considering the scans of high myopes with or without contact lenses. Although changes in RNFL measurements are relatively small, they may affect interpretation. Also, RGC thickness decreases with age, and by approximately 1% per 1 mm increase in axial length.

4.3.3 Practical Uses of Macular OCT

Early or Mild Glaucoma

In a patient with early or mild glaucoma the macular OCT scan may be particularly helpful. This is because in early glaucoma, defects may be very subtle or focal. On peripapillary OCT measurements, these may be easily averaged out as a focal defect and may not affect the overall value of global indices. Also, it may be difficult to determine if a focal defect in the RNFL is due to an artifact (such as loss of vitreous traction) or represents actual pathology. The macular OCT has the benefit of looking both at the contour and extent of a focal loss. Focal, arcuate-shaped losses are nearly pathognomonic for glaucomatous loss. Also, the hemisphere asymmetric analysis may highlight changes in early disease to the extent that sectoral losses do so on peripapillary OCT scans (▶ Fig. 4.3).

Patients with Paracentral Defects

Another use for macular OCT is to detect patients who have a paracentral defect. Patients with paracentral defects, which may be more commonly seen in patients with normal tension or low-tension glaucoma, have deficits that are difficult to

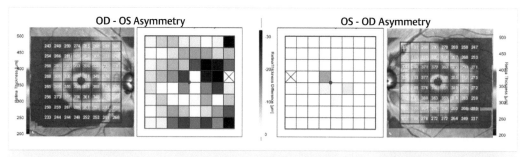

Fig. 4.3 Early stage glaucoma. This is a case example of a patient with asymmetric early stage glaucoma. Note the asymmetry seen in OD-OS asymmetry plot that demonstrates that the right eye macular thickness is thinner than the left. Clinicians should be aware that there are a variety of conditions that may lead to asymmetry between right and left macula thickness.

detect on ONH imaging alone or even with visual field testing. These dense focal defects may be subtle on OCT raw scans and may also be "averaged out" on the peripapillary OCT reports. Also, OCT artifacts—such as vitreous traction—may prevent their recognition. On the visual field, deficits may fall in between stimuli tested on 24–2 or 30–2 testing strategies. In a patient without other macular pathology, however, macular changes may be easier to decipher with analysis of the macular OCT scans, particularly, by focusing on the central annulus around the fovea. This is an area that typically has greater thickness than the center of the fovea due to displaced cell fibers and nuclei. Focal losses in this area can be from loss of RGCs. In ▶ Fig. 4.2 the Spectralis macular OCT shows a deep defect in the central total macular thickness in the annulus around the fovea. This OCT macular defect correlates to a paracentral visual field defect with the expected topographical map (inferotemporal macular OCT loss correlating to superonasal paracentral defect on the visual field).

Glaucoma Progression

Another area in which macular OCT can be very helpful is in the detection of progression. In the pathophysiology of glaucoma, progression seen on visual field testing typically occurs by widening or deepening of existing scotomas prior to new defects. Similarly, tracking the macular OCT maps over time, looking for changes in the subtraction maps, can be an effective way to detect possible progression. Further, defects of the RNFL in an arcuate pattern may give high confidence that there are changes occurring in these patients as a result of glaucoma. In ▶ Fig. 4.4, the OCT of a 78-year-old woman shows a macular defect that is progressively worsening over time. The subtraction map highlights a very thin arcuate line with decreased thickness over time. This can be followed back to a very small change on the OCT of peripapillary RNFL. This supports our concern that her glaucoma has progressed. Further intraocular pressure (IOP) reduction is considered for this

4

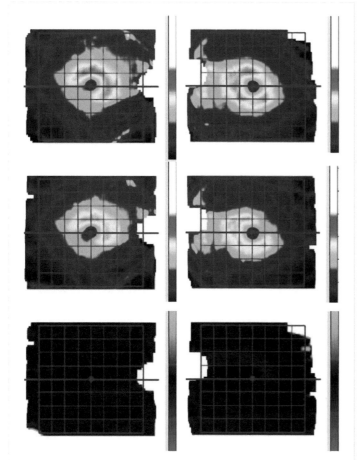

Fig. 4.4 Progression in advanced disease. In this example, macular optical coherence tomography (OCT) scans are performed at two different time points. This patient has loss of the perifoveal thickness in the inferotemporal location in the right eye and superotemporally in the left eye. At the *bottom*, the subtraction maps show subtle curvilinear defects (*red line*) in each eye that respects the horizontal.

4

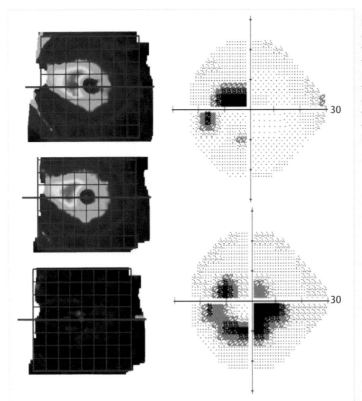

Fig. 4.5 Progressive normal tension glaucoma. On the *left*, the macular thickness maps at two different time points show a clear decrease in macular thickness on the retina thickness change plot (*bottom left*). Over this same time period, the visual field for this patient shows visual field loss in the superior and inferior paracentral area.

patient. ▶ Fig. 4.5 demonstrates how changes in macular OCT can correlate with automated perimetry.

Advanced Glaucoma

A very challenging circumstance is to determine if glaucoma is progressing in the patient with advanced glaucoma. Visual field testing tends to be less dynamic in these patients as it may be hard to determine if there is a change on testing. Further, any change would be very concerning as these patients have limited remaining vision. The macular OCT can be very helpful in this case. Unlike the peripapillary RNFL which may not be very dynamic as the values are near their "floor," the macular OCT may still be dynamic since there are more RGC nuclei in the parafoveal area. Even with substantial losses present in advanced glaucoma, there may be the ability to assess whether progressive losses are occurring.

4.4 Artifacts

Artifacts are common in OCT images of glaucoma patients. They can occur in nearly one out of four macular OCT images. Often, sources of artifacts are seen on the final report printout, but occasionally they are only seen on the raw data scans.[16] Special attention to the report as well as the raw data scans is important for proper interpretation. Fortunately, many report printouts have images that can aid in identifying potential artifacts.

4.4.1 Vitreous Traction/Adherence

Vitreous traction and/or adherence is a common source of artifact on OCT scans. For OCT around the ONH, vitreous traction can distort the RNFL. On OCT printouts this may be identified as sharp peaks in the contour of RNFL thickness. One can see how this can lead to "green disease" or the averaging out of sectors to normal values when in fact there is *low* thickness. You may even see peaks on the RNFL plot that are outside of the normal locations for the superior and inferior bundles.

In the macula (▶ Fig. 4.6), the vitreous traction and adherence can also be very disruptive to the segmentation used for interpretation. Similar to the RNFL scans, the segmentation software may inaccurately identify the anterior border of the

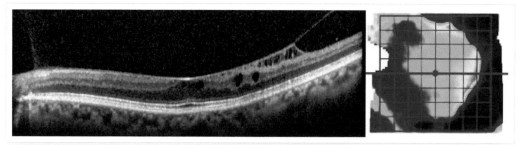

Fig. 4.6 Vitreomacular traction. This is an example of vitreomacular traction causing distortion of the anterior border of the retina and retinal cysts. Note that on the macular thickness map, on the right, the macula is thickest temporally due to this traction band.

retina and trace the posterior hyaloid. In the macula, however, the greatest amount of traction may be the center of the scan. This could leave the remaining areas, where there is no vitreous disturbance, open for standard interpretation. The user should also be on the lookout for traction that is causing macular cysts or lamellar holes in the scans.

Perhaps equally as problematic to interpretation of OCT imaging data as vitreous traction or vitreous adherence is what happens to thickness measurements when the vitreous is released. In patients who are followed over time with segmentation software creating subtraction plots to identify changes, users must be on the lookout for release of vitreous traction/adherence. Loss of vitreous traction can lead to a sudden collapse of the RNFL that was previously suspended by the adherent vitreous. This may be incorrectly interpreted as a sudden loss in thickness or progression of disease. Of course, this is not progressive glaucoma if the change in the plot is not from RGC death, but rather artifactual RGC thickening due to traction that reverses once the tissue is no longer under traction from the vitreous. There are also cases where vitreous traction/release has only affected the RNFL and not the macular OCT scans, allowing for continued interpretation of the macula for signs of progression.

4.4.2 Cystic Changes

Artifacts such as cystic changes of the macula can be seen in patients with advanced glaucoma. These may be due to vitreous traction/adherence to the internal limiting membrane, which would have a significant impact when the RNFL is not very thick. Importantly, it should be recognized that this may lead to a "normal" or near-"normal" appearing macular thickness as the cystic changes may mask decreases in retinal thickness and/or lead to inaccurate segmentation.

4.4.3 Epiretinal Membranes

Epiretinal membranes (ERMs) are also a very important finding to identify on OCT scans. ERM is a common ocular pathology that causes an OCT artifact. They are very common and like vitreous traction or adherence, the anterior border of the RNFL can become very jagged or irregular. Typically, ERMs affect the macular scan to a greater degree than the ONH, but in some cases the peripapillary RNFL scan can be subject to the edge of an ERM. This is typically the RNFL temporal to the ONH as ERMs are less common nasal to the optic nerve. ERM artifacts are similar to changes seen as a result of tractional membranes seen in conditions such as proliferative diabetic retinopathy.

4.4.4 Retinal Atrophy

Atrophy of the retina or RPE can also be a source of artifact. In the peripapillary region, atrophy leads to poor posterior border identification and often improper segmentation of the RNFL. Peripapillary atrophy can cause an enlarged blind spot or relative scotoma near the optic nerve on automated perimetry. In the macula there are many conditions that can lead to atrophy of the RPE or outer retina. RPE atrophy from age-related macular degeneration can lead to improper posterior border identification and affect total macular thickness measurements or even estimation of the GCC. Ultimately, atrophy can have a significant effect on segmentation. Some of these effects may be

4

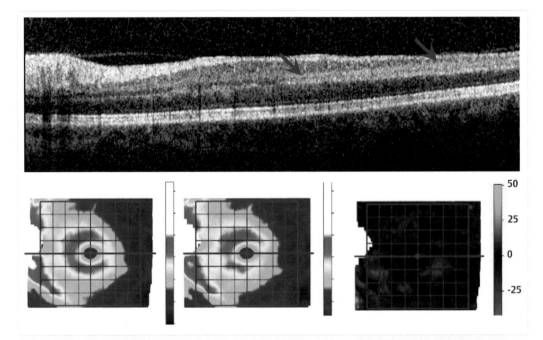

Fig. 4.7 Paracentral acute middle maculopathy. This patient shows interval arcuate loss inferiorly on the macula subtraction map. Close examination of the optical coherence tomography (OCT) line scans shows a hyperreflective inner nuclear layer (seen between the *red arrows*). This hyperreflective area represents paracentral acute middle maculopathy.

manually corrected on platforms that allow the user to adjust the posterior border of interest.

4.4.5 Other Macular Pathologies

A variety of other macular pathologies may influence the interpretation of macular OCT. Macular edema from diabetic or inflammatory causes can increase the retinal thickness. Although this is not an artifact itself, it can lead to segmentation error. Also, if the cystic changes are not recognized by the interpreter (note that the raw scans can be very helpful here) then one may misinterpret images as normal or miss progressive changes from glaucoma. Hemorrhage may also be associated with local thickening. Exudates and myelinated nerve fiber layers may cause a posterior shadow that can also lead to segmentation error.

There are overlapping disease patterns between glaucoma and retinal vessel occlusions: both can affect inner retinal thickness, and branch retinal vessel (vein or arterial) occlusions or paracentral acute middle maculopathy (PAMM) do not cross the horizontal (fovea-optic nerve line or horizontal raphe). Vascular occlusions typically cause an altitudinal defect and would cause an abrupt interval

change in a patient that is being followed for glaucoma. However, cases of PAMM can be more subtle, causing an arcuate pattern of loss. Detailed assessment of macular line scans is important to assess the OCT for changes in the middle macula (▶ Fig. 4.7). Patients with previous nonarteritic ischemic optic neuropathy (NAION) may have a similar pattern of altitudinal loss on OCT. This pattern, however, may confuse interpreters seeing a patient for the first time. It is important to look for other clinical signs that may favor the diagnosis of glaucoma (optic nerve cupping, glaucomatous change in fellow eye) or retinal vascular occlusion (retinal heme, the presence of risk factors for a vascular event).

4.4.6 Myopia

Certain patient characteristics may also influence OCT measurements and lead to artifacts. Certain populations may falsely be determined to have glaucoma, when in fact they do not have a progressive optic neuropathy. Myopic patients, for example, may have thinner RNFL and macular thickness measurements, which may lead to false classification of normal myopic patients as glaucomatous. Retinal nuclear layers and total retinal thickness are measurements that may be thinner in myopic patients. The longer axial length seen in myopic patients also leads to an optical artifact that is evident on peripapillary imaging where the optic nerve appears smaller. Although this magnification effect can be corrected for, it is not usually done so by the OCT machine and therefore may influence interpretation of ONH and RNFL parameters. When a normative database is used to compare a patient's OCT scan to reference, it should be remembered that there is no correction for high axial lengths. Therefore, in myopic patients, it may be best to compare OCT data to internal reference (i.e., the patient's opposite hemifield, fellow eye, or previous scan) and follow the patient longitudinally for progression. Comparison of patient's scans to a reference myopic normative database may be helpful to improve specificity for glaucoma diagnosis. Performance of macular GCC total or hemisphere measurements were similar to peripapillary RNFL thickness measurements when trying to distinguish patients with and without glaucoma in myopic patients.[17]

4.4.7 Active Uveitis

Active uveitis may be another confounder to OCT interpretation. Previous reports have shown that patients with active uveitis have increased RNFL thickness relative to controls or patients with inactive uvieits.[18] This results in two clinical scenarios in patients with uveitis and glaucoma that providers must exercise caution for: (1) a patient with uveitic glaucoma may be progressing despite having a "normal" appearing RNFL; and (2) a patient that transitions from active uveitis to inactive uveitis may show reversal of RNFL thickening (or volume loss) despite stability in the visual field. Overall, interpretation of OCT as a surrogate for glaucoma progression in patients with uveitis should be used with caution as uveitis activity may also influence RNFL thickness. Certainly, these patients may also have macular edema, complicating the interpretation of macular OCT for management of their glaucoma.

4.4.8 Acquisition Artifacts

Another cause of unintended artifacts is poor acquisition of OCT images. Media opacities such as corneal scar, cataract, or vitreous hemorrhage can reduce signal quality and lead to suboptimal images and segmentation. Posterior vitreous floaters may also cause shadows that can disturb image acquisition and lead to blank spaces in the acquired images. This leads to the OCT segmentation "guessing" the contour of the anterior and posterior borders of the OCT image, leaving gaps in the image.

The technician acquiring the image can also be responsible for artifacts in the OCT image. One common error, on some OCT platforms, is not placing the entire imaged retina (from anterior to posterior) in the image acquisition zone. This can lead to artificially truncating the anterior or posterior portions of the retina. The biggest issue here is if the doctor does not recognize this error and interprets the artifact as progression of glaucoma.

Another issue related to acquisition is poor centration in the scan field. For the optic nerve, poor centration can be very detrimental. The normal RNFL bundles are thickest superior and inferior; thus, any decentration will disturb this relationship, causing a shift in RNFL measurements. In the macula, decentration can also be a problem as the total macula field may not be on the OCT scan. Typically, macula parameters are not presented the same way peripapillary RNFL measurements are so problems with centration may be overcome by careful examination of the scans and reports.

Motion artifact can also degrade image quality. This can occur more commonly in macular OCT scans where the acquisition time is longer. Typically, toward the end of the macula scan, patients may fatigue and move, potentially causing a motion artifact. As OCT technology evolves and scans become faster, this will be less of an issue.

4.5 OCT Angiography

Early OCT angiography (OCT-A) studies have shown structural changes to be superior to angiographic metrics.[19] With ongoing research leading to improvements in algorithms and imaging resolution, OCT-A may improve on its currently diagnostic ability in glaucoma. There are ongoing studies looking at both peripapillary and macular OCT-A in glaucoma patients.

4.6 Conclusions

The use of macular OCT for the diagnosis and management of glaucoma will garner greater attention with time. As this imaging technology advances and our understanding of the first structural signals related to glaucoma onset or progression improves, we will undoubtedly find new uses for macular OCT in our management of glaucoma patients. Glaucoma specialists should be aware of the limitations of macular OCT due to artifacts and ocular comorbidities. At present, the macular OCT is an excellent companion to the peripapillary scan, not only offering similar interpretations in many cases, but also performing superiorly in cases of peripapillary artifacts or specific clinical scenarios.

References

[1] Kerrigan-Baumrind LA, Quigley HA, Pease ME, Kerrigan DF, Mitchell RS. Number of ganglion cells in glaucoma eyes compared with threshold visual field tests in the same persons. Invest Ophthalmol Vis Sci. 2000; 41(3):741–748

[2] Curcio CA, Allen KA. Topography of ganglion cells in human retina. J Comp Neurol. 1990; 300(1):5–25

[3] Ishikawa H, Stein DM, Wollstein G, Beaton S, Fujimoto JG, Schuman JS. Macular segmentation with optical coherence tomography. Invest Ophthalmol Vis Sci. 2005; 46(6):2012–2017

[4] Tan O, Chopra V, Lu AT, et al. Detection of macular ganglion cell loss in glaucoma by Fourier-domain optical coherence tomography. Ophthalmology. 2009; 116(12):2305–14.e1, 2

[5] Garway-Heath DF, Caprioli J, Fitzke FW, Hitchings RA. Scaling the hill of vision: the physiological relationship between light sensitivity and ganglion cell numbers. Invest Ophthalmol Vis Sci. 2000; 41(7):1774–1782

[6] Araie M, Saito H, Tomidokoro A, Murata H, Iwase A. Relationship between macular inner retinal layer thickness and corresponding retinal sensitivity in normal eyes. Invest Ophthalmol Vis Sci. 2014; 55(11):7199–7205

[7] Hood DC, Raza AS. Method for comparing visual field defects to local RNFL and RGC damage seen on frequency domain OCT in patients with glaucoma. Biomed Opt Express. 2011; 2(5):1097–1105

[8] Guedes V, Schuman JS, Hertzmark E, et al. Optical coherence tomography measurement of macular and nerve fiber layer thickness in normal and glaucomatous human eyes. Ophthalmology. 2003; 110(1):177–189

[9] Medeiros FA, Zangwill LM, Alencar LM, et al. Detection of glaucoma progression with stratus OCT retinal nerve fiber layer, optic nerve head, and macular thickness measurements. Invest Ophthalmol Vis Sci. 2009; 50(12):5741–5748

[10] Wollstein G, Schuman JS, Price LL, et al. Optical coherence tomography (OCT) macular and peripapillary retinal nerve fiber layer measurements and automated visual fields. Am J Ophthalmol. 2004; 138(2):218–225

[11] Kotowski J, Folio LS, Wollstein G, et al. Glaucoma discrimination of segmented cirrus spectral domain optical coherence tomography (SD-OCT) macular scans. Br J Ophthalmol. 2012; 96(11):1420–1425

[12] Kim NR, Lee ES, Seong GJ, Kim JH, An HG, Kim CY. Structure-function relationship and diagnostic value of macular ganglion cell complex measurement using Fourier-domain OCT in glaucoma. Invest Ophthalmol Vis Sci. 2010; 51(9):4646–4651

[13] Wang DL, Raza AS, de Moraes CG, et al. Central glaucomatous damage of the macula can be overlooked by conventional OCT retinal nerve fiber layer thickness analyses. Transl Vis Sci Technol. 2015; 4(6):4

[14] Rolle T, Manerba L, Lanzafame P, Grignolo FM. Diagnostic power of macular retinal thickness analysis and structure-function relationship in glaucoma diagnosis using SPECTRALIS OCT. Curr Eye Res. 2016; 41(5):667–675

[15] Sung KR, Sun JH, Na JH, Lee JY, Lee Y. Progression detection capability of macular thickness in advanced glaucomatous eyes. Ophthalmology. 2012; 119(2):308–313

[16] Asrani S, Essaid L, Alder BD, Santiago-Turla C. Artifacts in spectral-domain optical coherence tomography measurements in glaucoma. JAMA Ophthalmol. 2014; 132(4):396–402

[17] Kim NR, Lee ES, Seong GJ, et al. Comparing the ganglion cell complex and retinal nerve fibre layer measurements by Fourier domain OCT to detect glaucoma in high myopia. Br J Ophthalmol. 2011; 95(8):1115–1121

[18] Moore DB, Jaffe GJ, Asrani S. Retinal nerve fiber layer thickness measurements: uveitis, a major confounding factor. Ophthalmology. 2015; 122(3):511–517

[19] Triolo G, Rabiolo A, Shemonski ND, et al. Optical coherence tomography angiography macular and peripapillary vessel perfusion density in healthy subjects, glaucoma suspects, and glaucoma patients. Invest Ophthalmol Vis Sci. 2017; 58(13):5713–5722

4

5 Illustrative Case Examples

Julia A. Rosdahl, Ahmad A. Aref, Lawrence S. Geyman, Teresa C. Chen, Catherine M. Marando, Elli Park, Ki Ho Park, Yong Woo Kim, Hana L. Takusagawa, Atalie Carina Thompson, Andrew Williams, and Ian Conner

Summary

Case examples are presented to illustrate the use of optical coherence tomography (OCT) in the diagnosis and management of glaucoma. Examples from the spectrum of glaucoma stage are shown, from glaucoma suspect to advanced and progressing glaucoma, demonstrating the characteristic findings of OCT of the optic nerve and retinal nerve fiber layer (RNFL) (Chapter 3) and macula (Chapter 4), with structure–function correlations (Chapter 6) and from common devices (Chapter 7) as discussed in those chapters.

Keywords: glaucoma suspect, preperimetric glaucoma, early glaucoma, mild glaucoma, moderate glaucoma, severe glaucoma, OCT images

5.1 Overview

Optical coherence tomography (OCT) is a computerized imaging modality which is commonly used to diagnose and manage glaucoma, as well as other conditions in the eye. OCT imaging of the optic nerve, peripapillary retinal nerve fiber layer (RNFL), and macula are frequently employed for glaucoma patients.

As described in accompanying chapters, characteristic findings on OCT imaging of the optic nerve and RNFL include thinning of the neuroretinal rim following the inferior-superior-nasal-temporal (ISNT) rule, with inferior and superior quadrants affected earliest, followed by nasal, and finally temporal, in the course of glaucoma progression (Chapter 3). Characteristic findings on OCT imaging of the macula include losses in the ganglion cell layer, inner plexiform layer, and nerve fiber layer, and are often in an arcuate shape on thickness maps (Chapter 4). The structure–function correlations between the optic nerve head and visual fields that are characteristic of glaucoma are also demonstrated between structural OCT findings and functional automated visual field findings (Chapter 6). There are several widely used commercially available devices. Although the data from the devices are not directly interchangeable, they have been shown to have comparable diagnostic capabilities (Chapter 7).

Case examples illustrating the range of glaucoma severity are provided to show the reader how OCT is used in the clinical management of real-world glaucoma patients.

5.2 Early (Preperimetric) Glaucoma

The first case example (▶ Fig. 5.1) shows images from a 59-year-old African-American woman who has been followed for 4 years as a glaucoma suspect. Her intraocular pressure (IOP) has been in high teens to low twenties in both eyes with a central corneal thickness in the mid-400 s. Her visual fields are full. The OCT demonstrates normal RNFL thickness and ganglion cell analysis.

The next case example (▶ Fig. 5.2) shows the visual field and OCT image from the left eye of a 65-year-old African-American man with primary open-angle glaucoma (POAG). Based on the American Academy of Ophthalmology Preferred Practice[1] guidelines, the stage is mild due to optic nerve changes in the setting of a full visual field.

An example of a patient with progression on OCT testing is shown in ▶ Fig. 5.3. OCT images from a 56-year-old white woman with preperimetric glaucoma in the left eye shows RNFL thickness thinning temporally in the left eye, with progressive temporal thinning over 12 years of follow-up, seen also on the macular progression analysis. The patient was not tolerant of topical medications and has been observed off treatment. Visual field testing remains full in both eyes.

5.3 Mild-to-Moderate Glaucoma

▶ Fig. 5.4 shows a case of a 62-year-old white woman with normal tension glaucoma in her left eye. She received one treatment of selective laser trabeculoplasty (SLT) at the time of initial diagnosis and is currently on topical pressure lowering therapy. Her vision is 20/20 with corrective lenses with an IOP of 13 mmHg. Her examination is notable for 1 + nuclear sclerosis, and she has a cup to disc ratio of 0.5 with inferior temporal sloping. The OCT demonstrates inferotemporal thinning corresponding to the superior Seidel's scotoma, which

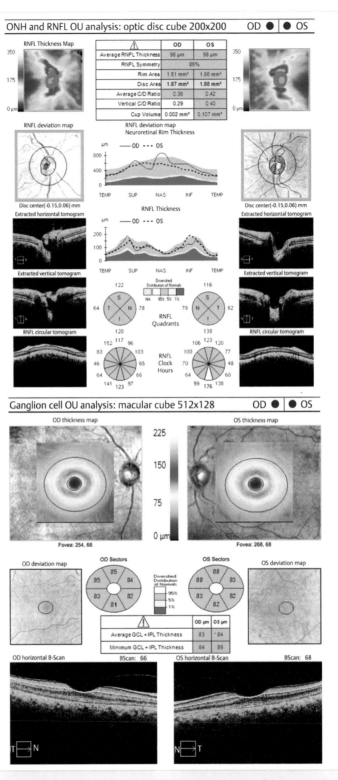

Fig. 5.1 Glaucoma suspect. This is a Cirrus optical coherence tomography (OCT) of the optic nerve (left panel) and macular ganglion cell analysis (right panel) from a 59-year-old African-American woman who has been followed for 4 years as a glaucoma suspect. The Cirrus OCT demonstrates normal retinal nerve fiber layer thickness and ganglion cell analysis. (Courtesy of Drs Andrew Williams and Ian Connor, University of Pittsburgh.)

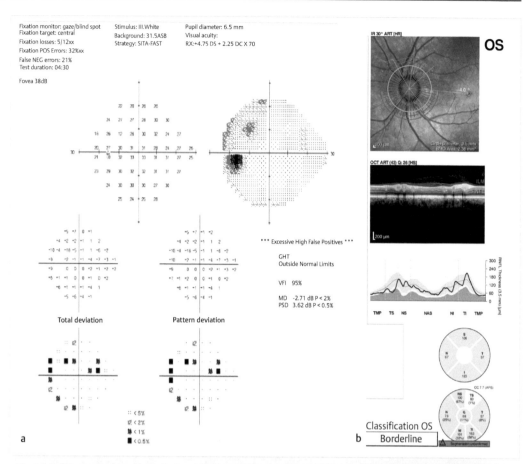

Fig. 5.2 Mild primary open-angle glaucoma (POAG) in the left eye. This is a case of a 65-year-old African-American man with POAG in his left eye. The Humphrey visual field **(a)** is unreliable with high fixation losses and false positive errors, and there appears to be some rim artifact temporally (Humphrey Visual Field, Carl Zeiss Meditec, Inc., Dublin, CA). The optical coherence tomography (OCT) of the optic nerve **(b)** demonstrates thinning of the retinal nerve fiber layer (RNFL) superotemporally, seen on the scan, the temporal-superior-nasal-inferior-temporal (TSNIT) plot, and the quadrant map with the borderline (yellow) classification (Spectralis OCT, Heidelberg Engineering, Heidelberg, Germany). Based on the American Academy of Ophthalmology Preferred Practice guidelines, the stage is mild due to optic nerve changes in the setting of a full visual field. (Courtesy of Dr Atalie Thompson, Duke Eye Center.)

can later develop into a superior arcuate scotoma if her glaucoma were to progress.

The next example (▶ Fig. 5.5) is a case of a 48-year-old Korean man with normal tension glaucoma in the left eye. Central corneal thickness measurements are normal, 583 OD and 592 OS. He is myopic (−9.50 −0.25 at 30 OD; −9.75 −1.00 at 180 OS), with long axial lengths (24.87 mm OD, 27.84 mm OS). Baseline IOPs were 11 to 14 mmHg OD and 12 to 14 mmHg OS. He is currently treated with topical pressure lowering therapy in the left eye, with recent readings of 11 mmHg OD and 12 mmHg OS. The OCT of the optic nerve demonstrates superior greater than inferior thinning and

the OCT of the macula demonstrates thinning of the superior and inferior macula. The visual field demonstrates inferior greater than superior nasal depressions on the pattern deviation analysis.

A case of a 71-year-old white man with pseudoexfoliation glaucoma of the left eye is shown in ▶ Fig. 5.6. This patient is status post combined cataract extraction and mitomycin C (MMC) trabeculectomy of left eye. His vision is 20/25–1 with corrective lenses with an IOP of 16 mmHg. His examination is notable for a superior bleb, pseudoexfoliation material on the anterior capsule, and a cup to disc ratio of 0.6. The OCT demonstrates superior and inferior thinning. The visual field

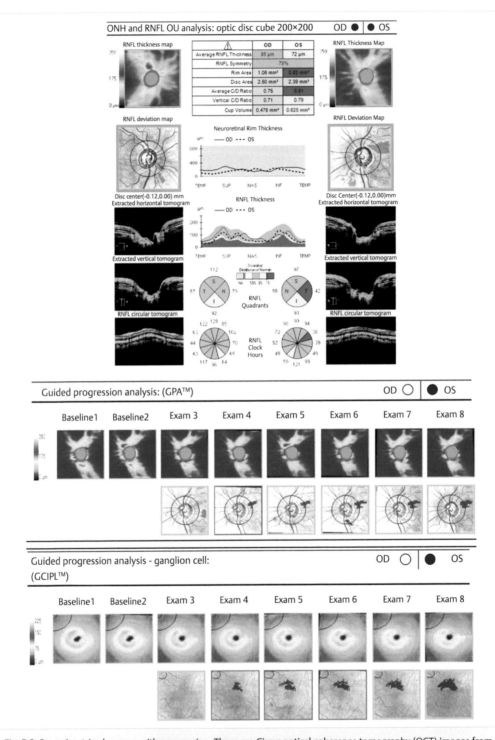

Fig. 5.3 Preperimetric glaucoma with progression. These are Cirrus optical coherence tomography (OCT) images from a 56-year-old white woman with preperimetric glaucoma in the left eye. Retinal nerve fiber layer thickness is thin temporally in the left eye (left panel). Guided progression analysis indicates temporal thinning over 12 years of follow-up (right panel, top), which is also reflected in the macular ganglion cell analysis (right panel, bottom). (Courtesy of Drs Andrew Williams and Ian Connor, University of Pittsburgh.)

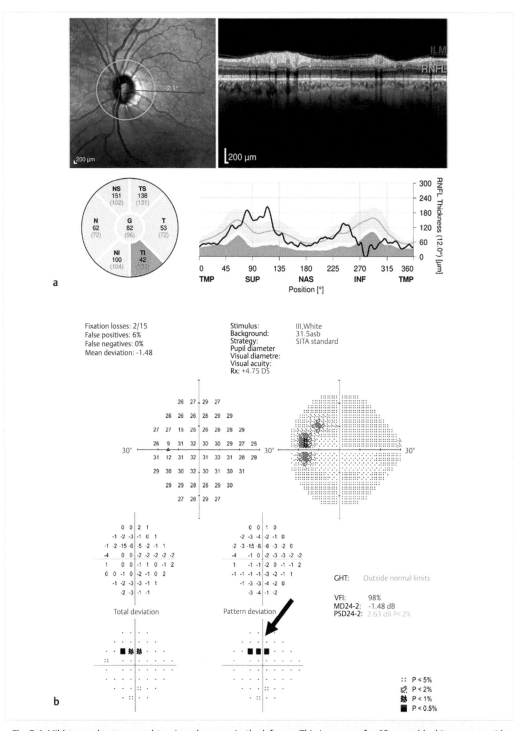

Fig. 5.4 Mild-to-moderate normal tension glaucoma in the left eye. This is a case of a 62-year-old white woman with normal tension glaucoma in her left eye. The optical coherence tomography (OCT) **(a)** demonstrates inferotemporal thinning (Spectralis OCT, Heidelberg Engineering, Heidelberg, Germany). The Humphrey visual field **(b)** is reliable with a mean deviation of −1.48 dB (Humphrey Visual Field, Carl Zeiss Meditec, Inc., Dublin, CA). Note the presence of a Seidel's scotoma (arrow), which can later develop into a superior arcuate scotoma if her glaucoma were to progress. (Courtesy of Drs Teresa Chen, Catherine Marando, and Elli Park of the Massachusetts Eye & Ear Infirmary.)

5

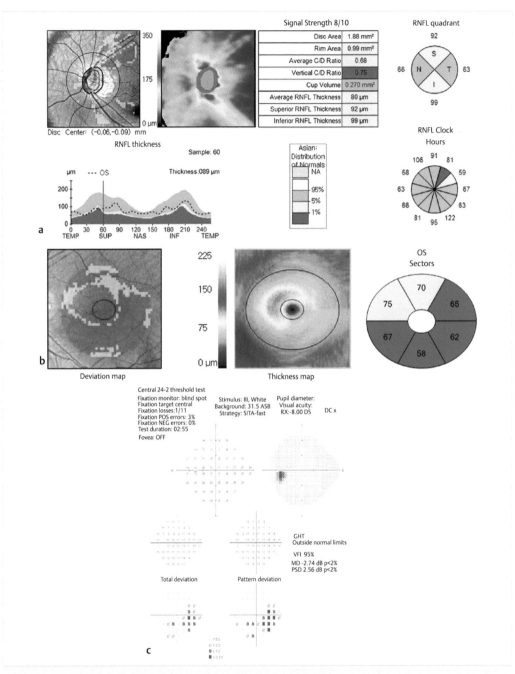

Fig. 5.5 Mild-to-moderate normal tension glaucoma. This is a case of a 48-year-old Korean man with normal tension glaucoma in the left eye. The optical coherence tomography (OCT) of the optic nerve **(a)** demonstrates greater thinning in the superior than inferior on the deviation map, thickness map, and quadrant plot; the temporal-superior-nasal-inferior-temporal (TSNIT) plot and sectoral plots highlight the superior thinning, in particular (Cirrus HD-OCT, Carl Zeiss Meditec, Inc., Dublin, CA). The OCT of the macula **(b)** demonstrates thinning of the superior and inferior macula on the deviation map, the thickness map, and the sectoral analysis. The visual field **(c)** is reliable and demonstrates greater nasal depressions in the inferior than superior on the pattern deviation analysis (Humphrey Visual Field, Carl Zeiss Meditec, Inc., Dublin, CA). (Courtesy of Drs Ki Ho Park and Yong Woo Kim of Seoul National University Hospital.)

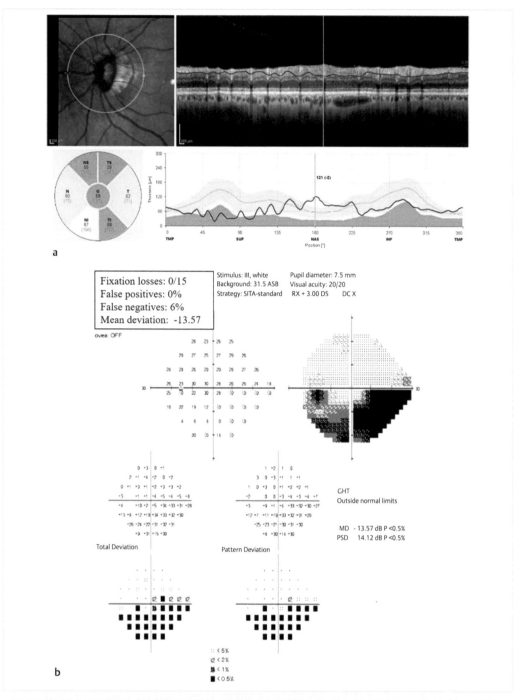

Fig. 5.6 Moderate-stage pseudoexfoliation glaucoma. This is a case of a 71-year-old white man with pseudoexfoliation glaucoma of the left eye. The optical coherence tomography (OCT) **(a)** demonstrates superior and inferior thinning (Spectralis OCT, Heidelberg Engineering, Heidelberg, Germany). The visual field **(b)** is reliable with a mean deviation of −13.57 dB (Humphrey Visual Field, Carl Zeiss Meditec, Inc., Dublin, CA). There is an inferior arcuate defect that spares central fixation. (Courtesy of Drs Teresa Chen, Catherine Marando, and Elli Park of the Massachusetts Eye & Ear Infirmary.)

demonstrates an inferior arcuate defect that spares central fixation. He is being treated with topical pressure lowering therapy.

A case of a 40-year-old Korean man with normal tension glaucoma in both eyes is shown in ▶ Fig. 5.7. Central corneal thickness measurements are normal, 582 OD and 587 OS. He is myopic (−7.75 −0.25 at 160 OD; −6.75 −1.00 at 180 OS), with long axial lengths (27.12 mm OD, 26.77 mm OS). He is currently treated with topical pressure lowering therapy in both eyes, with recent readings of 13 mmHg OU. The OCT of the optic nerve demonstrates superior and inferior thinning with relative sparing of the nasal quadrant. The OCT of the macula demonstrates diffuse thinning of the maculae with an area of relatively preserved macular thickness superiorly in the right eye. The visual fields demonstrate nasal defects superiorly and inferiorly with early arcuate extension OS, and superior nasal defect with inferior arcuate defect OD.

5.4 Severe Glaucoma

The American Academy of Ophthalmology Preferred Practice Patterns definition of severe glaucoma includes patients with either visual field abnormalities in both superior and inferior hemifields or a visual field defect within 5 degrees of fixation.

▶ Fig. 5.8 is an example of the former, showing images from a 72-year-old African-American woman with severe POAG. She presented with an IOP of over 30 mmHg in her left eye despite treatment with topical medical therapy. She underwent glaucoma filtering surgery and her disease has remained stable since that time. A fundus photo of the left eye demonstrates inferotemporal and superotemporal neuroretinal rim thinning. Visual field testing demonstrates superonasal and inferonasal defects. OCT imaging demonstrates superotemporal and inferotemporal RNFL thinning and an area of inferotemporal thinning of the ganglion cell layer–inner plexiform layer.

The next case is an example of severe stage glaucoma due to a paracentral defect: a 72-year-old white man with POAG of the right eye (▶ Fig. 5.9). His vision is 20/20 with corrective lenses with an IOP of 14 mmHg. His examination is notable for trace nuclear sclerosis, and a cup to disc ratio of 0.7 with inferior thinning to the rim. The OCT demonstrates inferotemporal thinning and borderline superonasal thinning. The visual field demonstrates a superior paracentral scotoma that is within 5

degrees of fixation. He is being followed closely on escalating topical pressure lowering therapy.

▶ Fig. 5.10 is another example of a case with paracentral involvement. The structure–function summary output is shown for a 67-year-old white man with severe-stage normal-tension glaucoma in both eyes. Visual field testing demonstrates a dense superior arcuate defect and a superior nasal step approaching fixation in both eyes. OCT of the RNFL and macular ganglion cell thickness demonstrates thin areas, more inferior than superior. The patient's testing has been stable on brinzolamide three times daily and latanoprostene bunod at bedtime.

5.4.1 Severe Stage Glaucoma, due to Significant Visual Field Constriction

Even in cases of glaucoma where there is significant visual field constriction, the OCT findings can still be useful in the clinical care of these patients.

▶ Fig. 5.11 shows a case of a 91-year-old white man with POAG of the right eye. His vision is 20/25-2 with corrective lenses with an IOP of 14 - mmHg. His examination is notable periocular skin hyperpigmentation, long eyelashes, 1 + nuclear sclerosis and trace cortical lens changes, and a cup to disc ratio of 0.8 with a superior notch and inferior thinning. The OCT demonstrates superior and inferior thinning and borderline temporal thinning. The visual field demonstrates superior and inferior arcuate scotomas which spare fixation. He was unfortunately lost to follow-up on maximum medical therapy and unreliable medication adherence.

Another example of severe glaucoma with visual field constriction is shown in ▶ Fig. 5.12, with the case of a 67-year-old Caucasian woman with severe POAG in each eye. She is being maintained on two topical combination therapies for a total of four IOP lowering agents. There is marked neuroretinal rim thinning of the left eye with a marked superior arcuate defect and a mild inferior arcuate defect on visual field testing. OCT imaging demonstrates prominent RNFL thinning and diffuse thinning of the ganglion cell layer–inner plexiform layer.

5.5 Glaucoma that Is Progressing

▶ Fig. 5.13 illustrates the OCT findings in a case of early glaucoma that is progressing: a 73-year-old

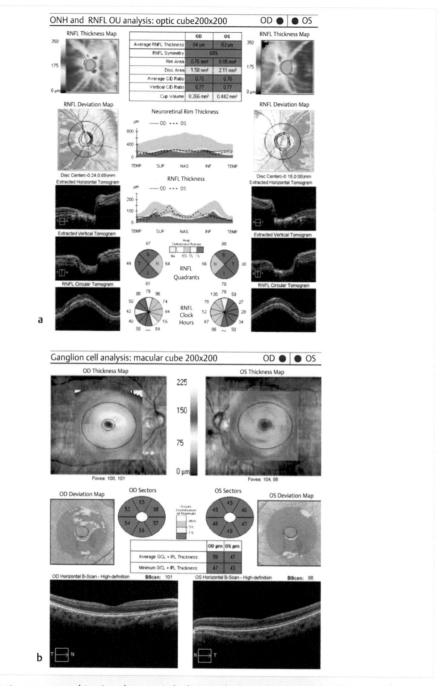

Fig. 5.7 Moderate-to-severe normal tension glaucoma in both eyes. This is a case of a 40-year-old Korean man with normal tension glaucoma in both eyes. The optical coherence tomography (OCT) of the optic nerve (**a**) demonstrates superior and inferior thinning on the thickness and deviation maps, as well as on the temporal-superior-nasal-inferior-temporal (TSNIT) and sectoral plots (Cirrus HD-OCT, Carl Zeiss Meditec, Inc., Dublin, CA). There is relative sparing of the nasal quadrant. The OCT of the macula (**b**) demonstrates diffuse thinning of the maculae on the thickness and deviation maps and the sectoral analyses; note the area relatively preserved in macular thickness superiorly in the right eye.

(Continued)

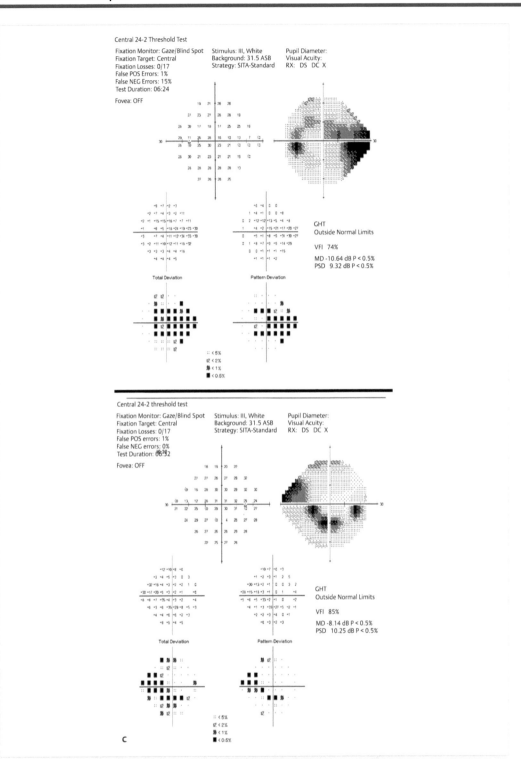

Fig. 5.7 *(Continued)* The visual fields **(c)** are reliable and demonstrate nasal defects superiorly and inferiorly with early arcuate extension OS, and superior nasal defect with inferior arcuate defect OD (Humphrey Visual Field, Carl Zeiss Meditec, Inc., Dublin, CA). (Courtesy of Drs Ki Ho Park and Yong Woo Kim of Seoul National University Hospital.)

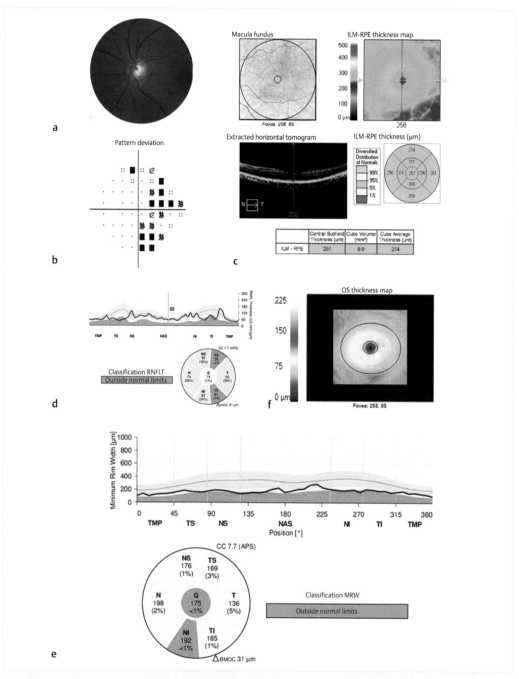

Fig. 5.8 Severe primary open-angle glaucoma (POAG) in the left eye. These clinical images are from a 72-year-old African-American woman with severe POAG. **(a)** A fundus photo of the left eye demonstrates inferotemporal and superotemporal neuroretinal rim thinning. **(b)** A Humphrey Visual Field (Carl Zeiss Meditec AG, Jena, Germany) pattern deviation plot demonstrates superonasal and inferonasal defects. **(c)** A *Macular Thickness Report* (Cirrus, Carl Zeiss Meditec AG, Jena, Germany) demonstrates no thinning of the total macular thickness. **(d)** A Glaucoma Module Premium Edition (GMPE) *RNFL Single Exam Report* (Spectralis, Heidelberg Engineering, Inc., Heidelberg, Germany) demonstrates superotemporal and inferotemporal RNFL thinning. **(e)** A GMPE *Bruch's Membrane Opening-Minimum Rim Width (BMO-MRW) Report* (Spectralis®) similarly notes neuroretinal rim thinning. **(f)** A *Ganglion Cell Analysis* (Cirrus, Carl Zeiss Meditec AG, Jena, Germany) demonstrates an area of inferotemporal thinning of the ganglion cell layer–inner plexiform layer as evident in the Sector Grid and Deviation Map. (Courtesy of Drs Ahmad Aref and Lawrence Geyman of the Illinois Eye & Ear Infirmary.)

5

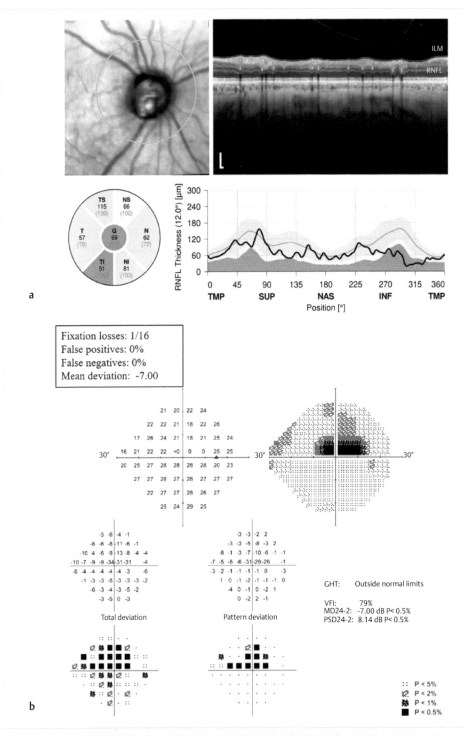

Fig. 5.9 Primary open-angle glaucoma (POAG) with a paracentral visual field defect. This is a case of a 72-year-old white man with POAG of the right eye. The optical coherence tomography (OCT) **(a)** demonstrates inferotemporal thinning and borderline superonasal thinning (Spectralis OCT, Heidelberg Engineering, Heidelberg, Germany). The visual field **(b)** is reliable with a mean deviation of −7.00 dB (Humphrey Visual Field, Carl Zeiss Meditec, Inc., Dublin, CA). There is a superior paracentral scotoma that is within 5 degrees of fixation. (Courtesy of Drs Teresa Chen, Catherine Marando, and Elli Park of the Massachusetts Eye & Ear Infirmary.)

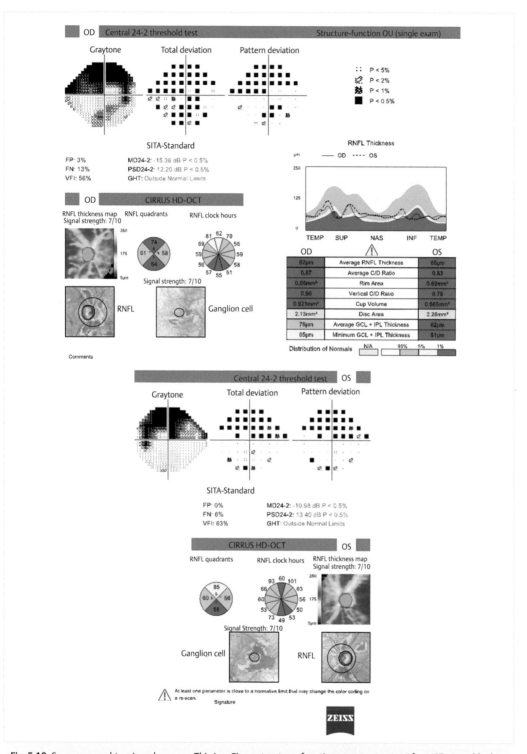

Fig. 5.10 Severe normal tension glaucoma. This is a Cirrus structure–function summary output for a 67-year-old white man with severe-stage normal-tension glaucoma in both eyes. Visual field testing demonstrates a dense superior arcuate defect and a superior nasal step approaching fixation in both eyes (top panel). Optical coherence tomography (OCT) of the retinal nerve fiber layer and macular ganglion cell thickness demonstrates thin areas, more inferior than superior. (Courtesy of Drs Andrew Williams and Ian Connor, University of Pittsburgh.)

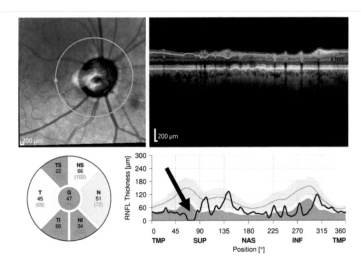

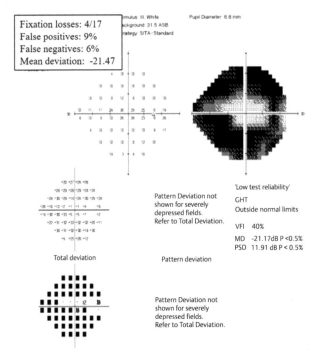

a

Fixation losses: 4/17
False positives: 9%
False negatives: 6%
Mean deviation: -21.47

'Low test reliability'

Pattern Deviation not shown for severely depressed fields. Refer to Total Deviation.

GHT
Outside normal limits

VFI   40%

MD   -21.17dB P <0.5%
PSD   11.91 dB P < 0.5%

Total deviation

Pattern deviation

Pattern Deviation not shown for severely depressed fields. Refer to Total Deviation.

b

Fig. 5.11 Severe primary open-angle glaucoma (POAG) with visual field constriction. This is a case of a 91-year-old white man with POAG of the right eye. The optical coherence tomography (OCT) **(a)** demonstrates superior and inferior thinning and borderline temporal thinning (Spectralis OCT, Heidelberg Engineering, Heidelberg, Germany). Note also the segmentation artifact in the OCT superiorly (arrow), whereby the retinal nerve fiber layer thickness is measured at 0 μm, which is physiologically impossible (see Chapter 8). The visual field **(b)** is moderately reliable with a mean deviation of −21.47 dB (Humphrey Visual Field, Carl Zeiss Meditec, Inc., Dublin, CA). There are superior and inferior arcuate scotomas which spare fixation. (Courtesy of Drs Teresa Chen, Catherine Marando, and Elli Park of the Massachusetts Eye & Ear Infirmary.)

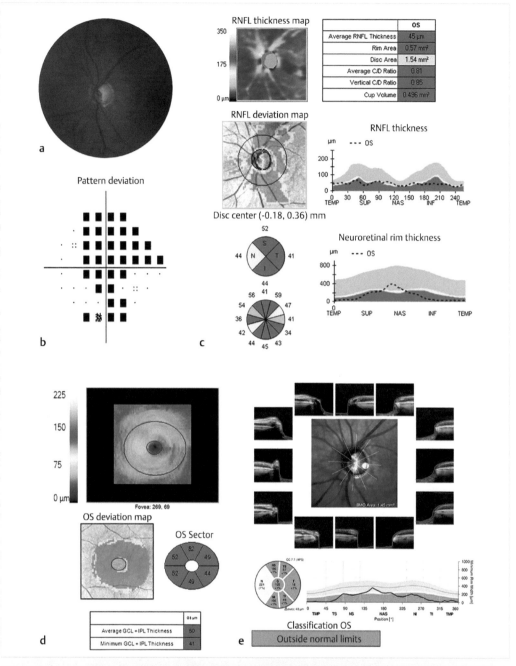

Fig. 5.12 Severe primary open-angle glaucoma (POAG) in both eyes. These clinical images are from a 67-year-old Caucasian woman with severe POAG in each eye. **(a)** A fundus photo of the left eye demonstrates marked neuroretinal rim thinning. **(b)** A Humphrey Visual Field (Carl Zeiss Meditec AG, Jena, Germany) pattern deviation plot demonstrates a marked superior arcuate defect with a mild inferior arcuate defect. **(c)** An *optic nerve head (ONH) and retinal nerve fiber layer (RNFL) analysis* (Cirrus, Carl Zeiss Meditec AG, Jena, Germany) demonstrates prominent RNFL thinning on the deviation map, sector grids, and thickness graph. The neuroretinal rim thickness graph similarly demonstrates marked thinning of the neuroretinal rim. The data table corroborates these findings. **(d)** A *Ganglion Cell Analysis* (Cirrus®) demonstrates diffuse thinning of the ganglion cell layer–inner plexiform layer as evidenced in the sector grid and deviation map. **(e)** A Glaucoma Module Premium Edition (GMPE) *Bruch's Membrane Opening-Minimum Rim Width (BMO-MRW) Report* (Spectralis, Heidelberg Engineering, Inc., Heidelberg, Germany) highlights inferior, superior, and temporal neuroretinal rim thinning. Twelve representative tomograms also demonstrate individual BMO-MRWs for each radial scan. (Courtesy of Drs Ahmad Aref and Lawrence Geyman of the Illinois Eye & Ear Infirmary.)

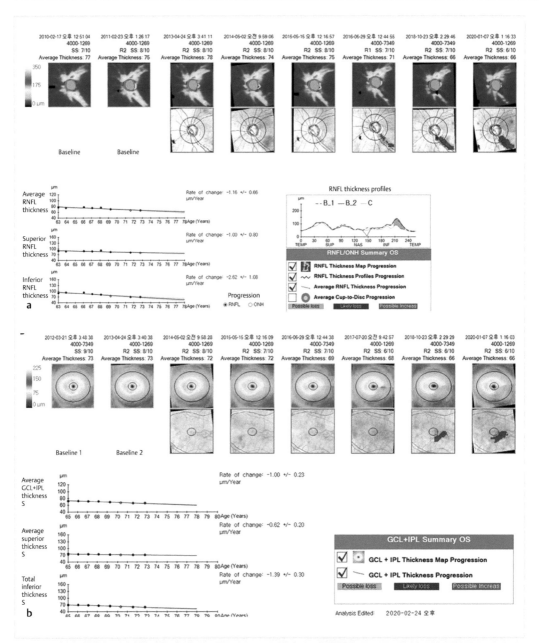

Fig. 5.13 Early normal tension glaucoma with progression in the left eye. This is a case of a 73-year-old Korean woman with normal tension glaucoma in both eyes. The optical coherence tomography (OCT) progression analysis of the left optic nerve is shown in **(a)** (Cirrus HD-OCT, Carl Zeiss Meditec, Inc., Dublin, CA). It demonstrates progressive losses of retinal nerve fiber layer (RNFL) inferiorly, seen on the thickness maps with the loss of the yellow and warm colors, and on deviation maps with the red-colored enlarging wedge. The loss of tissue is also demonstrated on the line graphs and on the temporal-superior-nasal-inferior-temporal (TSNIT) plot, with the area of loss highlighted in red. The OCT progression analysis of the left macula is shown in **(b)**. It demonstrates progressive loss of the inferior macula, seen on the thickness maps with the loss of the yellow, and on the deviation maps with the patches of yellow then red. As in **(a)**, the line graphs have a negative slope indicating loss of tissue over time. Note that the parafoveal location of the macular thinning is characteristic of early normal tension glaucoma.

(Continued)

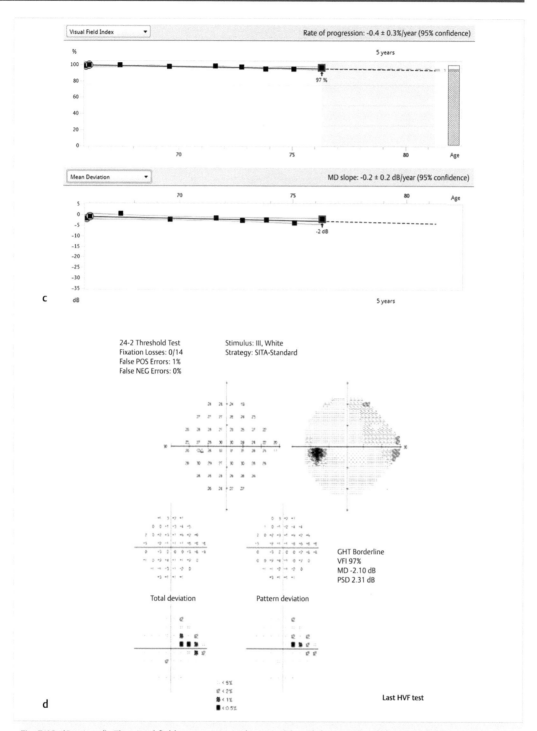

Fig. 5.13 *(Continued)* The visual field progression is shown in **(c)**, with line graphs of the visual field index and mean deviation demonstrating the loss of 2 dB over 11 years (Humphrey Visual Field, Carl Zeiss Meditec, Inc., Dublin, CA). A recent visual field **(d)** is reliable and demonstrates a paracentral depression superiorly corresponding to the changes seen on the RNFL and macular OCT progression analyses. (Courtesy of Drs Ki Ho Park and Yong Woo Kim of Seoul National University Hospital.)

5

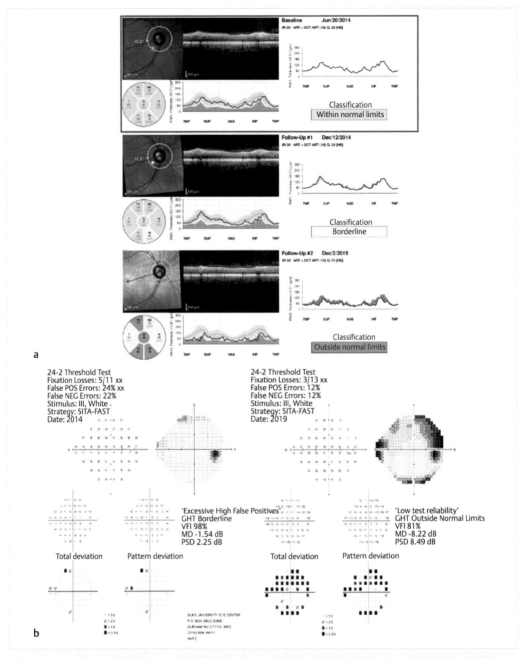

Fig. 5.14 Primary open-angle glaucoma (POAG) with progression in the right eye. This is a case of a 65-year-old African-American man with POAG in both eyes. His left eye is described in ▶ Fig. 5.2 and his right eye is described here. The optical coherence tomography (OCT) progression analysis of the right optic nerve is shown in (a) (Spectralis OCT, Heidelberg Engineering, Heidelberg, Germany). The baseline and 1-year follow-up scans are normal. He was lost to follow-up for 5 years, and the second follow-up scan demonstrates diffuse loss of retinal nerve fiber layer (RNFL) especially superiorly and inferiorly. The visual fields at baseline and after 5 years are shown in (b), demonstrating progressive visual field losses with superior greater than inferior depressions (Humphrey Visual Field, Carl Zeiss Meditec, Inc., Dublin, CA). (Courtesy of Dr Atalie Thompson, Duke Eye Center.)

Korean woman with normal tension glaucoma in both eyes. Central corneal thickness measurements are 527 OD and 521 OS. She is mildly hyperopic (+ 1.25 −0.75 at 90 OD; + 1.50 −0.50 at 90 OS), with axial lengths of 24.62 mm OD, 24.66 mm OS. She is currently treated with topical pressure lowering therapy in both eyes, with recent readings of 13 mmHg OD and 12 mmHg OS. The OCT progression analysis demonstrates progressive losses of RNFL inferiorly, seen on the thickness maps with the loss of the yellow and warm colors, and on deviation maps with the red-colored enlarging wedge. The loss of tissue is also demonstrated on the line graphs and on the TSNIT plot, with the area of loss highlighted in red. The OCT progression analysis of the left macula demonstrates progressive loss of the inferior macula, seen on the thickness maps with the loss of the yellow, and on the deviation maps with the patches of yellow then red. Note that the parafoveal location of the macular thinning is characteristic of early normal tension glaucoma. The visual field progression is shown with line graphs of the visual field index and mean deviation demonstrating the loss of 2 dB over 11 years. A recent visual field demonstrates a paracentral depression superiorly corresponding to the changes seen on the RNFL and macular OCT progression analyses.

Another example of progression is shown in images of the other eye of the patient shown in ▶ Fig. 5.2. The right eye of this 65-year-old African-American man with POAG in both eyes is described here (▶ Fig. 5.14). The OCT progression analysis of the right optic nerve shows the baseline and 1-year follow-up scans as normal. He was lost to follow-up for 5 years, and the second follow-up scan demonstrates diffuse loss of RNFL especially superiorly and inferiorly. The visual fields at baseline and after 5 years demonstrate progressive visual field losses with greater depressions in the superior than inferior.

▶ Fig. 5.15 illustrates progression in a case of secondary open-angle glaucoma. This is a case of a 65-year-old white man who was followed as a glaucoma suspect until an IOP spike. He had been followed from 2016 until 2018 when he had an episode of sudden IOP elevation to 57 OS. Examination revealed a diagnosis of Posner-Schlossman syndrome. A recent OCT report shows normal RNFL in the right eye and diffusely thin RNFL in the left. The RNFL progression analysis of the left eye demonstrates stable RNFL thickness from 2016 until 2018, after which there is diffuse thinning noted, with the change in thickness highlighted in red on the TSNIT progression plots. There is a subtle increase in thickness at one of the interval follow-ups consistent with an inflammatory process. Visual field testing of the left eye demonstrates superior and inferior depressions.

In the last example, OCT imaging reveals glaucomatous progression that slowed after surgical stabilization of the patient's glaucoma. ▶ Fig. 5.16 is a case of a 61-year-old white woman with POAG who was noted to have progressive OCT changes in her right eye. In 2018, a trabeculectomy was performed with stabilization of her IOP measurements and OCT measurements. A recent OCT report shows greater thinning in the inferior than superior in the right eye and normal RNFL in the left eye. The RNFL progression analysis of the right eye demonstrates greater RNFL thinning in the inferior than superior at the baseline in 2015, with suspicious changes noted in the superior bundle in 2018. Progressive losses were confirmed in the scan following the trabeculectomy surgery (2019) and have been stable since. Reliable visual field testing of the right eye demonstrates a dense superior altitudinal defect without involvement of the inferior hemifield.

5.6 Conclusions

The case examples shown in this chapter illustrate OCT imaging of the optic nerve, RNFL, and macula in patients with all stages of glaucoma, from those at risk who are followed as glaucoma suspects to patients with mild, moderate, and severe glaucoma. Characteristic findings in the optic nerve, RNFL, and macula described in earlier chapters can be seen in these examples, particularly in the management of glaucoma that is progressing.

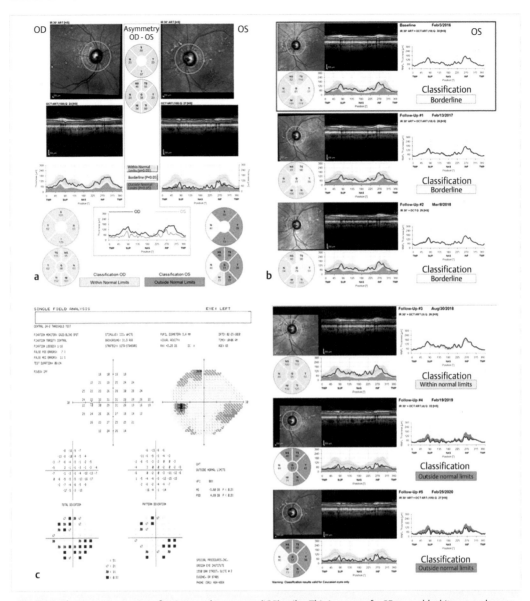

Fig. 5.15 Glaucoma progression after intraocular pressure (IOP) spike. This is a case of a 65-year-old white man who was followed as a glaucoma suspect until an IOP spike. He had been followed from 2016 until 2018 when he had an episode of sudden IOP elevation to 57 OS. Examination revealed a diagnosis of Posner-Schlossman syndrome. A recent optical coherence tomography (OCT) report (a) shows normal retinal nerve fiber layer (RNFL) in the right eye and diffusely thin RNFL in the left eye (Spectralis OCT, Heidelberg Engineering, Heidelberg, Germany). The RNFL progression analysis of the left eye (b) demonstrates stable RNFL thickness from 2016 until 2018, after which there is diffuse thinning noted, with the change in thickness highlighted in red on the temporal-superior-nasal-inferior-temporal (TSNIT) progression plots. Note the subtle increase in thickness at Follow-up #3 (green on the TSNIT progression plot) consistent with an inflammatory process. Reliable visual field testing of the left eye (c) demonstrates superior and inferior depressions (Humphrey Visual Field, Carl Zeiss Meditec, Inc., Dublin, CA). (Courtesy of Dr Hana Takusagawa of Oregon Eye Center.)

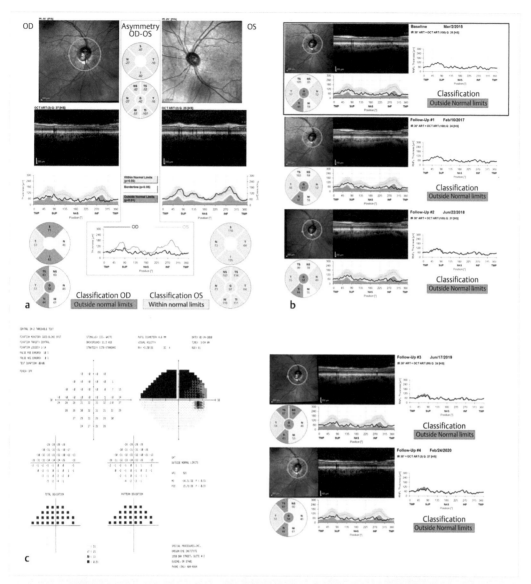

Fig. 5.16 Stabilization after trabeculectomy. This is a case of a 61-year-old white woman with primary open-angle glaucoma (POAG). She was noted to have progressive optical coherence tomography (OCT) changes in her right eye. In 2018, a trabeculectomy was performed with stabilization of her IOP measurements and OCT measurements. A recent OCT report (a) shows greater thinning in the inferior than superior in the right eye and normal retinal nerve fiber layer (RNFL) in the left eye (Spectralis OCT, Heidelberg Engineering, Heidelberg, Germany). The RNFL progression analysis of the right eye (b) demonstrates greater RNFL thinning in the inferior than superior at the baseline in 2015. In 2018, suspicious changes were noted in the superior bundle, with the change in thickness highlighted in red on the temporal-superior-nasal-inferior-temporal (TSNIT) progression plot. Progressive losses were confirmed in the scan following the trabeculectomy surgery (2019) and have been stable since. Reliable visual field testing of the right eye (c) demonstrates a dense superior altitudinal defect without involvement of the inferior hemifield (Humphrey Visual Field, Carl Zeiss Meditec, Inc., Dublin, CA). (Courtesy of Dr Hana Takusagawa of Oregon Eye Center.)

Reference

[1] American Academy of Ophthalmology Preferred Practice Patterns. Primary Open Angle Glaucoma PPP, November 2015. https://www.aao.org/preferred-practice-pattern/primary-open-angle-glaucoma-ppp-2015

5

6 Structure–Function Relationship

Felipe A. Medeiros

Summary

The relationship between structure and function of the optic nerve is a defining characteristic of glaucoma. This chapter describes how structure-function maps have been created and how they can aid the clinician in the care of glaucoma patients. The question of whether optical coherence tomography (OCT) damage precedes visual field loss in glaucoma is addressed. How structural changes are linked to functional changes in glaucoma is also discussed. Examples of structure-function relationships are provided.

Keywords: optical coherence tomography, visual field testing, perimetry, HVF 24–2, HVF 10–2

6.1 Introduction

Glaucoma is a progressive optic neuropathy characterized by typical changes in the optic nerve head (ONH) and retinal nerve fiber layer (RNFL).[1] These structural changes usually lead to functional losses as measured by perimetric examination. Both structural and functional changes result from a common pathophysiological process, namely, loss of retinal ganglion cells (RGCs) and their axons. An understanding of the structure–function relationship in glaucoma, that is, how the changes in the ONH and RNFL are related to perimetric losses, is central to clinical practice. With the development of sophisticated imaging technologies, such as optical coherence tomography (OCT), it has been possible to detect very small structural changes in the optic nerve, macula, and RNFL, to the micrometer scale. However, from a patient's standpoint, it is important to understand how such changes are related to, or predictive of, clinically relevant outcomes, as manifested by loss of vision.

6.2 Mapping Structural to Functional Loss in Glaucoma

In most patients with clearly defined glaucomatous damage, abnormalities on OCT imaging of the ONH and RNFL correspond topographically to abnormalities on standard automated perimetry (SAP), following a structure-to-function mapping. Several approaches have been used to derive such maps correlating regions of the ONH and RNFL to the locations tested by SAP. The most commonly used map was produced by Garway-Heath and colleagues.[2] The authors mapped localized RNFL defects seen on red-free photographs to the location of points on SAP in 63 patients with glaucoma. The authors then built a correspondence map of structure and function, which has been widely used in practice and is illustrated in ▶ Fig. 6.1. An appreciation of these maps can help clinicians understand the functional implications of certain patterns of structural damage. In other words, given a certain structural abnormality where should one expect to see a visual field defect? The assessment of structure–function correspondence helps to determine whether a particular finding on an imaging examination or on the visual field test has a higher chance of being true or may be a false-positive. This is illustrated on ▶ Fig. 6.2, which shows RNFL loss observed on spectral domain OCT (SD-OCT) and fundus photography in the inferior temporal region associated with the superior nasal visual field defect on SAP.

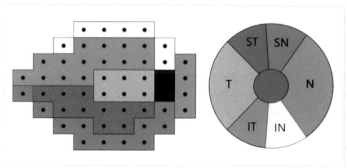

Fig. 6.1 Garway-Heath map illustrating the topographic correspondence between regions of the optic disc and visual field locations.

6

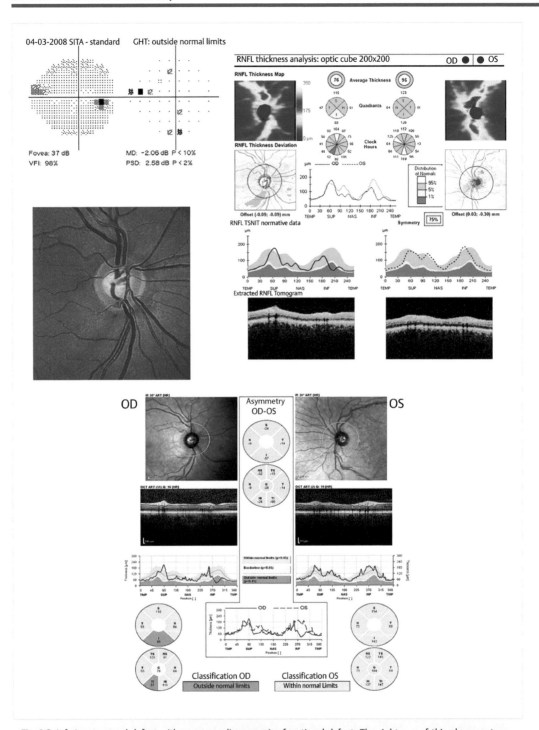

Fig. 6.2 Inferior structural defect with corresponding superior functional defect. The right eye of this glaucomatous patient shows an inferior localized retinal nerve fiber layer (RNFL) defect visible on the optic disc color photograph, as well as on the printouts of two different optical coherence tomography (OCT) devices. The inferior RNFL defect is associated with a superior nasal defect visible on standard perimetry.

Several authors have proposed variations of the structure–function maps using different techniques to map the locations of structural abnormality to visual field defects. In general, the results of all these modeling approaches yield similar results and, from a clinical standpoint, the differences do not bear much relevance. In a recent study, Mariottoni and colleagues[3] used artificial intelligence (deep learning) to map locations of damage on SD-OCT to SAP. The study included 26,499 pairs of SAP and SD-OCT from 15,173 eyes of patients with glaucoma or suspected of having the disease. Using a deep learning neural network, the authors showed how specific localized RNFL defects on SD-OCT could be mapped to specific locations on SAP.

Investigating central visual field defects and macular glaucomatous damage in patients with glaucoma, Hood et al[4] described the "macular vulnerability zone" (MVZ), a region that would correspond approximately to the sector between 300 and 330 degrees in the inferior RNFL thickness profile. They associated defects in the MVZ to superior paracentral visual field defects. ▶ Fig. 6.3 illustrates a glaucoma eye showing an inferior arcuate RNFL defect which extends to the macular region, affecting the MVZ. The SD-OCT macular examination shows central damage inferiorly. This corresponds to a superior visual field defect. Of note, the visual field defect was not prominent on the SAP 24–2 test greyscale, even though the pattern standard deviation (PSD) was statistically significantly outside normal limits, indicating the existence of a defect. On the 10–2 test, the defect is shown more extensively due to the higher density of points in the central region. Given that macular damage in glaucoma has been shown to occur more frequently than previously thought, this has led some investigators to suggest that 10–2 visual field tests should be performed routinely for glaucoma assessment. However, given inherent trade-offs in resources, and patient availability, such an approach may lead to a lack of enough 24–2 tests being acquired over time and inability to assess progression and, therefore, is not generally recommended.

Of note, superior localized RNFL defects resulting in small paracentral inferior visual field losses are relatively less common. Because of the relative anatomic positions of the optic nerve and macula, RNFL damage to the corresponding superior sector (30 to 60 degrees) actually tends to cause peripheral arcuate visual field defects inferiorly, rather than central macular defects. ▶ Fig. 6.4 illustrates a case where a dense inferior paracentral defect is seen, associated with a localized superior RNFL defect in an eye with glaucoma. However, it can be seen from the total and pattern deviation plots of the visual field that the defect is actually more extensive than the greyscale plot suggests, actually affecting most of the inferior hemifield of the 24–2 test.

Anatomically in the fovea, ganglion cell bodies are spatially displaced from their corresponding photoreceptors. This is relevant for structure–function mapping in the macular region because it creates a small spatial offset between the location of the photoreceptors that detect the centrally tested visual field locations (e.g., using the 10–2 test grid) and the location of expected corresponding RGC loss. This displacement has been previously studied by several authors and has recently been incorporated into processes for structure–function analysis in the macular region in glaucoma. According to Hood and co-authors,[4] improved concordance between structural and functional measures in the macula may be obtained by applying displacement of the visual field locations according to anatomical estimates of Henle fiber length. It should be noted, however, that for most eyes with glaucoma such differences have relatively little impact on actual clinical decision-making.

6.2.1 Does OCT Damage Precede Visual Field Loss in Glaucoma?

There has been a longstanding debate about whether signs of structural damage precede functional evidence of glaucomatous damage. Initial work by Quigley and colleagues suggested that up to 40% of RGCs could be lost before signs of damage are observed on standard achromatic perimetry.[5] In fact, signs of structural damage at the level of the ONH, RNFL, or macula may be seen very often before clearly detectable and statistically significant visual field defects are observed on SAP. This is illustrated in ▶ Fig. 6.5, where loss of RNFL was detected by OCT many years before the clear appearance of a reproducible visual field defect of SAP. It should be noted, however, that the idea that an eye must always lose 40% of its RGCs to develop a visual field defect is misleading. In fact, most often this is not the case. Previous histological work in monkeys has shown that visual field defects may appear in the presence of much smaller losses. The pattern of neural rim and RNFL

6

6

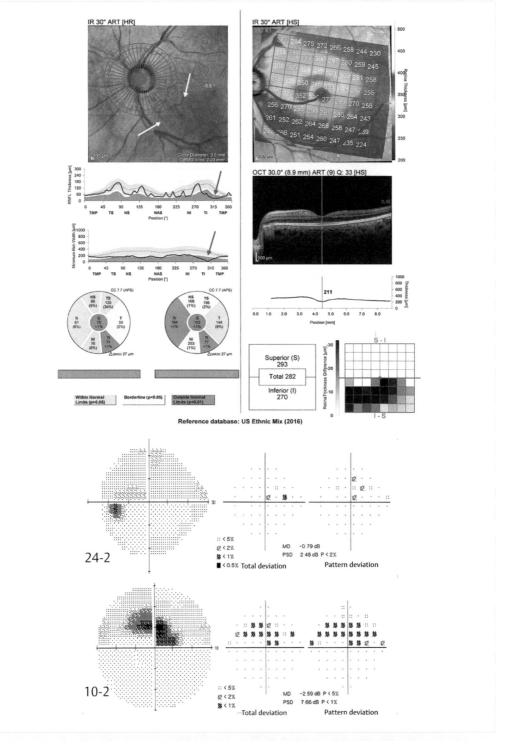

Fig. 6.3 Inferior structural defect with corresponding superior central functional defect. The optical coherence tomography (OCT) examination shows an inferior temporal retinal nerve fiber layer (RNFL) defect (*red arrows*), which is also visible on the confocal scanning image (*white arrows*). The arcuate defect extends to the macular area (*red curved lines*). The 24–2 visual field test shows a small superior nasal defect, with a statistically significant abnormal pattern standard deviation (PSD). However, the defect is more clearly delineated when evaluated by the 10–2 visual field test.

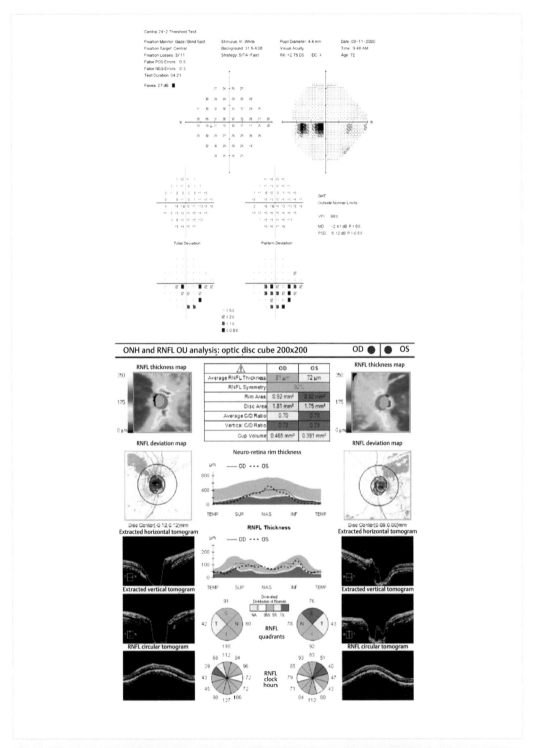

Fig. 6.4 Superior structural defect with corresponding inferior visual field defect. The optical coherence tomography (OCT) examination shows a superior localized retinal nerve fiber layer (RNFL) defect, which is seen on the color-coded map and deviation map, as well as in the summary parameters. The OCT RNFL loss is associated with a corresponding inferior paracentral defect shown on the visual field printout. Note that the inferior defect on perimetry is more extensive than what appears in the greyscale plot and actually involves most of the inferior arcuate area, as seen on the pattern deviation plot.

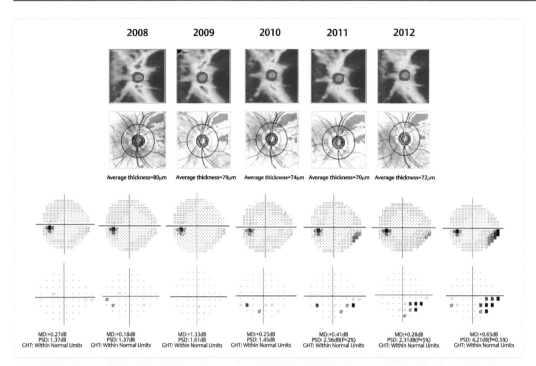

Fig. 6.5 Structural and functional defects over time. The series of optical coherence tomography (OCT) printouts show a retinal nerve fiber layer (RNFL) defect as early as 2008 which progresses over time. Note that a reproducible visual field defect only appears clearly 3 years later.

loss may be an important factor in determining how much loss of RGCs may need to occur before a visual field defect becomes detectable. Eyes with localized RNFL defects or rim notching will often present early localized visual field defects. In contrast, in eyes with diffuse loss of neuroretinal rim, SAP defects may not be detectable for a long time and these eyes are often found to have major structural damage by the time the first visual field defect becomes apparent. This occurs because SAP parameters usually target for detection of localized, rather than diffuse, visual field defects, in an attempt to reduce confounding effects of media opacities. This is illustrated in ▶ Fig. 6.6, which shows examinations from a 45-year-old patient with glaucoma. It is possible to see extensive and diffuse neuroretinal rim thinning and RNFL loss on the OCT. The visual field, however, shows normal PSD and glaucoma hemifield test, as well as unremarkable pattern deviation plot. However, the total deviation is indicative of diffuse loss of sensitivity, which is corroborated by the mean deviation (MD) with $P < 1\%$. Importantly, this young subject had no media opacities or other reasons for diffuse loss of sensitivity, indicating that such loss was related to the extensive diffuse structural

damage from glaucoma. Contrast these findings to those of previous examples shown in this chapter.

Of note, in some eyes, the reverse may occasionally happen, that is, visual field defects may be seen on standard perimetry in the absence of statistically significant abnormalities on imaging tests. In the Ocular Hypertension Treatment Study (OHTS) and European Glaucoma Prevention Study (EGPS), a significant proportion of eyes with ocular hypertension developed visual field loss as the earliest sign of glaucoma, as defined by the study endpoints. However, it is likely that most of these eyes actually already had signs of structural glaucomatous damage at baseline that were not clearly detected by subjective assessment of disc stereophotographs. Due to the wide normative range of RNFL thickness values, in some eyes it is possible to see the presence of repeatable visual field defects in the absence of clearly statistically significant OCT damage. Whether structural or functional change occurs first also depends on the chosen endpoints and how they are measured. Some disagreement might be always expected due to the asynchronous temporal relationship between RGC's functional and structural decline in the glaucomatous process. The concept of

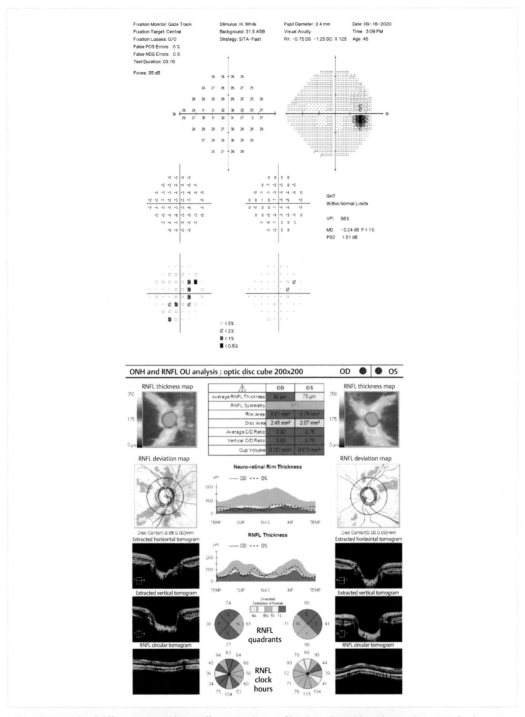

Fig. 6.6 Example of diffuse structural loss. Diffuse retinal nerve fiber layer (RNFL) loss detected on optical coherence tomography (OCT). The diffuse loss can be seen on the color-coded (RNFL thickness) map, deviation map, and also on summary parameters. The global average thickness was 62 μm, indicating very substantial neural tissue loss. The visual field printout shows normal pattern standard deviation (PSD) and glaucoma hemifield test (GHT). The greyscale plot and pattern deviation plot do not show clear abnormality. However, there is evidence of diffuse loss of sensitivity as seen on the total deviation plot and the depressed mean deviation with P < 1%. Note that this was a 45-year-old patient without any media opacities or conditions other than glaucoma.

"ganglion cell dysfunction" (rather than death) has also been proposed to explain why, in some patients, perimetric defects precede identifiable structural changes. In early stages of ganglion cell insult, cells may become dysfunctional, leading to a reduction in visual field sensitivity, so that "measured structure" may not be representative of functioning ganglion cell or axonal number. In spite of the above, there is no contradicting the fact that retinal nerve fiber layer abnormalities are present in many cases with normal visual fields. The reasons for this finding are more extensively explained in a few previous reports[6] and discussed below.

6.2.2 How Are Structural Changes Linked to Functional Changes in Glaucoma?

There have been many different models proposed to explain the link between structure and function in glaucoma, as measured by clinical tools. It is important to note that at a very basic microscopic level, a dead cell obviously cannot function and, therefore, structural loss is inexorably linked to functional loss. Therefore, it is important to understand that models explaining structure–function in glaucoma are limited by the idiosyncrasies of the methods that are used to measure structure and function in clinical practice. As both structural and functional changes result from a common pathophysiological process (loss of RGC somas and axons), it would be expected that both would be related to one another over the course of disease. However, the current structural and functional measurement methods show considerable variability, acquire measurements in different scales, and are susceptible to limitations that result in a suboptimal assessment of this relationship, which is dependent on the severity of the disease and the location being tested.

With OCT, structural assessment (ONH, RNFL, macula) aims at quantifying parameters such as rim area (mm^2), RNFL thickness (microns), or various inner retinal thickness measures (microns).

These represent absolute, linear, metrics of measurements and should be linearly related to RGC density. In contrast, visual field sensitivity with SAP is obtained in logarithmic units (decibels, dB). The dB is relative to a reference level (luminance of the stimulus vs. background luminance), and it is used to express a ratio rather than an absolute value. Thus, dB is a nonlinear measure, and a change of 3 dB represents a doubling or halving of light intensity. When dB increments are plotted against a linear scale, it shows that dB increments at different levels of intensity represent very different sized increments on a linear scale. For example, a 2 dB decrease from 38 to 36 dB is tenfold greater change in linear units than the same dB change at a sensitivity of 28 dB. The different units of measurements for structural and functional parameters are confounding factors when assessing structure–function relationship. There is strong evidence based on experimental and clinical studies that transforming dB to linear scale results in a clearer linear relationship between structure and function measurements. Nevertheless, it is important to understand that the logarithmic scale compresses the range of losses in early stages, while expanding the range in later stages. Although a linearization of the visual field data suggests that functional changes may occur at early stages of disease process, the simple linearization may not yield improvement in the detection of early functional losses because SAP data is originally acquired using staircase procedures based on logarithmic scale (decibels).[6] Thus, current implementations of SAP are not effective in detecting small amounts of RGC loss in early stages of disease. On the other hand, by expanding the range of the scale at later stages, SAP may be more sensitive to small RGC loss that do not seem to produce detectable changes in RNFL thickness.[6]

▶ Fig. 6.7 illustrates the relationship between RGC number and measurements of RNFL thickness as well as SAP MD. The data were obtained from human eyes using empirical formulas derived to estimate RGC counts.[6,7] Even though these formulas may have some limitations in predicting the actual RGC number on individual eyes, they can be

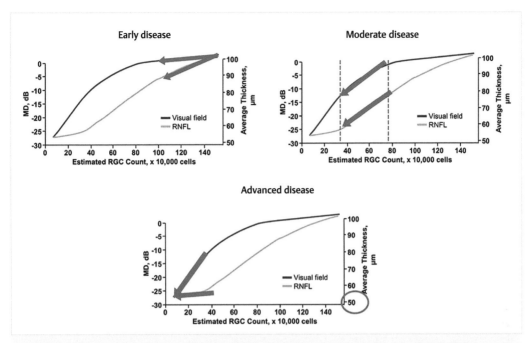

Fig. 6.7 The relationship between retinal ganglion cell (RGC) number, retinal nerve fiber layer (RNFL) thickness, and visual field mean deviation. This figure illustrates the relationship between RGC number and measurements of optical coherence tomography (OCT) RNFL thickness and standard automated perimetry (SAP) mean deviation (MD). The data were obtained from human eyes using empirical formulas derived to estimate RGC counts. It can be seen that the relationship between RGC counts and MD is nonlinear, whereas the relationship between RGC counts and RNFL thickness is mostly linear until OCT measurements reach the "floor" level. In early disease (*left plot*), large losses of RGCs are associated with only relatively small changes in MD, as measured in dB. In late disease (*right plot*), even relatively small RGC losses are associated with large changes on SAP MD. In moderate stages (*middle plot*), changes in MD and RNFL appear to occur at similar rates in response to RGC loss, explaining greater concordance between changes in structure and function that is frequently seen at this stage.

extremely helpful to illustrate the concepts being discussed here. From ▶ Fig. 6.7, it can be seen that the relationship between RGC counts and MD is nonlinear. In early disease (left plot), large losses of RGCs will be associated with only relatively small changes in MD, as measured in dB. Again, this occurs due to the logarithmic nature of MD. In contrast, there is a relatively linear relationship between RGC loss and RNFL thickness change in early disease. This explains, at least in part, why it is so common to see eyes that have RNFL damage in the absence of detectable visual field defects in perimetry. In late disease (right plot), even relatively small RGC losses are associated with large

changes on SAP MD. In other words, to lose 1 dB in visual field sensitivity an eye does not need to lose much additional RGCs once the disease is advanced. This may explain, at least in part, why it becomes so difficult to control glaucoma and stop visual field progression once the disease is advanced. It may also explain why even some small losses of RGCs, which may be due to natural aging, may still produce an impact on visual fields once there is severe damage. At this stage, OCT measurements have generally reached what we call "floor effect." This usually corresponds to average RNFL thickness measurements of around 30 to 50 μm and corresponds to residual tissue, such as glia. In fact, eyes with "absolute" glaucoma, where there is total loss of RNFL, do not generally have OCT measurements of RNFL that go down to zero. Once the OCT measurements reach the floor level, detection of further progression on OCT becomes very limited, explaining why in many eyes with severe glaucoma progression is better detected with visual field. In intermediate stages (middle plot), there is frequently a concordance between changes in RNFL and changes in SAP MD. Note that this only occurs throughout a relatively small portion of the range. When this factor is added to issues of variability of tests, quality, etc., this explains why disagreements in structure and function are so common.[8] Recent work has suggested that disagreements can be reduced by painstakingly assessing the relationship between small locations in the visual field and OCT, rather than relying on summary parameters. Although that may be true in principle, these studies have been done in very small and highly selected samples and the clinical relevance of these findings is unclear.[9] Also, assessment of change using summary parameters still provides the most important metric for glaucoma monitoring which is the rate of change.

Even though the disagreement between structural and functional changes may seem puzzling, it can be easily understood when considering the properties of the tests available to measure structure and function, such as their different scales, variability, and dynamic range, as described above.[5] If methods for assessing structural and functional progression were to agree perfectly, there would be no need for using both in monitoring progression. One test would suffice. Importantly, in order to justify decision-making based on results of OCT only, these results need to be of demonstrable clinical relevance and predictive of outcomes that are clinically relevant for patients. It is crucial to demonstrate that progressive structural changes are actually predictive of outcomes that are clinically relevant for patients. Several studies have shown consistent data in this regard. OCT abnormalities have been identified up to 8 years before field loss in some patients.[10] Using SD-OCT, rates of RNFL thinning were shown to be significantly faster in eyes that eventually developed a visual field defect compared to those that did not, with each 1 μm per year faster RNFL loss associated with a greater than two times higher risk of developing a future field defect. Measurement of progressive structural change has also been shown to be predictive of further visual field progression in eyes with established perimetric defects, at least in early to moderate disease. Progressive RNFL thinning has also been shown to be associated with quality-of-life outcomes in patients with glaucoma, as measured by the National Eye Institute Visual Function Questionnaire (NEI VFQ-25).

Studies of the structure–function relationship in glaucoma have also attempted to identify when to use one versus another test during the course of the disease. For the reasons discussed above, imaging measurements seem to have most utility for detecting change in early stages of the disease, while perimetry seems to perform better when visual field losses are already present. It should be noted that recent evidence from a very large cohort study has shown that many cases of progression in advanced glaucoma may be detected by SD-OCT despite absence of apparent deterioration on visual fields.[11] This is illustrated in ▶ Fig. 6.8. In addition, in the evaluation of patients with moderate or severe glaucoma, there may be regions of interest that have relatively well-preserved nerve tissue and that can be used for follow-up.

As a matter of fact, the disagreement between the tests can be used to our advantage, by improving the chances of detecting progressive changes over time. However, the difficulty lies in how best to integrate their results, without increasing the chance of false-positives. Several methods of combining structural and functional measurements have been proposed, including using sophisticated statistics and by a single combined structure-function index.[12] These combined measurements have been shown to outperform isolated measurements of structure and function for diagnosis and assessment of disease progression and are finding their way into clinical practice.

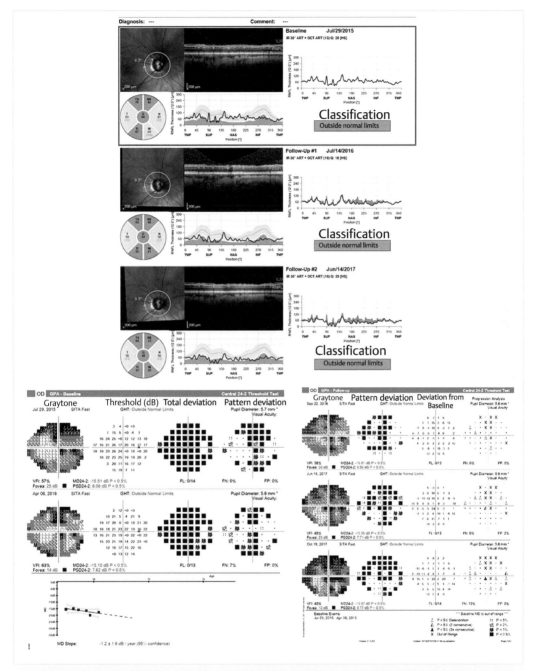

Fig. 6.8 Example from a patient with advanced glaucomatous damage. Eye with advanced glaucomatous damage showing significant progressive optical coherence tomography (OCT) retinal nerve fiber layer (RNFL) loss.

References

[1] Weinreb RN, Aung T, Medeiros FA. The pathophysiology and treatment of glaucoma: a review. JAMA. 2014; 311 (18):1901–1911

[2] Garway-Heath DF, Poinoosawmy D, Fitzke FW, Hitchings RA. Mapping the visual field to the optic disc in normal tension glaucoma eyes. Ophthalmology. 2000; 107(10):1809–1815

[3] Mariottoni EB, Datta S, Dov D, et al. Artificial intelligence mapping of structure to function in glaucoma. Transl Vis Sci Technol. 2020; 9(2):19

[4] Hood DC, Raza AS, de Moraes CG, Liebmann JM, Ritch R. Glaucomatous damage of the macula. Prog Retin Eye Res. 2013; 32:1–21

[5] Quigley HA, Addicks EM, Green WR. Optic nerve damage in human glaucoma. III. Quantitative correlation of nerve fiber loss and visual field defect in glaucoma, ischemic neuropathy, papilledema, and toxic neuropathy. Arch Ophthalmol. 1982; 100(1):135–146

[6] Medeiros FA, Zangwill LM, Bowd C, Mansouri K, Weinreb RN. The structure and function relationship in glaucoma: implications for detection of progression and measurement of rates of change. Invest Ophthalmol Vis Sci. 2012; 53 (11):6939–6946

[7] Harwerth RS, Wheat JL, Fredette MJ, Anderson DR. Linking structure and function in glaucoma. Prog Retin Eye Res. 2010; 29(4):249–271

[8] Abe RY, Diniz-Filho A, Zangwill LM, et al. The relative odds of progressing by structural and functional tests in glaucoma. Invest Ophthalmol Vis Sci. 2016; 57(9):OCT421–OCT428

[9] Hood DC, Tsamis E, Bommakanti NK, et al. Structure-function agreement is better than commonly thought in eyes with early glaucoma. Invest Ophthalmol Vis Sci. 2019; 60 (13):4241–4248

[10] Kuang TM, Zhang C, Zangwill LM, Weinreb RN, Medeiros FA. Estimating lead time gained by optical coherence tomography in detecting glaucoma before development of visual field defects. Ophthalmology. 2015; 122(10):2002–2009

[11] Jammal AA, Thompson AC, Mariottoni EB, et al. Rates of glaucomatous structural and functional change from a large clinical population: the Duke Glaucoma Registry Study. Am J Ophthalmol. 2020; 222:238–247

[12] Medeiros FA, Lisboa R, Weinreb RN, Girkin CA, Liebmann JM, Zangwill LM. A combined index of structure and function for staging glaucomatous damage. Arch Ophthalmol. 2012; 130 (9):1107–1116

6

7 Comparison of Common Devices

Lawrence S. Geyman and Ahmad A. Aref

Summary

Various optical coherence tomography (OCT) devices produced by different manufacturers are available to aid in clinical assessment of glaucomatous individuals, and a comparison of commonly used devices is discussed here. This chapter outlines differences in the imaging specifications, analysis techniques, normative databases, and diagnostic capabilities among the Cirrus 6000 (Carl Zeiss Meditec AG, Jena, Germany), Standard and Glaucoma Module Premium Editions of the Spectralis (Heidelberg Engineering GmbH, Heidelberg, Germany), Avanti RTVue XR (Optovue, Inc., Fremont, CA, USA), and 3D OCT (Topcon Corporation, Tokyo, Japan) imaging platforms. Differences are highlighted according to measurement and analysis of retinal nerve fiber layer, optic nerve head, and macular parameters.

Keywords: glaucoma, imaging, optical coherence tomography, retinal nerve fiber layer, optic nerve head, macula, Cirrus, Spectralis, Avanti, Topcon

7.1 Retinal Nerve Fiber Layer Thickness

All of these optical coherence tomography (OCT) devices offer a scanning pattern that provides data on retinal nerve fiber layer (RNFL) thickness. The scan patterns offered by the devices can be divided into circle scans and volume scans. Circle scans measure *circumpapillary* RNFL (cpRNFL) thickness using a dedicated circular scanning pattern centered on the optic nerve head (ONH). Devices employing this strategy include the Spectralis (Heidelberg Engineering, Inc., Heidelberg, Germany), the Avanti RTVue XR (Optovue, Inc., Fremont, CA, USA), and the 3D OCT-2000 (Topcon Corp., Tokyo, Japan). In contrast, volume scans (also known as cube scans) secondarily derive a calculation circle to measure cpRNFL thickness. The volume scan, however, affords the benefit of providing a thickness map detailing the RNFL thickness across the entire scanned area. Devices employing this strategy include the Cirrus 6000 (Carl Zeiss Meditec AG, Jena, Germany), and the 3D OCT-2000 and OCT-1 Maestro2 (Topcon Corp., Tokyo, Japan). Devices may also be divided on the

basis of their scanning and/or analytical axis, with some aligned to the horizontal axis and others to the fovea-disc (FoDi) axis. Although the chosen axis may affect RNFL thickness measurements, aligning analyses to the FoDi axis may not improve glaucoma detection.[1]

Studies comparing the RNFL metrics of multiple devices have shown that, although they have been shown to be comparable, the diagnostic capabilities of devices may exhibit slight differences, including throughout a range of disease stages and myopia.[2,3,4,5] Diagnostic capabilities generally increase with more advanced stages of glaucoma and are least with preperimetric and mild glaucoma. (See subsequent subsections for details on each device.)[5] Note that literature cited in the following sections includes studies on single devices; as such, direct comparisons of study outcomes cannot be made across devices. ▶ Table 7.1 highlights the main differences among the various platforms in imaging the RNFL and ONH.

7.1.1 Cirrus 6000 (Carl Zeiss Meditec AG, Jena, Germany)

Imaging Specifications

The Cirrus 6000 is the latest OCT model from Carl Zeiss Meditec AG. Imaging specifications[6] include scanning speeds of 100,000 A-scans per second, an improvement over the prior model, the Cirrus 5000, which attains scanning speeds of 27–68,000 A-scans per second. For RNFL metrics, the device employs a 6.0×6.0 mm volume scan comprising 40,000 data points (200 horizontal B-scans each comprising 200 A-scans). The scan pattern is manually centered over the ONH. The software then derives a calculation circle with diameter estimated to be 3.46 mm and comprising 256 data points.[7] The calculation circle is automatically centered over the ONH by identifying the Bruch's membrane opening (BMO) and then identifying the center of corresponding enclosed area.

Analysis

The Cirrus 6000 offers a comprehensive analysis report, the *ONH and RNFL Analysis*[6] (▶ Fig. 7.1c and ▶ Fig. 7.2c). The report displays an RNFL thickness map, where cooler colors (blue and green)

7

Table 7.1 Comparison of imaging devices for retinal nerve fiber layer and optic nerve head analysis in glaucoma

cpRNFL & ONH	Cirrus	Spectralis			Avanti RTVue XR		3D OCT-1 Maestro2	3D OCT-2000	
Speed (A-scans/sec)	Cirrus 5000: 27K–68K; Cirrus 6000: 100K	OCT1: 40K; OCT2: 85K			70K		50K		
Shape & scan name*	Cube "Optic Disc Cube 200 × 200"	Cube "ONH"	Circle "RNFL"	Circle + Radial "ONH-RC" (GMPE only)	Cube "3D Disc"	Circle + Radial "ONH"	Cube	Cube "3D 6.0 × 6.0"	Circle "Circle 3.40"
Size (cube)	6 × 6 mm	15 × 15 degrees			6 × 6 mm		6 × 6 mm	6 × 6 mm	
Data points (cube)	40,000 (200 B-scans of 200 A-scans)	37,376 (73 B-scans of 512 A-scans)			51,813 (101 B-scans of 513 A-scans)		65,536 (128 B-scans of 512 A-scans)	65,536 (128 B-scans of 512 A-scans)	
Length (radial)				15 degrees		3.4 mm			
Diameter, mm (circle)†	3.46		3.45	3.5/4.1/4.7		3.4 (1.3–4.9 mm in 0.3 mm increments)	3.4		
Data points (circle or radial)	256		768	Radial: 768; Circle: 768		Radial: 455 (12 scans); Circle: 4.3–4.9 mm: 965, 3.4–4.0 mm: 775, 2.5–3.1 mm: 587, 1.3–2.2 mm: 425	1024		
Centration of scan	Manual	Manual		BMOC	Manual		Manual		
Axis of cube scan	Horizontal	Horizontal			Horizontal		Horizontal		
Centration of analysis	BMOC	BMOC	FoDi	FoBMOC	BMOC	BMOC	RPEOC	ONH center‡	ONH center‡
Axis of analysis	Horizontal	Horizontal			Horizontal		Horizontal	Horizontal	

(Continued)

Table 7.1 (Continued) Comparison of imaging devices for retinal nerve fiber layer and optic nerve head analysis in glaucoma

cpRNFL & ONH	Cirrus	Spectralis (Cube)	Spectralis (Circle)	Spectralis (Circle+Radial)	Avanti RTVue XR (Cube)	Avanti RTVue XR (Circle+Radial)	3D OCT-1 Maestro2 (Cube)	3D OCT-2000 (Cube)	3D OCT-2000 (Circle)
Speed (A-scans/sec)	Cirrus 5000: 27K–68K; Cirrus 6000: 100K	OCT1: 40K; OCT2: 85K			70K		50K		
Shape & scan name*	Cube "Optic Disc Cube 200×200"	Cube "ONH"	Circle "RNFL"	Circle+Radial "ONH-RC" (GMPE only)	Cube "3D Disc"	Circle+Radial "ONH"	Cube	Cube "3D 6.0×6.0"	Circle "Circle 3.40"
Delineation of optic disc Margin	BMO		Not reported.	BMO		BMO	RPEO		
Calculation of neuroretinal rim thickness	MRA§	Not reported.		MRW	Not reported.		Not reported.		
Plane of rim & cup area calculation	BMO¶	Not reported.				BMO + 150 μm	RPE edge + 120 μm		
Anterior boundary of cup volume	BMO + 200 μm	Not reported.				BMO + 150 μm	RPE edge + 120 μm		

Abbreviations: BMO, Bruch's membrane opening; FoBMOC, fovea-Bruch's membrane opening center; FoDi, Fovea-disc; MRA, minimal rim area; MRW, minimum rim width; ONH, optic nerve head; RNFL, retinal nerve fiber layer; RPE, retinal pigment epithelium; RPEO, retinal pigment epithelium opening; RPEOC, retinal pigment epithelium opening center.

Notes: *Several of the devices offer wide scans that simultaneously image the optic nerve head and macular regions. In this table, only the scan types that dedicatedly image the optic nerve head region are named.

†Diameters of circle and/or radial scans are often given in either degrees or estimated millimeters; for consistency, estimated millimeters are reported when available.

‡The optic nerve head center is identified based on an infrared fundus image using a proprietary method. The centration is further optimized through registration to a color fundus photograph.

§Note that although the calculation of neuroretinal rim thickness on the Cirrus® employs a minimum rim area-reduction algorithm, it is a vector (i.e., a width) that represents the neuroretinal rim thickness (Section 7.2.1, Analysis).

¶Note that the rim and cup area values ultimately derive from the neuroretinal rim thickness calculation, and as such, do not correspond to the plane of the BMO in the way that do the values of the Avanti RTVue XR or the 3D-OCT series.

7

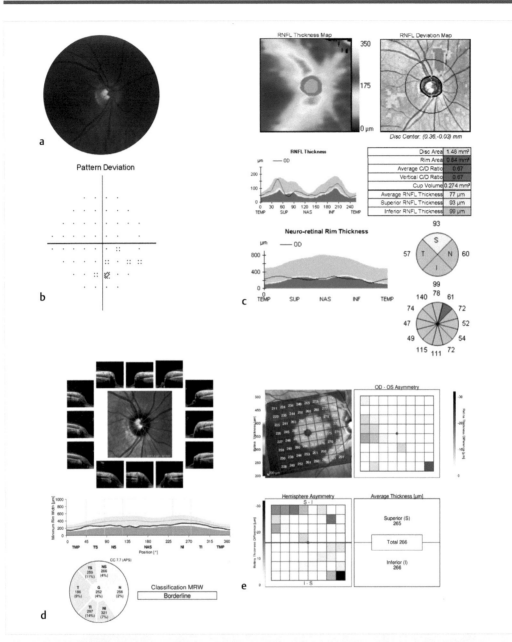

Fig. 7.1 Mild pigmentary glaucoma. Clinical images were obtained in a 46-year-old Caucasian male with mild pigmentary glaucoma in each eye. His disease is controlled with a topical prostaglandin analogue. (a) A fundus photo of the right eye demonstrates possible superior neuroretinal rim thinning. (b) A Humphrey visual field (Carl Zeiss Meditec AG, Jena, Germany) pattern deviation plot demonstrates no significant defects. (c) An *ONH and RNFL Analysis* (Cirrus, Carl Zeiss Meditec AG, Jena, Germany) demonstrates superior retinal nerve fiber layer (RNFL) thinning on the deviation map, further evidenced by thinning on the two sector grids and circumpapillary RNFL (cpRNFL) thickness graph. The neuroretinal rim thickness graph exhibits mild thinning, corroborated by other optic nerve head metrics, such rim area, average cup-to-disc ratio, and vertical cup-to-disc ratio. (d) A Glaucoma Module Premium Edition (GMPE) *Bruch's Membrane Opening-Minimum Rim Width (BMO-MRW) Report* (Spectralis, Heidelberg Engineering, Inc., Heidelberg, Germany) highlights superonasal and nasal neuroretinal rim thinning. For each radial scan, 12 representative tomograms also demonstrate individual BMO-MRWs. (e) The *Asymmetry Analysis Single Exam Report OU* (Spectralis®) highlights hemisphere asymmetry, notably superior thinning relative to inferior. Note the orientation of the grid along the fovea-disc axis.

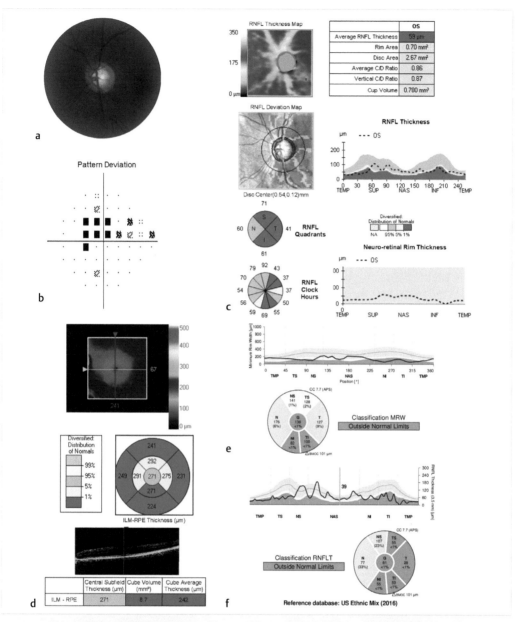

Fig. 7.2 Severe primary open-angle glaucoma. Clinical images were obtained in a 66-year-old Caucasian male with severe primary open-angle glaucoma in each eye. He has undergone glaucoma filtering surgery in his right and is being treated with three topical intraocular pressure lowering agents in his left eye. (**a**) A fundus photo of the left eye demonstrates marked neuroretinal rim thinning. (**b**) A Humphrey visual field (Carl Zeiss Meditec AG, Jena, Germany) pattern deviation plot demonstrates paracentral loss with an early superonasal defect. (**c**) An *ONH and RNFL Analysis* (Cirrus, Carl Zeiss Meditec AG, Jena, Germany) demonstrates prominent circumpapillary RNFL (cpRNFL) thinning on the deviation map, sector grids, and thickness graph. The reuroretinal rim thickness graph is colored gray as the disc area size is outside of the limits of the normative database, highlighting the importance of considering the inclusion and exclusion criteria of these databases. (**d**) A *Macular Thickness Report* (Cirrus®) demonstrates fairly marked thinning of the total retinal thickness. (**e**) A Glaucoma Module Premium Edition (GMPE) *Bruch's Membrane Opening-Minimum Rim Width (BMO-MRW) Report* (Spectralis, Heidelberg Engineering, Inc., Heidelberg, Germany) highlights inferior and borderline superior neuroretinal rim thinning. (**f**) A GMPE *RNFL Single Exam Report* (Spectralis®) demonstrates inferior, superior, and temporal cpRNFL thinning. Note the reference database that specifies its provenance from a United States-specific cohort, as is the case in the GMPE.

represent thinner RNFL and warmer colors (red and yellow) represent thicker RNFL. Thickness colors range from 0 (blue) to 350 μm (white). Adjacent to the thickness map is displayed a deviation map, which compares regions of the thickness map to an age-matched normative database. Pixels are binned into "superpixels" of 16 pixels (4×4 pixels) for a total of 2,500 superpixels analyzed.[6]

The deviation map is color-coded with respect to deviation from the normative database, whereby yellow signifies an RNFL thickness seen in the bottom 1 to 5% of normals, and red signifies an RNFL thickness seen in the bottom 1% of normals. Given that 5% of normals will have yellow- or red-range RNFL thickness, out of 2,500 superpixels analyzed, approximately 125 of these can be expected to be highlighted even in normals.

In addition to the RNFL thickness and deviation maps, cpRNFL thickness measured from the calculation circle is displayed in sector grids (both four- and twelve-sector) and a thickness graph (colloquially known as a "TSNIT" graph). The thickness graph plots cpRNFL thickness as a function of the position along the optic disc circumference, with 0 degree located at the horizontal axis. The cpRNFL thickness values are compared to an age-matched normative database, with the same yellow–red percentile deviation scheme as the deviation map. For review, the calculation circle tomogram is also displayed, as is a single B-scan of the volume scan.

In the data table, the average cpRNFL thickness (around the calculation circle) and the inter-eye asymmetry are displayed. The symmetry analysis is a correlation coefficient, converted to a percentage, that compares the 256 data points of the right eye calculation circle to the corresponding points of the left eye.

Normative Database

The Cirrus RNFL and Macula Normative Database[6] included males or females aged 18 years or older with a normal Humphrey 24–2 SITA Standard visual field in both eyes. Ocular exclusion criteria included: best-corrected visual acuity in either eye worse than 20/40; refractive error (spherical equivalent) outside of −12.00 D to + 8.00 D; presence or history of intraocular pressure ≥ 22 mmHg in either eye; a diagnosis of glaucoma or glaucoma suspect in either eye; an occludable angle or a history of angle-closure in either eye; presence or history of disc hemorrhage in either eye; presence of RNFL defect in either eye; presence of amblyopia in either eye; previous laser or incisional surgery; any active

infection of anterior or posterior segments; or evidence of diabetic retinopathy, diabetic macular edema, or other vitreoretinal disease. Systemic exclusion criteria included: history of diabetes, leukemia, AIDS, uncontrolled systemic hypertension, dementia, or multiple sclerosis; a life-threatening or debilitating disease; current or recent (within the past 14 days) use of an agent with photosensitizing properties by any route. Images were obtained of those with a signal strength of 5 or lower, large motion artifact, > 10% area of data loss, and/or a floater obstructing appropriate view.

The Cirrus RNFL and Macula Normative Database[6] comprises 284 subjects: 134 males and 150 females, aged 19 to 84. Only 28 subjects were aged 70 to 79, and only 3 subjects were 80 years of age or older. Thus, results in patients aged 70 or above should be interpreted with caution. The normative database also exhibits the following ethnic breakdown: 43% Caucasian, 24% Asian, 18% African-American, 12% Hispanic, 1% Indian, and 2% mixed ethnicity.

Among all variables studied, age was found to have the greatest effect on the RNFL thickness metrics. For this reason, all results are corrected for age.

Diagnostic Capability

Numerous studies have evaluated the reliability and diagnostic capabilities of cpRNFL metrics on the Cirrus, generally on prior models with similar imaging specifications and analytics, albeit with slower scanning speeds. Overall, the area under the receiver operating characteristic curve (AUC, listed parenthetically) to distinguish all-stage glaucoma from normal reaches a maximum for average (0.964, 0.950, 0.921, 0.88), superior (0.933, 0.906, 0.891, 0.88), and inferior (0.953, 0.952, 0.924, 0.87) cpRNFL thickness.[2,3,7,8] AUCs to distinguish mild glaucoma from normal were greatest for inferior (0.923, 0.895, 0.857), average (0.940, 0.893, 0.856), and superior (0.872, 0.859, 0.842) cpRNFL thickness.[3,7,8] Considering the specific case of preperimetric glaucoma, the parameters with the best discriminating capability were average (0.752) and inferior (0.744) cpRNFL thickness.[9]

Additional studies have evaluated the diagnostic capability of cpRNFL thickness in myopic eyes. The parameters with the highest discriminating capabilities reside in the average (0.899) and inferior (0.906) cpRNFL thickness in highly myopic glaucomatous eyes and the average cpRNFL thickness (0.920) in nonhighly myopic eyes.[10]

7.1.2 Spectralis (Heidelberg Engineering GmbH, Heidelberg, Germany)

Standard Edition

Imaging Specifications

The Spectralis is a spectral-domain OCT (SD-OCT) from Heidelberg Engineering GmbH. The OCT1 model attains scanning speeds of up to 40,000 A-scans per second, whereas the latest OCT2 model attains speeds of up to 85,000 A-scans per second. The Standard Edition[11] of the Spectralis offers a circle scan, labeled the "RNFL" scan, in order to measure cpRNFL thickness. The circle scan diameter subtends 12 degrees, estimated to extend across 3.45 mm and consisting of 768 data points.[12] The scan pattern is manually centered over the ONH, though the software will automatically place the circle scan over the approximate center of the ONH (2.6 degrees nasal and 2.1 degrees) for assistance.

In addition to the circle scan, the Standard Edition[11] offers a volume scan, labeled the "ONH" scan, which consists of a 15 degrees × 15 degrees cube comprising 37,376 data points (73 horizontal B-scans, each consisting of 512 A-scans). The volume scan is manually centered and generates a thickness map of the RNFL.

Analysis

The principal report of the Spectralis circle scan is the *RNFL Single Exam Report*,[11] which may be created for one eye or both eyes (▶ Fig. 7.3c). Similar information may also be viewed immediately during the imaging session with the *Thickness Profile Tab*. The *RNFL Single Exam Report* displays sector grids (four- and six-sector, symmetric about the vertical axis) and a thickness graph. In the sector grids, the mean RNFL thickness is indicated for each sector, as well as the global mean of all RNFL thickness values for that eye. The thickness graph plots cpRNFL thickness as a function of the position along the optic disc circumference, with 0 degree located at the intersection of the fovea-disc (FoDi) axis to the circle scan, *not* the horizontal axis.

Sector grids and the cpRNFL thickness graph adhere to a green–yellow–red significance scheme, whereby green color includes values present in 95% of normal subjects, yellow color indicates values present in the bottom 1 to 5% of normal subjects, and red color indicates values present in the bottom 1% of normal subjects.

An overall classification bar displays a yellow or red color if any sector in either sector grid displays a yellow or red color, respectively. In addition, a confocal scanning laser ophthalmoscopy (cSLO) image with overlaid circle scan pattern and FoDi axis, plus a circle scan tomogram, are available for review.

If a macula scan is also obtained, one may generate a combined *RNFL and Asymmetry Analysis Single Exam Report*,[11] details of which are found in the following sections.

Normative Database

The Reference Database[11] for the Standard Edition derives from an international cohort and includes 201 healthy subjects of European descent (111 males and 90 females). There is no normative database for the Standard Edition that includes a US population. The mean age of the European cohort is 48.2 ± 14.5 years, with an age range of 18 to 78 years. Refractive errors ranged from + 5.00 D to −7.00 D. All subjects manifested the following characteristics: normal intraocular pressure, normal visual field, normal optic disc appearance, and a lack of history of glaucoma. RNFL thickness was found to decrease with age. Thus, all reference data were adjusted with respect to age.

Diagnostic Capability

Numerous studies have evaluated the capabilities of the Spectralis Standard Edition. Overall, the area under the receiver operating characteristic curve (AUC) to distinguish all-stage glaucoma from normal reaches a maximum for global (0.952), inferotemporal (0.947), inferior (0.905), superior (0.925), and superotemporal (0.911) cpRNFL thickness.[13] The AUC to distinguish mild glaucoma from normal reaches a maximum for global (0.895), inferotemporal (0.888, 0.858), inferior (0.861, 0.855), and superotemporal (0.873, 0.810) cpRNFL thickness.[13,14]

Glaucoma Module Premium Edition

Imaging Specifications

The Glaucoma Module Premium Edition[15] (GMPE) offers a novel "ONH-RC" scan (▶ Fig. 7.4e). This scan consists of three circle scans of estimated diameters 12, 14, and 16 degrees (estimated to be 3.5, 4.1, and 4.7 mm, respectively), and 24 radial scans of length 15 degrees, all automatically centered on the optic nerve using the Anatomic Positioning System (APS) (see below).[16] Each circle scan and each radial scan

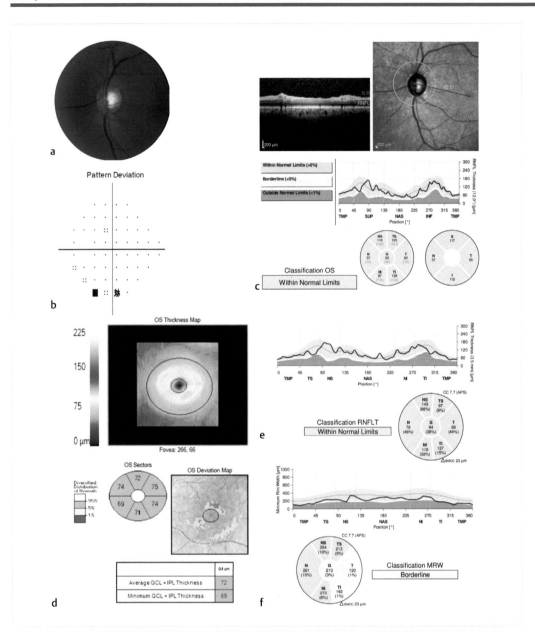

Fig. 7.3 Mild primary open-angle glaucoma. Clinical images were obtained in a 62-year-old African-American male with mild primary open-angle glaucoma in each eye. Based on the patient's clinical presentation, including intraocular pressures elevated to the mid-20 s in each eye, the decision was made to start therapy with a prostaglandin analogue. **(a)** A fundus photo of the left eye demonstrates a grossly intact neuroretinal rim. **(b)** A Humphrey visual field (Carl Zeiss Meditec AG, Jena, Germany) pattern deviation plot demonstrates no significant defects. **(c)** An *RNFL Single Exam Report* (Spectralis, Standard Edition, Heidelberg Engineering, Inc., Heidelberg, Germany) with representative tomogram (top-left) and confocal scanning laser ophthalmoscope image with superimposed circle scan (top-right). Note that the circle scan is oriented along the fovea-disc axis with the subtended angle displayed. The thickness graph and two sector grids demonstrate no circumpapillary RNFL (cpRNFL) thinning; as such, the classification bar is colored green, indicating that the values are all within the top 95% of normal values. **(d)** A *Ganglion Cell Analysis* (Cirrus, Carl Zeiss Meditec AG, Jena, Germany) demonstrates mild areas of thinning of the ganglion cell layer-inner plexiform layer as evident in the deviation map. **(e)** A Glaucoma Module Premium Edition (GMPE) *RNFL Single Exam Report* (Spectralis®) utilizing a Garway-Heath sector divisions demonstrates no cpRNFL thinning. **(f)** A GMPE *Bruch's Membrane Opening-Minimum Rim Width (BMO-MRW) Report* (Spectralis®) demonstrates borderline temporal and inferotemporal BMO-MRW thinning, despite no cpRNFL thinning evident on the *RNFL Single Exam Report* in either the Standard Edition or GMPE.

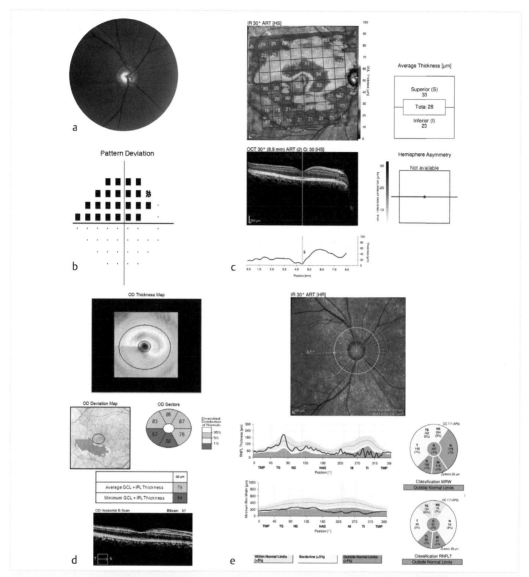

Fig. 7.4 Severe juvenile open angle glaucoma. Clinical images were obtained from a 49-year-old Hispanic male with a history of severe juvenile-onset open-angle glaucoma in each eye. The patient has previously undergone aqueous shunt implantation in his right and requires adjunctive therapy with four topical intraocular pressure lowering agents in each eye. **(a)** A fundus photo of the right eye demonstrates inferotemporal neuroretinal rim thinning. **(b)** A Humphrey visual field (Carl Zeiss Meditec AG, Jena, Germany) pattern deviation plot demonstrates a dense superior arcuate defect. **(c)** A ganglion cell layer (GCL) thickness map with overlying thickness grid, available on numerous reports on the Glaucoma Module Premium Edition (GMPE) (Spectralis, Heidelberg Engineering, Inc., Heidelberg, Germany), exhibits inferotemporal thinning. In the average thickness display, the average inferior thickness is decreased compared to the superior thickness. In this report, hemisphere asymmetry is not reported. **(d)** A *Ganglion Cell Analysis* (Cirrus, Carl Zeiss Meditec AG, Jena, Germany) corroborates the aforementioned Spectralis® report and demonstrates an area of inferotemporal thinning of the ganglion cell layer-inner plexiform layer. In this report, a deviation map is available for viewing. **(e)** Data from a GMPE *RNFL Single Exam Report* (Spectralis®) and a *Bruch's Membrane Opening-Minimum Rim Width (BMO-MRW) Report* (Spectralis®) demonstrate prominent inferior thinning of their respective metrics. Note the scan pattern in the confocal scanning laser ophthalmoscope image that includes a combination of radial and circle scan patterns. There are three circle scan diameters, with inner 12-degree scan, the default for generating analysis reports. Also note that the scan is automatically centered on the optic nerve head and aligned to the fovea-BMO center (FoBMOC) axis via the Anatomic Positioning System (APS).

consist of 768 data points. The GMPE also offers the standard circle scan and volume scan available in the Standard Edition.

One unique component of the GMPE is the APS.[15] Using the APS, the ONH-RC scan itself, as opposed to the postscan analysis grid, is fixed to two structures: the foveal center and the Bruch's membrane opening center (BMOC). All ONH-RC scans are thus automatically centered on the optic disc based on the BMOC. In addition, a line is drawn to connect these two centers to create an axis along which all scans are aligned, termed fovea-to-Bruch's membrane opening center axis (FoBMOC). Because the ONH-RC scan consists of circle and radial scans (i.e., not a volume scan), small errors in alignment across longitudinal scans may lead to discrepancies in RNFL measurements. For this reason, proper alignment is paramount and accordingly ensured by the APS. Of importance, note that this differs from the Standard Edition circle scan, which is manually centered—thus inter-scan alignment cannot be guaranteed.

Analysis

GMPE analytics demonstrate both similarities and differences to those in the Standard Edition. The *RNFL Thickness Tab* and the corresponding *RNFL Thickness Report*[15] display sector grids (four- and six-sector) and a thickness graph, as in the Standard Edition. Data displayed may stem from any of the three circle scan diameters (though the inner circle is the default). However, the sector grids adhere to the Garway-Heath division, differing from those used in the Standard Edition (▶ Fig. 7.3e and ▶ Fig. 7.2f). In this model, the temporal sector subtends 90 degrees (315 to 45 degrees), the superior-temporal sector subtends 40 degrees (45 to 85 degrees), the superior-nasal sector subtends 40 degrees (85 to 125 degrees), the nasal sector subtends 110 degrees (125 to 235 degrees), the inferior-nasal sector subtends 40 degrees (235 to 275 degrees), and the inferior-temporal sector subtends 40 degrees (275 to 315 degrees).

For the sector grid, the mean RNFL thickness is indicated for each sector, as well as the global mean of all RNFL thickness values for that eye. The thickness graph displays RNFL thickness as a function of the position along the optic disc circumference, with 0 degree located at the intersection of the fovea-disc (FoBMOC) axis to the circle scan, *not* the horizontal axis.

Sector grids and the thickness graph adhere to an identical significance color scheme as the

Standard Edition. The remainder of the data and layout are similar to that in the Standard Edition. Of note, a *Hood Report* may be generated, the cpRNFL specifics of which are discussed later in Section 7.1.4, *Analysis*.

Normative Database

An RNFL thickness normative database[15] is available for the United States version of the GMPE and thus deviation maps and normative comparisons may be created with cpRNFL data. The US normative database includes 330 eyes of 330 normal subjects (146 male and 184 female) with a racial and ethnic composition representative of the US population and age range of 20 to 90 years. Inclusion criteria included healthy eyes without prior intraocular surgery (except cataract surgery or LASIK); an absence of clinically significant vitreoretinal disease, optic nerve disease, or history of glaucoma; intraocular pressure ≤21 mmHg; best-corrected visual acuity ≥ 0.5; refraction range + 6.00 D to −6.00 D; astigmatism ≤ 2.00 D; normal visual fields in a glaucoma hemifield test and mean deviation within normal limits; and a clinically normal appearance of the optic disc. As RNFL thickness was found to decrease with increasing age and decreasing BMO area, all reference data were adjusted with respect to age and BMO area.

Diagnostic Capability

Numerous studies have evaluated the capabilities of the Spectralis GMPE cpRNFL thickness metrics, chiefly using the area under the receiver operating characteristic curve (AUC), which are listed parenthetically. The capability of the GMPE to distinguish all-stage glaucoma from normal reaches a maximum for global (0.954, 0.86) and inferotemporal (0.929) cpRNFL thickness metrics.[16,17] Its capability to discriminate mild glaucoma from normal peaks for global (0.76) cpRNFL thickness and that for preperimetric glaucoma peaks for inferonasal (0.860), global (0.839), and inferotemporal (0.767) cpRNFL thickness.[16,17] The AUC to distinguish all-stage glaucoma from normal in *myopic* eyes remains excellent using the global cpRNFL thickness.[18]

7.1.3 Avanti RTVue XR (Optovue, Inc., Fremont, CA, USA)

Imaging Specifications

The Avanti RTVue XR is an SD-OCT from Optovue, Inc. Specifications[19] include scanning speeds of

70,000 A-scans per second and the inclusion of two scans: a volume scan (labeled "3D Disc") and a circle + radial scan (labeled "ONH"). The volume scan images a 6.0 × 6.0 mm area, manually centered over the ONH, and consists of 51,813 data points (101 horizontal B-scans consisting of 513 A-scans). The circle + radial scan is a manually centered scan and consists of 13 circle scans of increasing diameter and 12 radial scans. The radial scans are of length 15 degrees and each comprise 455 data points. The circle scans have diameters ranging from 1.3 to 4.9 mm (increasing by 0.3 mm increments) and comprise 425 to 965 data points, depending on the circle diameter.

Analysis

The principal RNFL thickness report is the *ONH Report*[19] (▶ Fig. 7.5c), which displays thickness values calculated along a 3.4-mm calculation circle (i.e., the cpRNFL). The report displays sector grids of various sizes (two-hemisphere, four-quadrant, and eight-sector, symmetric about the vertical and horizontal axes) with their respective cpRNFL thickness values. The eight-sector display also includes an enclosed thickness map. The average global, superior, and inferior cpRNFL thickness values, plus the difference between superior and inferior cpRNFL thickness, are displayed in a data table. In addition, a thickness graph plots cpRNFL thickness as a function of the position along the optic disc circumference, with 0 degree located along the horizontal axis.

Sector grids and the thickness graphs adhere to a green-yellow-red significance scheme, whereby green color includes values present in 95% of normal subjects, yellow color indicates values present in the bottom 1 to 5% of normal subjects, and red color indicates values present in the bottom 1% of normal subjects.

A cSLO image with overlaid thickness map and circle scan (corresponding to the diameter used for cpRNFL thickness measurements), plus a representative tomogram of the aforementioned circle scan, are available for review. If circle + radial scans are obtained for both eyes, an *OU Report* may be generated, which additionally displays inter-eye differences of various metrics.

Normative Database

The RTVue Normative Database[19] for the circle + radial ("ONH") scan of the Avanti RTVue XR consists of 649 eyes from 366 subjects, with a mean age of 49.9 and an age range of 19 to 84 years. Ethnicity percentages included Caucasian (34%), Asian (22%), Hispanic (12%), African Descendant (19%), Indian/Middle Easterner (12%), Pacific Islander (0%), and other (1%). Mean sphere was −0.46 ± 1.9 D (range −7.75 D to + 5.50 D).

Inclusion criteria included: age ≥ 18, refractive error of + 8.00 D to −8.00 sphere and + 2.00 to −2.00 D cylinder, and best-corrected visual acuity of 20/30 or better in each eye. Exclusion criteria included: a history of leukemia, AIDS, dementia, or multiple sclerosis; concomitant use of hydroxychloroquine or chloroquine; a family history of glaucoma among first-degree relatives; intraocular pressure of ≥ 22 mmHg or greater in either eye; a visual field demonstrating positive results (>30% false-negative responses, >30% false-positive responses, or > 30% fixation losses, pattern standard deviation of $p < 5\%$ or worse, and/or a glaucoma hemifield test outside normal limits); active ocular disease including degenerative myopia; previous diagnosis of glaucoma or glaucoma suspect; congenital intraocular surgery or laser treatment (other than refractive surgery or uncomplicated cataract surgery greater than 6 months prior); and/or an anatomically narrow angle.

Correlational analyses revealed that decreased RNFL thickness was associated with increasing age and decreasing optic disc size. For this reason, all clinical data comparisons to the normative database are adjusted for age and optic disc size.

Diagnostic Capability

As measured by the area under the receiver operating characteristic curve (AUC, listed parenthetically in the following section), the capabilities of the Avanti SD-OCT to distinguish all-stage glaucoma from normal reach a maximum for average (0.968, 0.919, 0.87, 0.879) and inferior (0.947, 0.884, 0.86) cpRNFL thickness.[2,3,20,21] The capability to distinguish mild or preperimetric glaucoma from normal remains excellent though slightly decreased compared to that for all-stage glaucoma.[3,22] Of note, in highly myopic eyes, the diagnostic capability of cpRNFL has been shown to decline compared to emmetropic eyes.[4]

7.1.4 3D OCT (Topcon Corporation, Tokyo, Japan)

Imaging Specifications

The 3D OCT series from Topcon Corporation includes the 3D OCT-2000 and the 3D OCT-1 Maestro2, the

7

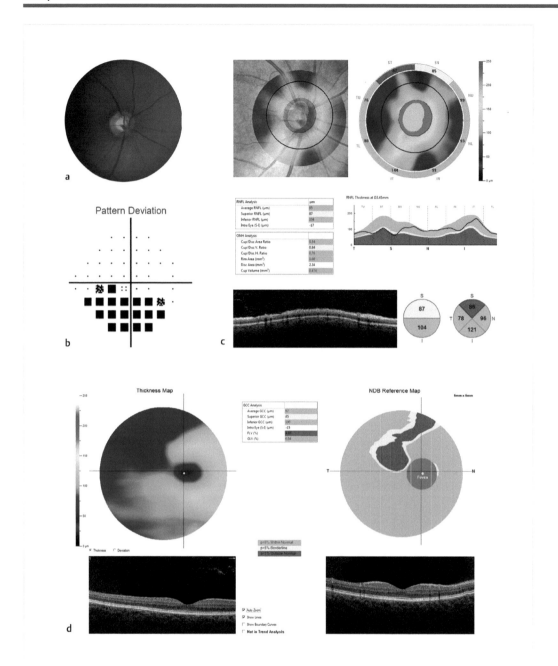

Fig. 7.5 Moderate primary open-angle glaucoma. Clinical images were obtained from a patient suffering from moderate primary open-angle glaucoma in each eye. **(a)** A fundus photo of the right eye demonstrates inferotemporal and superotemporal neuroretinal rim thinning. **(b)** Humphrey visual field (Carl Zeiss Meditec AG, Jena, Germany) pattern deviation plot demonstrates an inferior arcuate defect. **(c)** An *ONH Report* (Avanti RTVue XR, Optovue, Inc., Fremont, CA, USA) demonstrates superior circumpapillary RNFL (cpRNFL) thinning on the sector grids and thickness graph. **(d)** A *GCC Report* (Avanti RTVue XR®) demonstrates prominent superior thinning of the ganglion cell complex (GCC) on the normative database (NDB) reference map, corroborated in the GCC Analysis Table. In addition, the focal loss volume (FLV%) value suggests significant GCC loss. (Figure used with permission from David Huang, MD, PhD, and Liang Liu, MD, Center for Ophthalmic Optics & Lasers (www.CooLab.net), Casey Eye Institute, Oregon Health & Science University.)

latter being the latest model in this series. The OCT-2000[23] attains scanning speeds of 50,000 A-scans per second. The OCT-2000 offers two scans: a volume scan, labeled "3D 6.0 × 6.0," and a circle scan, labeled "Circle 3.40." The volume scan consists of a manually centered 6.0 × 6.0 mm scan consisting of 65,536 data points (128 horizontal B-scans, each consisting of 512 A-scans). The volume scan derives a peripapillary calculation circle of 3.4 mm diameter. The standalone circle scan consists of a 3.4-mm-diameter circle with 1,024 data points and is automatically centered using the optic disc auto-search function, which identifies the optic disc center through registration to both infrared and color fundus photographs.

The 3D OCT-1 Maestro2[24] is the latest SD-OCT model from Topcon Corporation. The device attains scanning speeds of 50,000 A-scans per second. The OCT-1 Maestro2 offers a single scan: a manually centered 6.0 × 6.0 mm volume scan consisting of 65,536 data points (128 horizontal B-scans, each consisting of 512 A-scans). The software derives a peripapillary circle of 3.4 mm diameter composed of 1,024 data points and automatically centered on the optic disc using the retinal pigment epithelium (RPE) edge as the optic disc margin.

Analysis

The 3D OCT-1 Maestro2 includes an updated normative database and the most up-to-date glaucoma analytics from Topcon Corporation. As such, focus will be placed on the OCT-1 Maestro2. Analytics of the OCT-2000 are comparable though lack several new features found in the OCT-1 Maestro2.

Various displays and reports are available on the OCT-1 Maestro2.[24] The OCT-1 Maestro2 includes an *OCT Data View* that simultaneously displays a color fundus photo centered on the ONH, a calculation circle tomogram, an RNFL thickness map, a thickness graph, and a sector grid (twelve-sector). The thickness graph plots cpRNFL thickness as a function of the position along the optic disc circumference, with 0 degree located at the horizontal axis. A second fundus photo may display an array of images, including a red-free photo, an infrared photo, or any reference image.

A 6.0 × 6.0 mm volume scan begets a *3D Disc Report*, for either one or both eyes. The *3D Disc Report* includes a fundus photograph, thickness map, sector grids (four- and twelve-sector), and thickness graph plotting cpRNFL as a function of the position along the optic disc circumference, with 0 degree located at the horizontal axis. The

average RNFL thickness is reported as well, which represents the average of the *cpRNFL* thickness from the calculation circle, *not* the overall RNFL thickness from the thickness map.

Clinical data follow the typical scheme whereby those in the bottom 1% of the normative database are colored red and those in the bottom 1 to 5% are colored yellow. In addition, data in the top 1 to 5% are colored orange and those in the top 1% are colored magenta. With a 3D Wide scan, one may generate a comprehensive report including metrics of the cpRNFL, ONH, and macula.

A *Hood Report* may also be generated. This report displays a thickness map, sector grids (four- and twelve-sector), and thickness graph (with reversed, *nasal-to-nasal* orientation). An *en face* 52.0-μm slab is displayed along with a horizontal tomogram image of the cpRNFL calculation circle. Additional macular metrics are displayed (discussed in Section 7.3.4, *Analysis*).

Normative Database

The US version of the 3D OCT-2000 does not include a normative database. On the contrary, the OCT-1 Maestro2 includes a normative database[24] for the US version and will be discussed. The database includes 399 eyes of 504 subjects, with a mean age of 46.3 ± 16.3 years (range 18 to 88).[25] Females consitituted 57% of the subjects. The demographic stratification was as follows: 59% Caucasian, 20% African-American, 18% Hispanic/Latino, 13% Asian, 2% Native American/Pacific Islander, 1% American Indian/Alaskan Native, and 6% other. The population had a mean sphere of −1.441 D ± 2.537 (range −12.5 D to + 4.0 D), a cylinder of 0.565 D ± 0.691 (range 0 to 5.0 D), and a manifest refractive spherical equivalent of −1.159 D ± 2.418 (range −11.00 to + 4.50 D).

Peripapillary RNFL thickness was found to be greatly associated with disc area and minimally associated with age. As such cpRNFL thickness values are all adjusted for age and disc area. If no birth date is provided or if the disc area is unavailable, no comparison with reference data is performed. If either the age or the disc area are outside of the range of the database (18 to 90 years for age, and 1.03 to 3.85 mm[2] for disc area), the clinical data are compared by extrapolation.

Diagnostic Capability

A few studies have evaluated the capabilities of the 3D OCT series, though chiefly of the OCT-2000.

Overall, using the area under the receiver operating characteristic curve (AUC), the capability of the OCT-2000 to distinguish all-stage glaucoma from normal is greatest for the global and inferior cpRNFL thickness metrics (AUC 0.957 and 0.955, respectively).[3] AUC values representing the capability to distinguish mild glaucoma from normal remained excellent though less than those regarding all-stage glaucoma.[3]

7.2 Optic Nerve Head

Metrics on the ONH are varied and differ among the available OCT devices. Metrics may be grouped into the following measurement categories: (1) area (disc, rim, and cup); (2) volume (cup volume); (3) ratios (vertical linear, area, among others); and (4) neuroretinal rim thickness. Among these, the calculation of neuroretinal rim thickness is the most nuanced and specific to each particular device. For this reason, neuroretinal rim thickness measurements may not necessarily be compared across devices and caution should be exercised when doing so. The reader should refer to the subsection for each device for details on the calculation of ONH metrics. ▶ Table 7.1 highlights the main differences among the various platforms in imaging the RNFL and ONH.

7.2.1 Cirrus 6000 (Carl Zeiss Meditec AG, Jena, Germany)

Imaging Specifications

As mentioned in Section 7.1.1, *Imaging Specifications*, the Cirrus 6000 employs a single 6.0 × 6.0 mm volume scan to calculate both RNFL thickness and ONH metrics. Please refer to that section for further details on the imaging specifications of the Cirrus 6000 device.

Analysis

The Cirrus employs a custom algorithm[26] to calculate the neuroretinal rim thickness. The software identifies the optic disc border by using the edge of Bruch's membrane, that is, the BMO. Optic disc area is calculated as the area enclosed by and along the plane of the BMO. It samples the BMO at 180 points, creating equally spaced segments 2 degrees in length. At each point, a vector is drawn from the BMO to the inner limiting membrane (ILM). This vector forms the height of a trapezoid, bounded by the 2 degrees BMO segment (the "floor"), a

corresponding 2 degrees ILM segment (the "roof"), and two "sides" adjoining the edges of the BMO and ILM segments. The vector is rotated about the BMO until the area of its corresponding trapezoid is minimized. At this minimum area, the vector length is considered optimized and is defined as the neuroretinal rim thickness. This process is completed for all 180 vectors, such that a thickness graph of neuroretinal rim thickness may be plotted for the entire circumference of the ONH.

To calculate the remaining ONH metrics, the device algorithm rotates all 180 optimized vectors into the plane of the BMO. The area between these optimized vectors is summed to calculate the optic rim area. The optic cup area is calculated as the optic disc area minus the optic rim area. The square root of the ratio of the optic cup area to disc area yields the average cup-to-disc ratio. The vertical cup-to-disc ratio is a unitless metric calculated as the ratio of the optic cup diameter to the optic disc diameter in the vertical meridian.

Optic cup volume is calculated as the volume enclosed by the following boundaries: anterior boundary defined as the retinal pigment epithelium (RPE) plane plus 200 µm, and posterior boundary defined as the internal limiting membrane (i.e., vitreoretinal interface). With this algorithm, the anterior border remains fixed, whereas the posterior border deepens with worsening disease.

All of the aforementioned calculated metrics are available on the *ONH and RNFL Analysis*[6] report (▶ Fig. 7.1c and ▶ Fig. 7.2c).

Normative Database

The Cirrus Optic Nerve Head Normative Database[6] was derived from post-hoc analysis of the RNFL thickness normative database. The inclusion and exclusion criteria are thus the same as those employed for the RNFL and macula normative database (Section 7.1.1, *Normative Database*). ONH metrics include disc area, rim area, average cup-to-disc area, vertical cup-to-disc area, and cup volume. Among all variables studied, age and disc area were found to have the greatest effect on the ONH metrics. For this reason, all clinical results are compared with age-matched and optic disc area-matched normative data.

Diagnostic Capability

Numerous studies have evaluated the diagnostic accuracy of the ONH metrics of the Cirrus device, generally on prior models with similar imaging specifications and analytics, albeit with slower scanning speeds. The diagnostic capability, represented by the AUC (listed parenthetically), to distinguish all-stage glaucoma from normal was greatest for rim thickness (0.963), rim area (0.962, 0.845), and vertical cup-to-disc ratio (VCDR) (0.951, 0.864).[7,8] The capability to distinguish mild glaucoma from normal was greatest for rim thickness (0.914), rim area (0.912, 0.805), and VCDR (0.890, 0.792).[7,8] AUCs in the case of preperimetric glaucoma were overall low, with the greatest being rim area (AUC 0.767) and VCDR (0.714).[9] ONH parameters in myopic eyes overall fare poorly in their diagnostic capabilities and have been shown to perform inferiorly to cpRNFL and, in particular, macular metrics.[27]

7.2.2 Spectralis (Heidelberg Engineering, Inc., Heidelberg, Germany)

Standard Edition

The Standard Edition of the Spectralis does not generate ONH metrics. ONH metrics are available in the GMPE.

Glaucoma Module Premium Edition

Imaging Specifications

ONH metrics are derived from the same ONH-RC scan used to calculate RNFL thickness (Section 7.1.2, *GMPE Imaging Specifications*).

The ONH metric calculated by the ONH-RC is the Bruch's membrane opening–minimum rim width[15] (BMO-MRW). To calculate this variable, the software samples the BMO at 48 discrete points (two for each of the 24 radial scans, given each radial line intersects the BMO at two points). For each point, a line is drawn from the BMO to the ILM. The *shortest* distance from the BMO to the ILM, among all distances sampled, is termed the BMO-MRW for that point. This process is then completed for all 48 points.

Analysis

There are multiple tabs and reports that display BMO-MRW information.[15] The *BMO Overview Tab* (available immediately after imaging) and the *BMO Overview Report* (available at any time) display a cSLO image with six overlaid radial scans and their corresponding 12 (two for each radial scan) tomograms of BMO-MRW segments (upper half of ▸ Fig. 7.1d).

On the *BMO Rim Analysis Tab* or the *Minimum Rim Width Analysis Report*, a sector grid (six-sector, Garway-Heath division) and a BMO-MRW graph are displayed (bottom half of ▸ Fig. 7.1d). The mean BMO-MRW and corresponding percentile (compared to the normative database) are indicated for each sector, as well as the global mean of all BMO-MRW values. The BMO-MRW graph displays BMO-MRW values as a function of the position along the optic disc circumference, with 0 degree located at the FoBMOC axis, *not* the horizontal axis.

Clinical data adhere to a green-yellow-red significance scheme, whereby green color includes values present in 95% of normal subjects, yellow color indicates values present in the bottom 1 to 5% of normal subjects, and red color indicates values present in the bottom 1% of normal subjects. An overall classification bar displays a yellow or red color if any sector of the sector grid displays a yellow or red color, respectively.

The *Minimum Rim Width & RNFL Analysis Single Exam Report*, exhibited in ▸ Fig. 7.3e–f and ▸ Fig. 7.4e, displays BMO-MRW and cpRNFL thickness data on one report.

Normative Database

As with cpRNFL thickness, a BMO-MRW Normative Database[15] is available for the United States version of the GMPE and thus deviation maps and normative comparisons may be made with BMO-MRW data. The US cohort includes 368 eyes of 368 subjects (165 male and 203 female) with racial and ethnic composition representative of the US population, with the age range of 20 to 90 years. Inclusion criteria included healthy eyes without prior intraocular surgery (except cataract surgery or LASIK); an absence of clinically significant vitreoretinal disease, optic nerve disease, or history of glaucoma; intraocular pressure ≤ 21 mmHg; best-corrected visual acuity ≥ 0.5; refraction range + 6.00 D to −6.00 D; astigmatism ≤ 2.00 D; normal visual fields in a glaucoma hemifield test and mean deviation within normal limits; and a clinically normal appearance of the optic disc. BMO-MRW was found to decrease with increasing age and increasing BMO area. Thus, all reference data were adjusted with respect to age and BMO area.

Diagnostic Capability

Numerous studies have evaluated the capabilities of the Spectralis GMPE BMO-MRW metrics, usually of the global BMO-MRW. Overall, diagnostic capability, represented by the AUC (listed parenthetically), to distinguish all-stage glaucoma from normal reaches a maximum for inferotemporal (0.946), global (0.929), and superotemporal (0.924) BMO-MRW.[16] The diagnostic capability of global BMO-MRW to distinguish mild glaucoma from normal remains fair,[17] and that in the case of preperimetric glaucoma reaches a maximum for superotemporal (0.835) and global (0.821) BMO-MRW.[16] Overall, BMO-MRW has been shown to be comparable if not superior to cpRNFL thickness in its diagnostic capabilities, particularly in the setting of myopia.[16,18]

7.2.3 Avanti RTVue XR (Optovue, Inc., Fremont, CA, USA)

Imaging Specifications

The Avanti RTVue XR calculates several ONH metrics.[19] It utilizes the "3D Disc" volume scan to establish the optic disc margin by identifying the edge of the Bruch's membrane, that is, the BMO. Although each subsequent circle + radial scan must be manually centered, the optic disc margin, as determined by the initial "3D Disc" volumes scan, remains constant and thus permits more accurate longitudinal comparisons.

Analysis

ONH metrics are displayed on the *ONH Report*,[19] which also displays RNFL thickness metrics (▶ Fig. 7.5c). Displayed in the data table are the following metrics: cup-to-disc area ratio, cup-to-disc vertical ratio, cup-to-disc horizontal ratio, rim area, disc area, and cup volume.

To calculate the cup-to-disc ratios (CDR), the software calculates a best-fit ellipse based on the optic disc margin. It then uses the longest diameter of the ellipse as the *vertical* line from which it calculates the vertical cup-to-disc ratio. The line perpendicular to this is used for the horizontal cup-to-disc ratio.

The optic disc area is calculated as the area encircled by and along the plane of the BMO. The cup area is calculated as the area encircled by the ILM (i.e., the vitreoretinal interface) along a plane 150 μm anterior to the plane of the BMO. Optic rim area is then calculated as disc area minus cup area; rim area is therefore, by extension, measured at 150 μm anterior to the BMO plane. Optic cup volume is calculated as the volume enclosed with the following boundaries: anterior boundary defined as 150 μm anterior the BMO plane, and posterior boundary defined as the ILM (i.e., vitreoretinal interface). Beware that the plane used to calculate the optic cup parameters on OCT angiography (OCTA) devices manufactured by Optovue is the BMO plane itself (i.e., *without* the anterior 150 μm shift)—the measurements between these two devices are not interchangeable.

Normative Database

The RTVue Normative Database[19] for ONH metrics consists of the same population as that for RNFL metrics (Section 7.1.3, *Normative Database*).

Diagnostic Capability

The diagnostic capability of ONH metrics, measured by the AUC (listed parenthetically), to distinguish all-stage glaucoma from normal reaches a maximum for vertical cup-to-disc ratio (0.854, 0.810) and cup-to-disc area ratio (0.832, 0.786).[20,21] These values remain fair in the case of preperimetric glaucoma though decline for eyes with large optic discs.[22] Overall, ONH metrics have been shown to be somewhat comparable, though at times inferior, to cpRNFL metrics in their diagnostic capabilities.[20]

7.2.4 3D OCT (Topcon Corporation, Tokyo, Japan)

Imaging Specifications

The imaging specifications[24] for the ONH metrics derive from the same scans as those used to derive cpRNFL metrics. This holds true for both the 3D OCT-2000 and the OCT-1 Maestro2. The OCT-1 Maestro2 reports the following parameters: rim area, disc area, linear CDR, vertical CDR, and cup volume. Disc area is defined as the area enclosed by the edge of the RPE. The plane from the edges of the RPE is termed the "base plane" and all other parameters are obtained relative to this plane. The cup area and volume are calculated along and deep to, respectively, a plane 120 μm perpendicular and anterior to the base plane. The rim area is then calculated as the disc area minus the cup area; rim area is therefore, by extension, measured at 120 μm anterior to the base plane.

The linear cup-to-disc ratio ("LCDR") is calculated as the square root of the cup area-to-disc area ratio. The vertical cup-to-disc ratio is calculated as the ratio of the height of a rectangle circumscribed around the cup area to the height of a rectangle circumscribed around the disc area.

Analysis

The OCT-1 Maestro2 includes a *3D Disc Report*,[24] which includes a table displaying the following metrics: rim area, disc area, linear CDR, vertical CDR, and cup volume. The calculations for these metrics are explained above in Section 7.2.4, *Imaging Specifications*. In addition, a graph of rim-to-disc (R/D) ratio per polar angle around the disc center is displayed for both eyes. This metric represents the ratio of the rim length (equal to disc radius minus cup radius) to the disc diameter. For review, *en face* and tomogram images of the reference planes used to calculate the ONH are displayed, to allow the viewer to identify any calculation errors. Clinical data for ONH parameters follow an identical color scheme to that for cpRNFL thickness (see corresponding section above).

With a 3D Wide scan, one may generate a comprehensive report including data on cpRNFL thickness, ONH metrics, and macular parameters (Section 7.3.4, *Analysis*).

Normative Database

Normative data for the ONH metrics stem from the same database as that used for the cpRNFL metrics (Section 7.1.4, *Normative Database*).

ONH parameters were found to be associated with disc area, though not significantly with age. Nonetheless, all ONH parameters are adjusted for disc area and age. If no birth date is provided or if the disc area is unavailable, no comparison with reference data is performed. If either the age or the disc area is outside of the range of the database (18 to 90 years for age, and 1.03 to 3.85 mm^2 for disc area), the clinical data are compared by extrapolation.

Diagnostic Capability

There are no studies evaluating the diagnostic capabilities of the ONH parameters of the OCT-2000 or the OCT-1 Maestro2.

7.3 Macula

Macular metrics have seen several advancements in recent years, namely, the development and adoption of ganglion cell analysis algorithms. These algorithms seek to calculate the thickness of the ganglion cell layer (GCL) (plus adjacent layers). Macular metrics may be divided into three categories: total thickness, lamellar thickness, and asymmetry analyses. Devices may employ one or multiple categories of analysis.

Studies on individual devices are discussed in the following sections. There have been a few notable studies comparing devices to one another, with results generally demonstrating that the devices are comparable in their diagnostic capabilities, including in highly myopic eyes.[3,5] Diagnostic capabilities generally increase in more advanced stages of glaucoma.[5] There is some evidence that ganglion cell metrics may be most useful in myopic eyes and that diagnostic capabilities of macular parameters are less influenced by nerve fiber layer defect location.[5] Note that literature cited in the following sections by and large includes studies on single devices; as such, direct comparisons of study outcomes (particularly diagnostic capabilities) cannot be made across devices. ▶ Table 7.2 highlights the main differences among the various platforms in imaging macular parameters.

7.3.1 Cirrus 6000 (Carl Zeiss Meditec AG, Jena, Germany)

Imaging Specifications

To image the macula, the Cirrus device employs a 6.0 × 6.0 mm volume scan comprising 40,000 data points (200 horizontal B-scans, each comprising 200 A-scans), identical to the volume scan employed for optic nerve metrics (Section 7.1.1, *Imaging Specifications*).[6]

Analysis

The Cirrus SD-OCT generates a principal report titled *Ganglion Cell Analysis*[6] (▶ Fig. 7.3d and ▶ Fig. 7.4d), whereby the retina is segmented into the GCL and the inner plexiform layer (IPL). The software places an elliptical annulus automatically centered on the fovea to calculate the GCL plus IPL (GCIPL) thicknesses along the annulus.

Displayed on this report are a thickness map and a deviation map. The deviation map compares the thickness map to a normative database, with corresponding yellow and red colors signifying a GCIPL thickness seen in the bottom 1 to 5% and bottom 1% of normal subjects, respectively.

To further analyze the data, the software overlays onto the thickness map an ellipse, of area 14.13 mm^3 and with the following dimensions: a vertical inner and outer radius of 0.5 and 2.0 mm, respectively, and a horizontal inner and outer

7

Table 7.2 Comparison of imaging devices for macular analysis in glaucoma

Macula	Cirrus	Spectralis		Avanti RTVue XR	3D OCT-2000 & 3D OCT-1 Maestro2
Shape & scan name	Cube	Cube "P. Pole" (Standard Ed.)	Cube "PPoleH" (GMPE)	Cube "GCC"	Cube "3D Macula"
Size	6 × 6 mm	30° × 25°	30° × 25°	7 × 7 mm	6 × 6 mm
Layers	GCL-IPL	Any one layer	Any one layer	RNFL-GCL-IPL	RNFL-GCL-IPL
Data points (Cube)	40,000 (200 B-scans of 200 A-scans) 65,536 (512 B-scans of 128 A-scans)	46,848 (61 B-scans of 768 A-scans)	46,848 (61 B-scans of 768 A-scans)	14,928 (15 *vertical* B-scans of 933 A-scans *plus* 1 *horizontal* B-scan of 933 A-scans)	65,536 (128 B-scans of 512 A-scans)
Centration of scan	Manual	Fovea	Fovea	1 mm temporal to fovea	Manual
Axis of scan	Horizontal	7 degrees upward nasal	FoBMOC	Horizontal	Horizontal
Centration of analysis	Fovea	Fovea	Fovea	Fovea	Fovea
Axis of analysis	Horizontal	7 degrees upward nasal	FoBMOC	Horizontal	Horizontal
Shape of analysis	Annulus	ETDRS & 8 × 8 Grid	Annulus	*No analysis grid*	Superpixel grid *and* ETDRS grid

Abbreviations: ETDRS, Early Treatment Diabetic Retinopathy Study; FoBMOC, fovea-Bruch's membrane opening center; GCL, ganglion cell layer; IPL, inner plexiform layer; RNFL, retinal nerve fiber layer.

radius of 0.6 and 2.4 mm, respectively. The annulus is then divided into six sectors, symmetric about the horizontal axis. The average GCIPL thickness for each sector is displayed in a sector grid. In addition, a data table displays the (global) average GCIPL thickness and minimum GCIPL thickness of the annulus. Representative horizontal and vertical tomogram images are also displayed for review.

A conventional *Macular Thickness Analysis* is also available (▶ Fig. 7.2d), which displays an identical report as that for GCIPL thickness, though it measures total retinal thickness and overlays an Early Treatment in Diabetic Retinopathy Study (ETDRS) grid in lieu of the aforementioned annulus.

Normative Database

The Macula Normative Database[6] consists of the same cohort as the RNFL normative database, though with 282 subjects given poor image quality in two scans. The database consisted of 133 males and 149 females, with an identical ethnic breakdown as the RNFL normative database. The macular normative database images were analyzed with an ETDRS grid and average values for variables were calculated for each subfield (Section 7.1.1, *Normative Database*).

Correlation analyses demonstrated that the central subfield had nearly no dependence on age, whereas the remaining subfields demonstrated a very mild negative correlation with age. Macular thickness results are therefore not matched for age.

Diagnostic Capability

The diagnostic capability, represented by the AUC curve (listed parenthetically), to distinguish all-stage glaucoma from normal was greatest for average (0.931, 0.888), inferotemporal (0.946), inferior (0.937, 0.908), superotemporal (0.932), and minimum (0.949) GCIPL thicknesses.[3,8] AUCs to distinguish mild glaucoma from normal were greatest for the minimum (0.904), inferotemporal (0.936), superotemporal (0.842), inferior (0.882, 0.853), and average (0.885, 0.844) GCIPL thicknesses.[3,8] The discriminating ability of GCIPL in preperimetric eyes remains fair, though less than that for mild glaucoma, with the best parameters being inferotemporal (0.823) and minimum (0.821) GCIPL thickness.[9]

Additional studies have evaluated the diagnostic capabilities of GCIPL thickness in myopic eyes. The parameters with the highest diagnostic accuracy include inferotemporal (0.852) and minimum (0.830) GCIPL thickness in highly myopic glaucomatous eyes and minimum GCIPL thickness (0.908) in nonhighly myopic glaucomatous eyes.[10] When considering myopic preperimetric glaucoma, inferotemporal (0.752) GCIPL thickness demonstrates the highest discriminating capability, greater than that of cpRNFL thickness and ONH parameters.[27]

7.3.2 Spectralis (Heidelberg Engineering, Inc., Heidelberg, Germany)

Standard Edition

Imaging Specifications

The Standard Edition[11] of the Spectralis offers a volume scan of the macula, termed the "PPole" scan. The scan images a 30 × 25 degree area of the retina and consists of 46,848 points (61 B-scans of 768 A-scans). The scan is automatically centered on the fovea though the B-scans are angled 7 degrees upward nasally, in order to approximate the fovea–disc axis.

Analysis

Following image acquisition, both a *Thickness Map Tab* and a *Posterior Pole Tab* may be displayed.[11] The *Thickness Map Tab* displays a cSLO image with an overlaid ETDRS grid centered on the fovea. For both the current examination and a reference examination, a thickness map and adjacent ETDRS grid are displayed. On the thickness map, warmer colors indicate thicker retina and cooler colors indicate thinner retina. The ETDRS grid displays the average retinal thickness for each grid section. A third pair of thickness map and ETDRS grid displays changes in retinal thickness between the reference examination and the current examination. On this thickness "change" map, greener hues suggest thickening, whereas redder hues suggest thinning. The thickness of either the full retina or any retinal layer may be analyzed.

The *Posterior Pole Tab* (▸ Fig. 7.4c) displays a 24 × 24 degree grid divided into 64 3 × 3 degree square cells (i.e., an 8 × 8 cell grid). The grid is centered on the fovea and aligned along the scanning angle (7 degrees upward nasally), though the centration and axis may be adjusted manually. The grid is superimposed on a cSLO image with overlaid retinal thickness map, with warmer colors indicating thicker retina and cooler colors indicating thinner retina.

On the same report are also displayed an asymmetry grid and a thickness map for both the current examination and a reference examination. The thickness of the entire retina or of any single retinal layer may be analyzed. The asymmetry grid displays the asymmetry in retinal thickness between the superior and inferior hemispheres for each square cell. In the upper half of the grid, the difference in retinal thickness between a superior cell and its paired inferior cell is displayed. In the lower half of the grid, the difference in retinal thickness between an inferior cell and its paired superior cell is displayed. The darker the grid cell shading, the greater the asymmetry in retinal thickness. An X-marked cell signifies that the average retinal thickness could not be calculated and thus asymmetry could not be derived.

The *Asymmetry Analysis Single Exam Report OU* displays similar data to the thickness map and Posterior Pole Tabs, though it also includes an inter-eye asymmetry grid (▸ Fig. 7.1e). As with the hemispheric asymmetry, darker cell shading indicates a greater degree of asymmetry. In addition, the report displays the average superior, inferior, and global retinal thickness.

Reports may be combined depending on which scans were obtained. The *RNFL & Asymmetry Analysis Single Exam Report* and *Posterior Pole Assessment Report* allow for the simultaneous presentation of cpRNFL and macular thickness data in one report.

Normative Database

There is no normative database for retinal thickness data in the Standard Edition.

Diagnostic Capability

Overall, the area under the AUC representing the capability to distinguish glaucoma from normal reaches a maximum for inferior (0.833), total (0.832), and superior (0.825) macular thickness, depending on the staging criteria used.[14] Neither right-left nor hemispheric asymmetry were found to demonstrate particularly strong diagnostic capabilities.[14]

Glaucoma Module Premium Edition

Imaging Specifications

The GMPE offers two volume scans, the "PPoleH" scan (horizontal) and the "PPoleV" scan (vertical).[15] Generally speaking, it is the horizontal scan that is used for clinical data acquisition and thus will be covered. The "PPoleH" scan images a 30 × 25 degree area of the retina and consists of 46,848 points (61 B-scans of 768 A-scans). The scan is automatically centered on the fovea and aligned along the FoBMOC axis using the Anatomic Positioning System (Section 7.1.2, *Imaging Specifications*).

Analysis

The GMPE may display information on macular parameters through multiple reports.[15] Both the *Thickness Map Tab* and the *Posterior Pole Tab* (▶ Fig. 7.4c), available in the Standard Edition, may be generated. In addition, a *Deviation Map Tab* or *Report* may be displayed—these are unique to the GMPE. The *Deviation Map Tab* or *Report* displays an elliptical annulus divided into equally spaced six sectors (symmetrical about the horizontal axis) with inner diameters of 0.618 mm in horizontal and 0.531 mm in the vertical, and outer diameters of 1.857 mm in the horizontal and 1.590 mm in the vertical. The annulus is centered on the fovea and aligned to the FoBMOC axis. A deviation map requires a normative database for comparison which is pending for the United States (Section 7.3.2, *Normative Database*).

The *Deviation Map Tab* or *Report* displays a cSLO image with overlaid thickness map and sector grid. As the GMPE contains a normative database (Section 7.3.2, *Normative Database*), a displayed deviation map illustrates the differences in retinal thickness map between the current examination and the normative database. In addition, a sector grid (six-sector, elliptical, symmetric about the horizontal) displays the mean retinal thickness and corresponding percentile (compared to the normative database) for each sector, as well as the global mean of all retinal thickness values. The thickness of either the RNFL, the GCL, the IPL, or all retinal layers may be displayed. At right, a thickness map, deviation map, and elliptical sector grid display data on a default retinal layer, typically the full retinal thickness, for comparison.

As in the Standard Edition, multiple data may be combined into a single report. The RNFL data, BMO-MRW data, and retinal thickness asymmetry data may be combined into an *MRW, RNFL & Asymmetry Analysis Single Exam*. The most comprehensive report is titled the *Glaucoma Overview Report* and includes data on the RNFL thickness, BMO-MRW, retinal thickness asymmetry, and GCL thickness.

The *Hood Glaucoma Report* is also available and incorporates data on RNFL thickness, BMO-MRW, and GCL thickness. It overlays the points of 10–2 and 24–2 Humphrey visual field (Carl Zeiss Meditec AG, Jena, Germany) onto the GCL and RNFL thickness maps, respectively.

Normative Database

Unlike the Standard Edition, the GMPE includes a normative database[15] for retinal thickness metrics, thus allowing for the creation of deviation maps. Only an international normative database exists; although a normative database derived from a United States cohort is pending, it is anticipated to include a similar demographic breakdown as the international database.

For the international database, the retinal thickness database included 255 eyes of 255 subjects (110 males and 145 females) of European descent. The mean age was 52.3 years with an age range of 20 to 87 years. Inclusion criteria included healthy eyes without prior intraocular surgery (except cataract surgery or LASIK); an absence of clinically significant vitreoretinal disease, optic nerve disease, or history of glaucoma; intraocular pressure ≤ 21 mmHg; best-corrected visual acuity ≥ 0.5; refraction range + 6.00 D to −6.00 D; astigmatism ≤ 2.00 D; normal visual fields in a glaucoma hemifield test and mean deviation within normal limits; and a clinically normal appearance of the optic disc.

Retinal thickness was found to decrease with increasing age and increasing fovea-to-BMO-center distance. Thus, all reference data were adjusted with respect to age and fovea-to-BMO-center distance.

Diagnostic Capability

Several studies have evaluated the capabilities of the ganglion cell analysis in the Spectralis device. In one comprehensive study, authors compared the diagnostic capabilities of various layer segmentations and analysis grids. Results demonstrated that the highest AUCs resided in the GCL thickness, GCIPL thickness (GCL + IPL), and ganglion cell complex thickness (GCC, consisting of

7

the RNFL + GCL + IPL), particularly for the inferior quadrants of analysis grids.[28] An additional study further demonstrated that the standalone GCL metric displays excellent diagnostic capability (AUC 0.945 at the central macula), overall superior to that of IPL.[29]

7.3.3 Avanti RTVue XR (Optovue, Inc., Fremont, CA, USA)

Imaging Specifications

The Avanti RTVue XR offers a 7.0 × 7.0 mm volume scan[19] (labeled "GCC") to sample the ganglion cell complex (GCC), consisting of the RNFL, GCL, and IPL. The scan consists of 14,928 data points (15 *vertical* B-scans of 933 A-scans plus 1 horizontal B-scan of 933 A-scans). The scan is manually centered though it is automatically placed 1 mm temporal to the fovea for assistance.

Analysis

GCC metrics are available for review on the *GCC Report*[19] (▶ Fig. 7.5d). The report displays a thickness map (6 mm in diameter) and a normative database (NDB) map, which displays differences between the thickness map and a normative database. A green color includes values present in 95% of normal subjects, yellow color indicates values present in the bottom 1 to 5% of normal subjects, and red color indicates values present in the bottom 1% of normal subjects. A deviation map is also available which displays the percentage deviations from NDB-derived normal thickness (−50% to + 50%).

A data table displays average global, superior, and inferior GCC thicknesses, as well as the superior-minus-inferior hemisphere difference. Unlike cpRNFL thickness measurements, which is calculated along a calculation circle, the GCC thickness measurements are derived from the *entire* 6-mm-diameter thickness map. Two additional parameters are reported: focal loss volume (FLV) and global loss volume (GLV). To calculate these parameters, the software calculates several derived GCC maps.[30] The fractional deviation (FD) map is calculated as the GCC map minus the normal reference map divided by the normal reference map. Thus, the FD map represents the percentage of GCC loss. The pattern map is calculated as the GCC map divided by the average GCC thickness. Thus, the pattern map represents a normalized GCC. The pattern deviation (PD) map is

calculated as the pattern map minus the normal reference map. Thus, the PD map represents the deviation from normal, though using relative, normalized GCC values as opposed to absolute values.

Using these three maps, the FLV and GLV are calculated. In summary, the FLV represents *significant* GCC loss, whereas the GLV represents *total* GCC loss. The FLV is calculated as the sum of FD values with significant GCC loss, defined as a corresponding PD value more than 1.65 standard deviations below the normal average (i.e., the bottom 5%). The GLV is calculated as the sum of the FD values that are negative (implying GCC loss). An *ONH/GCC Report* may also be generated to combine the RNFL, ONH, and GCC data into one report.

Normative Database

The RTVue Normative Database[19] for GCC metrics included 656 eyes from 364 subjects. Ethnicity percentages included Caucasian (34%), Asian (22%), Hispanic (12%), African Descendant (19%), Indian/Middle Easterner (12%), Pacific Islander (0%), and other (1%). Mean sphere was −0.46 ± 1.9 D (range −7.75 D to + 5.50 D). Inclusion and exclusion criteria are identical to those for the RNFL thickness and ONH metric population. See corresponding section above for further details. Correlational analyses revealed that gender had a significant effect on GCC thickness. For this reason, all clinical data comparisons to the normative database are adjusted for gender.

Diagnostic Capability

The diagnostic capability, represented by the AUC (listed parenthetically), to distinguish all-stage glaucoma from normal reaches a maximum for inferior (0.925, 0.826) and average (0.932, 0.814) GCC, and remains moderately high for GLV and FLV (0.819 and 0.804, respectively).[3,20] The diagnostic capability to distinguish mild glaucoma remains excellent though it declines slightly from that in all-stage glaucoma.[3] Ganglion cell parameters overall displayed greater diagnostic capabilities than metrics of total macular thickness.[20] In preperimetric glaucoma, the GCC metric retains a moderate diagnostic capability, with a maximum AUC of 0.89 (FLV), though this may decline for large optic discs.[22] In contrast to average cpRNFL thickness, GCC metrics retained high diagnostic capability even in highly myopic eyes, with AUCs of 0.935 and 0.940 for average GCC and GLV, respectively.[4]

7

7.3.4 3D OCT (Topcon Corporation, Tokyo, Japan)

Imaging Specifications

The 3D OCT series, including both the OCT-2000 and the OCT-1 Maestro2, offer a 6.0 × 6.0 mm volume scan termed the "3D Macula" scan. The volume scan consists of 128 B-scans each comprising 512 A-scans, for a total of 65,536 discrete data points.[24] The scan is manually centered and is oriented along a horizontal axis. The analysis grid is automatically centered on the fovea and is oriented along the horizontal axis.

Analysis

Glaucoma-focused macular analytics have been updated in the OCT-1 Maestro2 coupled with the newest version of the IMAGEnet software.[24] When a 3D Macula scan is obtained, thicknesses of the GCL + (approximately the GCL plus the IPL) or the GCL + + (approximately the NFL, GCL, and IPL) may be analyzed in the *OCT Data View*. Analysis grids of differing shapes and sizes may be superimposed on the area-in-question.

For more comprehensive analytics, several reports of macular data may be generated. The *3D Macula Report* displays the following for *both* GCL + and GCL + + analyses: a thickness map, a sector grid (six-sector), and an asymmetry map (superior-inferior hemisphere). The sector grid consists of an annulus with outer diameter equal to 6 mm and inner diameter equal to 1 mm (thus mimicking the dimensions of an ETDRS grid). In the sector grid, values represent the average thickness within each sector. In addition, data on superior, inferior, and average thickness (from the sector grid) are displayed for each parameter. Color and red-free fundus photos with superimposed 3D Macula scans, plus vertical and horizontal tomogram images, are displayed for review. Clinical data for ONH parameters follow an identical green-yellow-red color scheme to that for cpRNFL thickness (Section 7.1.4, *Analysis*).

If a 3D Wide scan is obtained, a *3D Wide Report* may be generated. This report includes data on cpRNFL thickness and ONH parameters, as well as macular metrics. These include thickness maps for total retinal, GCL + + or GCL +, and RNFL thicknesses, as well a sector grid (six-sector) and ETDRS grid, both of which are centered on the fovea.

A 3D Wide scan may also generate a *Hood Report*, the cpRNFL metrics of which are discussed in Section 7.1.4, *Analysis*. The *Hood Report* additionally displays a GCL + thickness map, an RNFL probability map with superimposed 24–2 visual field data points, and a GCL + probability map with superimposed 10–2 visual field data points.

Normative Database

Normative data for the macular metrics stem from the same database as that used for the cpRNFL and ONH metrics (Section 7.1.4, *Normative Database*). Ganglion cell parameters were found to be associated with age. Thus, GCL + thickness and GCL + + thickness are adjusted for age prior to comparison with the normative database.[24] If no birth date is provided, no comparison with reference data is performed. If the age is outside of the range of the database (18 to 90 years), clinical data are compared by extrapolation.

Diagnostic Capability

Overall, the AUC, representing the capability to distinguish all-stage glaucoma from normal is greatest for the average and inferior GCL + + thickness metrics (AUC 0.919 and 0.901, respectively).[3] The AUC representing the capability to distinguish mild glaucoma from normal similarly reaches a maximum for average and inferior GCL + + thicknesses (AUC 0.884 for both).[3]

7.4 Progression Analysis

7.4.1 Cirrus 6000 (Carl Zeiss Meditec AG, Jena, Germany)

The Cirrus device offers a *Guided Progression Analysis*[6] (GPA) to assist with qualitative and quantitative analysis of glaucomatous progression. The GPA compares various optic nerve metrics and GCIPL thickness across three to eight examinations. The first two are registered as baseline examinations to be used as points of comparison. Up to six subsequent high-quality (signal strength ≥ 6) comparison examinations are displayed and compared to the two baseline examinations. The software will align all scans to the first baseline scan (including the second baseline scan) based on the location of the blood vessels. If this is not possible (e.g., motion artifact), the software will attempt to align the images based on the location of the optic disc.

In the upper portion of the GPA report, the software displays thickness maps for all examinations and deviation maps for the nonbaseline examinations, for either RNFL or retinal thickness data. The deviation maps compare the nonbaseline examinations to the baseline examinations. A region-of-interest will be colored yellow (signifying "possible loss") or red (signifying "likely loss") when one subsequent examination or two subsequent examinations, respectively, demonstrates significant loss relative to the two baseline examinations. A region-of-interest will be colored lavender when there is an increase in thickness relative to the two baseline examinations.

Average cpRNFL thickness (global, superior, and inferior—all derived from the calculation circle), average cup-to-disc ratio, and GCIPL thickness (global, superior, and inferior) may be graphed chronologically, one data point for each examination. Data points are highlighted when a change has occurred in comparison to the two baseline examinations greater than expected for usual test-retest variability. A data point will be colored yellow ("possible loss") or red ("likely loss") when one subsequent examination or two subsequent examinations, respectively, demonstrate significant loss relative to the two baseline examinations. A data point will be colored lavender when there is an increase in thickness relative to the two baseline examinations. A best-fit curve is plotted with its associated rate of change and 95% confidence interval (displayed as an error).

A summary table displays an overview of progression for various variables. RNFL and ONH metrics include thickness maps, thickness graphs, average cpRNFL thickness, and average cup-to-disc ratio. A yellow, red, or lavender checkmark next to any of these four variables indicates "possible loss," "likely loss," and "possible increase," respectively.

For RNFL thickness, an additional thickness graph is displayed, plotting the RNFL as a function of the position along the optic disc circumference, with 0 degree located at the horizontal axis. Any significant changes between the most recent examination and the two baseline examinations are highlighted using a yellow-red-lavender color scheme, indicating "possible loss," "likely loss," and "possible increase," respectively. A change will be labeled as significant if at least 14 adjacent A-scans along the circle scan demonstrate this change.

7.4.2 Spectralis (Heidelberg Engineering, Inc., Heidelberg, Germany)

Standard Edition

The Standard Edition[11] displays a *Progression Tab* that may be viewed during the imaging session.

The *Progression Tab* plots the average global or sectoral RNFL thickness of the circle scan. The shade of each data point corresponds with the quality of that particular scan. The yellow region includes values seen in the bottom 1 to 5% of normals, and the red region includes values seen in the bottom 1% of normals. The yellow and red regions are adjusted for age.

The *RNFL Change Report* displays successive RNFL circle scan examinations (▶ Fig. 7.6). The report will display a sector grid (six-sector) and a cpRNFL thickness graph for each visit. Importantly, the cpRNFL thickness graphs of each successive examination is compared to a baseline examination. Differences at any point of the thickness graph are highlighted using the yellow-red color scheme to denote *any* (not only statistically significant) changes from baseline. The *RNFL Trend Report* plots for successive sector grids a linear graph of average global and sectoral RNFL thickness over time.

Glaucoma Module Premium Edition

The GMPE[15] displays a *Progression Tab*, similar in appearance to the Standard Edition. The GMPE *Progression Tab* plots the global average RNFL thickness (of either the 3.4-, 4.1-, or 4.7-mm circle scans) or the BMO-MRW over time. The yellow region includes values seen in the bottom 1 to 5% of normals, and the red region includes values seen in the bottom 1% of normals. The yellow and red regions are adjusted for age and BMO area. After five or more data points are present, a best-fit regression line is plotted with 95% confidence level lines and a corresponding slope and p-value. The GMPE also has the capability of displaying the same *RNFL Change Report* and *RNFL Trend Report* available in the Standard Edition.

7.4.3 Avanti RTVue XR (Optovue, Inc., Fremont, CA, USA)

A *Nerve Fiber ONH/GCC Change Analysis Report*[19] displays various metrics to assess for change in examinations across time. For each examination, the report displays an NDB map and a thickness map with surrounding sector grid (eight-sector). The sector grid values are calculated along the calculation circle. In addition, a thickness graph plots cpRNFL thickness with a separate curve for each examination date. A data table displays GCC, RNFL, and ONH color-coded metrics for each examination date (details in Sections 7.1.3, *Analysis*, and

7

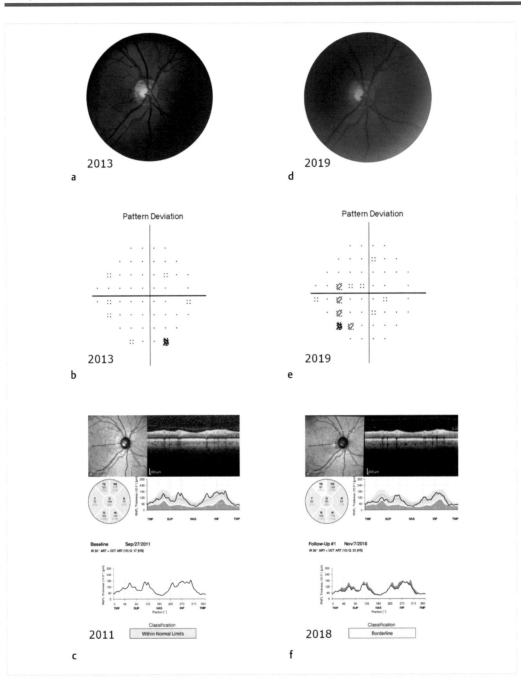

Fig. 7.6 Glaucoma suspect. Clinical images were obtained from a 66-year-old Hispanic female who was initially diagnosed as a glaucoma suspect in 2013. She was lost to follow-up for 5 years and returned for care in 2018. She was diagnosed with moderate primary open-angle glaucoma at that time and started on topical medical therapy. **(a)** A fundus photo from 2013 of the right eye demonstrates no gross neuroretinal rim thinning. **(b)** A Humphrey visual field (Carl Zeiss Meditec AG, Jena, Germany) pattern deviation plot from 2013 with no significant, contiguous defects. **(c)** A Standard Edition *RNFL Single Exam Report* (Spectralis, Heidelberg Engineering, Inc., Heidelberg, Germany) from 2011 demonstrates no circumpapillary RNFL (cpRNFL) thinning. **(d)** A fundus photo from 2019 of the right eye demonstrates minimal change from 2013. **(e)** A Humphrey visual field (Carl Zeiss Meditec AG) pattern deviation plot from 2019 demonstrates contiguous inferonasal defects. **(f)** An *RNFL Change Report* (Spectralis) from 2018 demonstrates cpRNFL thinning compared to the baseline examination in 2011. The thinning, denoted by the red shadowing on the thickness graph, is prominent superotemporally.

7.3.3, *Analysis*). Finally, average cpRNFL thickness (calculated along the calculation circle) and average GCC thickness (calculated from the *entire* 6-mm thickness map) are plotted chronologically. Using simple linear regression, a line is plotted with corresponding slope, 95% confidence interval, and p-value. Color coding with yellow or red color signifies data observed in the bottom 1 to 5% and bottom 1% of normal subjects, respectively.

7.4.4 3D-OCT (Topcon Corporation, Tokyo, Japan)

The latest image software[24] on the OCT-1 Maestro2 includes a *Trend View* that may be displayed during an imaging session. The *Trend View* displays multiple images and data points across time and may be applied to either the 3D Disc, 3D Macula, or 3D Wide scans of the OCT-1 Maestro2. The data that may be displayed depend on which scans have been obtained. In the *Trend View*, two images each from up to four examinations (including one baseline examination) may be populated for each eye, to be displayed simultaneously. Each image may be overlaid with various grids and analyses, for example, a four-quadrant cpRNFL sector grid or a cpRNFL thickness graph. In addition, the following data may be plotted across time: global cpRNFL thickness (centered on the optic disc) or total retinal, GCL+, or GCL++ thicknesses (centered on the macula). The data may be parsed into various analyses, such as average or sectoral data. A regression line is automatically calculated with its corresponding slope and p-value displayed.

The *3D Disc Trend Analysis Report* displays a fundus photo, an RNFL thickness map, and a shadowgram from up to four examinations (including one baseline examination). A shadowgram represents a fundus photograph that has been modified to accentuate shadowing from vasculature. Superior, inferior, and average cpRNFL thickness values, as well as disc area, rim area, cup volume, and RPH (reference plane height, set to 120 μm by default; Section 7.2.4, *Imaging Specifications*) are displayed for each of the included examinations as well. Also displayed is a cpRNFL thickness graph plotting curves for all examinations, as well as a graph of average, superior, and inferior cpRNFL thickness values across the included examinations.

A *3D Wide Trend Analysis Report* for one eye displays a fundus photo, RNFL thickness map, and GCL+thickness map for up to four examinations (including one baseline examination). Also displayed is a graph plotting superior, inferior, and average cpRNFL thickness, and a second graph plotting GCL+thickness, all across multiple examinations. For the latest examination, the report includes the following: cpRNFL thickness graph, ONH metrics (rim area, disc area, linear CDR, vertical CDR, and cup volume), cpRNFL sector grids (four- and twelve-sector), and a GCL+sector grid (six-sector). Data may also be plotted for both eyes on the same report.

References

[1] Hwang YH, Lee JY, Kim YY. The effect of head tilt on the measurements of retinal nerve fibre layer and macular thickness by spectral-domain optical coherence tomography. Br J Ophthalmol. 2011; 95(11):1547–1551

[2] Leite MT, Rao HL, Zangwill LM, Weinreb RN, Medeiros FA. Comparison of the diagnostic accuracies of the Spectralis, Cirrus, and RTVue optical coherence tomography devices in glaucoma. Ophthalmology. 2011; 118(7):1334–1339

[3] Akashi A, Kanamori A, Nakamura M, Fujihara M, Yamada Y, Negi A. Comparative assessment for the ability of Cirrus, RTVue, and 3D-OCT to diagnose glaucoma. Invest Ophthalmol Vis Sci. 2013; 54(7):4478–4484

[4] Shoji T, Nagaoka Y, Sato H, Chihara E. Impact of high myopia on the performance of SD-OCT parameters to detect glaucoma. Graefes Arch Clin Exp Ophthalmol. 2012; 250 (12):1843–1849

[5] Kansal V, Armstrong JJ, Pintwala R, Hutnik C. Optical coherence tomography for glaucoma diagnosis: an evidence based meta-analysis. PLoS One. 2018; 13(1):e0190621

[6] Cirrus HD-OCT User Manual—Models 500, 5000. Jena, Germany: Carl Zeiss Meditec, Inc.; 2015

[7] Mwanza JC, Oakley JD, Budenz DL, Anderson DR, Cirrus Optical Coherence Tomography Normative Database Study Group. Ability of cirrus HD-OCT optic nerve head parameters to discriminate normal from glaucomatous eyes. Ophthalmology. 2011; 118(2):241–8.e1

[8] Blumberg DM, Dale E, Pensec N, et al. Discrimination of glaucoma patients from healthy individuals using combined parameters from spectral-domain optical coherence tomography in an African American population. J Glaucoma. 2016; 25(3):e196–e203

[9] Kim MJ, Jeoung JW, Park KH, Choi YJ, Kim DM. Topographic profiles of retinal nerve fiber layer defects affect the diagnostic performance of macular scans in preperimetric glaucoma. Invest Ophthalmol Vis Sci. 2014; 55(4):2079–2087

[10] Choi YJ, Jeoung JW, Park KH, Kim DM. Glaucoma detection ability of ganglion cell-inner plexiform layer thickness by spectral-domain optical coherence tomography in high myopia. Invest Ophthalmol Vis Sci. 2013; 54(3):2296–2304

[11] SPECTRALIS Product Family User Manual. Software Version 6.8. Heidelberg, Germany: Heidelberg Engineering GmbH; August 2017

[12] Silverman AL, Hammel N, Khachatryan N, et al. Diagnostic accuracy of the Spectralis and Cirrus reference databases in differentiating between healthy and early glaucoma eyes. Ophthalmology. 2016; 123(2):408–414

[13] Wu H, de Boer JF, Chen TC. Diagnostic capability of spectral-domain optical coherence tomography for glaucoma. Am J Ophthalmol. 2012; 153(5):815–826.e2

7

[14] Dave P, Shah J. Diagnostic accuracy of posterior pole asymmetry analysis parameters of spectralis optical coherence tomography in detecting early unilateral glaucoma. Indian J Ophthalmol. 2015; 63(11):837–842

[15] SPECTRALIS Glaucoma Module Premium Edition User Manual. Software Version 6.12. Heidelberg, Germany: Heidelberg Engineering GmbH; May 2019

[16] Gmeiner JM, Schrems WA, Mardin CY, Laemmer R, Kruse FE, Schrems-Hoesl LM. Comparison of Bruch's membrane opening minimum rim width and peripapillary retinal nerve fiber layer thickness in early glaucoma assessment. Invest Ophthalmol Vis Sci. 2016; 57(9):OCT575–OCT584

[17] Enders P, Adler W, Kiessling D, et al. Evaluation of two-dimensional Bruch's membrane opening minimum rim area for glaucoma diagnostics in a large patient cohort. Acta Ophthalmol. 2019; 97(1):60–67

[18] Malik R, Belliveau AC, Sharpe GP, Shuba LM, Chauhan BC, Nicolela MT. Diagnostic accuracy of optical coherence tomography and scanning laser tomography for identifying glaucoma in myopic eyes. Ophthalmology. 2016; 123(6):1181–1189

[19] RTVue XR Avanti User Manual. Fremont, CA, USA: Optovue, Inc.; 2018

[20] Rao HL, Zangwill LM, Weinreb RN, Sample PA, Alencar LM, Medeiros FA. Comparison of different spectral domain optical coherence tomography scanning areas for glaucoma diagnosis. Ophthalmology. 2010; 117(9):1692–1699, 1699.e1

[21] Huang JY, Pekmezci M, Mesiwala N, Kao A, Lin S. Diagnostic power of optic disc morphology, peripapillary retinal nerve fiber layer thickness, and macular inner retinal layer thickness in glaucoma diagnosis with fourier-domain optical coherence tomography. J Glaucoma. 2011; 20(2):87–94

[22] Rao HL, Addepalli UK, Chaudhary S, et al. Ability of different scanning protocols of spectral domain optical coherence tomography to diagnose preperimetric glaucoma. Invest Ophthalmol Vis Sci. 2013; 54(12):7252–7257

[23] 3D OCT-2000 Instruction Manual. Tokyo, Japan: Topcon Corporation; November 2009

[24] IMAGEnet 6 Ophthalmic Data System User Manual. In. Version 2.2, Revision A. Oakland, NJ, USA: Topcon Healthcare Solutions; August 2019

[25] Chaglasian M, Fingeret M, Davey PG, et al. The development of a reference database with the Topcon 3D OCT-1 Maestro. Clin Ophthalmol. 2018; 12:849–857

[26] Mwanza JC, Huang LY, Budenz DL, Shi W, Huang G, Lee RK. Differences in optical coherence tomography assessment of Bruch membrane opening compared to stereoscopic photography for estimating cup-to-disc ratio. Am J Ophthalmol. 2017; 184:34–41

[27] Seol BR, Jeoung JW, Park KH. Glaucoma detection ability of macular ganglion cell-inner plexiform layer thickness in myopic preperimetric glaucoma. Invest Ophthalmol Vis Sci. 2015; 56(13):8306–8313

[28] Chien JL, Ghassibi MP, Patthanathamrongkasem T, et al. Glaucoma diagnostic capability of global and regional measurements of isolated ganglion cell layer and inner plexiform layer. J Glaucoma. 2017; 26(3):208–215

[29] Moghimi S, Fatehi N, Nguyen AH, Romero P, Caprioli J, Nouri-Mahdavi K. Relationship of the macular ganglion cell and inner plexiform layers in healthy and glaucoma eyes. Transl Vis Sci Technol. 2019; 8(5):27

[30] Tan O, Chopra V, Lu AT, et al. Detection of macular ganglion cell loss in glaucoma by Fourier-domain optical coherence tomography. Ophthalmology. 2009; 116(12):2305–14.e1, 2

7

8 Artifacts and Masqueraders

Teresa C. Chen, Catherine M. Marando, and Elli Park

Summary

All spectral domain optical coherence tomography (SD-OCT) machines have artifacts. Our job as physicians is to spot these artifacts in order to make an accurate diagnosis. Although tools and technologies can help the physician diagnose or monitor glaucoma, we still need to critically assess any test results to see if it can be used for treatment decisions.

SD-OCT plays a key role in the diagnosis and management of glaucoma. These high-resolution cross-sectional scans of the eye allow ophthalmologists to detect structural changes with axial resolutions of 5 to 7 μm at the peripapillary retina, optic nerve head, and macula. However, like any technology, optical coherence tomography (OCT) is imperfect, and the images it generates may sometimes contain artifacts. These artifacts can arise from errors in scan acquisition, subsequent analysis, or from ocular pathology unrelated to glaucoma. Regardless of the cause, artifacts represent false data and can be misleading to those unfamiliar with them. Therefore, it is important for ophthalmologists to be able to identify artifacts when they occur and to interpret OCT information within the context of the entire patient.

First, this chapter will discuss the types of artifacts that ophthalmologists may encounter when using OCT to diagnose and manage glaucoma. Second, the chapter will describe how these artifacts can give rise to the phenomenon of "OCT diseases" and will review relevant clinical examples of red and green disease. Lastly, the chapter will discuss future directions, such as three-dimensional parameters and OCT angiography, and the role that artifacts will play.

Keywords: artifact, decentration, poor signal, segmentation error, floor effect, OCT diseases

8.1 Incidence of Artifacts in OCT Imaging

Artifacts are unintended and undesired, yet inescapable, features of optical coherence tomography (OCT) scans. These artifacts occur frequently in clinical practice. In fact, between 7.1 and 46.3%[1,2] of peripapillary retinal nerve fiber layer (pRNFL) thickness scans from spectral domain optical coherence tomography (SD-OCT) demonstrate some form of artifact. The SD-OCT instrument is also capable of generating high-density volume scans of the macula and optic nerve head (ONH). These cube scans carry frequent artifacts as well, with rates ranging between 6.0 and 90.9%[3,4] for the macula and 12.1 and 84.0%[5,6] for the ONH. Notice the wide range of percentages of reported artifact rates. These variabilities may arise from differences in scan protocols, scan locations, OCT machines, enrollment criteria, study methodologies, and artifact definitions used throughout the literature. These differences make it difficult to compare numbers between any two studies. The high frequency of artifacts may seem intimidating. However, by keeping in mind the principles of this chapter, the clinician will be able to avoid common pitfalls from OCT artifacts.

8.2 Etiologies of Peripapillary RNFL OCT Artifacts

Peripapillary RNFL thickness is the OCT parameter that is most commonly used when following glaucoma patients. Therefore, the following section describes common artifacts that present in scans of the peripapillary RNFL.

8.2.1 Artifacts from Errors in Scan Acquisition

Decentration

Decentration artifact (► Fig. 8.1) is the most common type of artifact seen in peripapillary RNFL circular B-scans, occurring in 27.8% of Spectralis (Heidelberg Engineering, Heidelberg, Germany) B-scans, where a technician needs to manually center the RNFL circular scan over the optic nerve and when decentration is defined as imperfect alignment of the circular scan over the ONH by at least 10%.[2] Decentration artifacts are less of an issue in machines where the software automatically determines the optic nerve location (e.g., Cirrus, Carl Zeiss Meditec, Dublin, CA). Since the RNFL normally thins farther away from the ONH, decentration may cause artifactually increased or decreased measurements of RNFL thickness for a given sector or clock hour, depending on whether the measured region is closer or farther away from

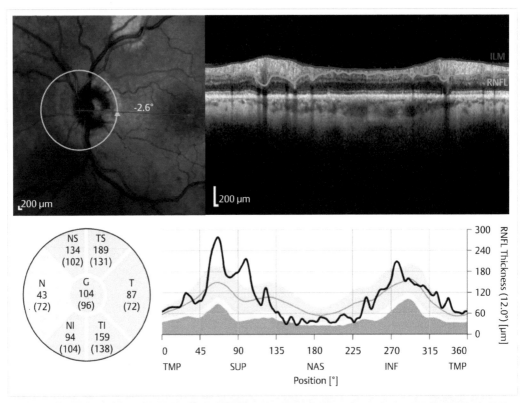

Fig. 8.1 Decentration artifact. This is a retinal nerve fiber layer (RNFL) optical coherence tomography (OCT) of the left eye. Note that the scan circle is displaced nasally (top left panel). Recall that the RNFL is thinner further from the nerve head. In this case, the nasal RNFL is erroneously thin and the temporal RNFL is erroneously thick (Spectralis OCT, Heidelberg Engineering, Heidelberg, Germany).

the optic disc, respectively. For instance, if the scan circle is shifted superiorly, then the superior quadrant will appear artifactually thin (farther from the nerve head) and the inferior quadrant will appear artifactually thick (closer to the nerve head). It is evident that superior decentration may make it appear to the clinician as though the patient has glaucomatous thinning in the superior quadrant, when in fact there was no change at all.

Poor Signal

Poor signal (▶ Fig. 8.2 and ▶ Fig. 8.6) is another common type of artifact seen in OCT scans, presenting in 5.1% of peripapillary RNFL circle scans taken with the Spectralis SD-OCT machine (Heidelberg Engineering, Heidelberg, Germany).[2] Poor signal often looks grainy or static-like, which makes it difficult to discern the layers of the retina. When the OCT attempts to segment these blurry or grainy images, it is difficult and sometimes impossible for the software to locate the boundaries of the retinal layers, thereby leading to false measurements.

Signal can be degraded by any of the ocular structures that the OCT light beam must pass in order to image the retina. This includes the cornea, anterior chamber, lens, and vitreous. The most common causes of poor signal include dry eyes[7] and cataract.[8] These conditions make it difficult for the OCT machine to take a clear picture of the back of the eye, just as it would be difficult for a camera to take a good photo of an object through frosted glass. Stein and associates sought to establish the effects of dry eye by taping normal subjects' eyelids open to prevent blinking over the course of the testing period. They found significant reductions in both signal strength and RNFL thickness strictly by preventing blinking (Stratus OCT, version 3.0; Carl Zeiss Meditec, Inc., Dublin, CA).[7] Also using the Stratus OCT, Mwanza and associates found a 9.3 and 24.1% increase in peripapillary RNFL thickness and signal strength, respectively, in 45 glaucomatous and normal eyes after cataract removal.[8] These studies demonstrate that poor signal due to dry eyes and cataract may significantly

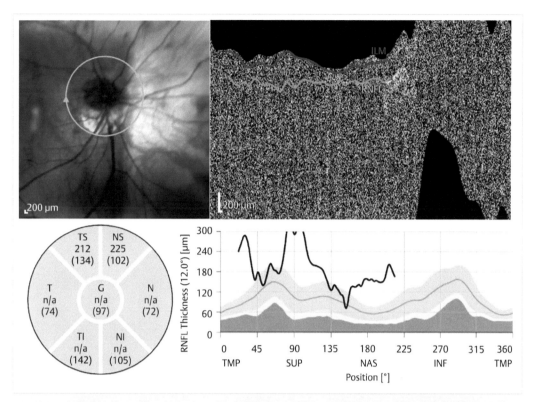

Fig. 8.2 Poor signal and cut edge. This is a retinal nerve fiber layer (RNFL) optical coherence tomography (OCT) of the right eye. This scan has a grainy quality due to poor signal, making it impossible for the OCT software to accurately segment the anterior and posterior RNFL boundaries. The OCT has arbitrarily assigned anterior and posterior boundaries for the superior and nasal quadrants, and neglects to give any data for the remaining quadrants due to a cut edge artifact (Heidelberg Engineering, Heidelberg, Germany). (Reproduced with permission from Park EA, Budenz DL, Lee RK, Chen TC. Red and Green Disease in Glaucoma. In: Budenz DL, ed. Atlas of Optical Coherence Tomography for Glaucoma. Springer; 2020: 145.)

Table 8.1 Quality score. Different OCT machines have different methods for defining the quality of the scan generated. This is a list of the quality score range and minimum acceptable score for the most commonly used OCT machines

Model (instrument)	Quality score range	Minimum acceptable score
Carl Zeiss Meditec (Cirrus)	0 to 10	>6
Topcon Medical Systems (3D OCT 1000)	0 to 160	>60
Heidelberg Engineering (Spectralis)	0 to 40	>15
Optovue (RTVue)	0 to 100	>30

Abbreviation: OCT, optical coherence tomography. Reproduced with permission from Park EA, Budenz DL, Lee RK, Chen TC. Red and Green Disease in Glaucoma. In: Budenz DL, ed. Atlas of Optical Coherence Tomography for Glaucoma. Springer; 2020:171.

impair accurate OCT measurement of RNFL thickness, and that strategies such as blinking and administration of artificial tears can improve signal quality if a scan needs to be retaken. Other less common causes of poor signal include anterior chamber cell or flare, posterior capsular opacification, and vitreous hemorrhage. In fact, it is even important to make sure that the OCT lens is cleaned, so as to avoid "smudge artifact" from dirty equipment degrading signal quality.

OCT machines automatically generate a quality score to reflect the signal strength of each scan. The range of scores differs among instruments, and each manufacturer defines a separate minimum acceptable value (▶ Table 8.1). For the Spectralis SD-OCT, quality scores range from 0 to 40, and a score less than 15 is considered poor. On the other hand, the Cirrus SD-OCT quality scores range from 0 to 10, and a score less than 6 is considered poor.

Motion Artifact

Motion artifact (▶ Fig. 8.3) presents in 0.2% of RNFL circular peripapillary B-scans taken with the Spectralis SD-OCT machine (Heidelberg Engineering, Heidelberg, Germany).[2] These artifacts result from subtle eye motions that occur during eye fixation, such as tremor, drifts, and microsaccades, or from larger movements, such as those due to head motion, heartbeat, respiration, or blinking. Eye-tracking technology can minimize errors from the former. Larger movements, however, can produce

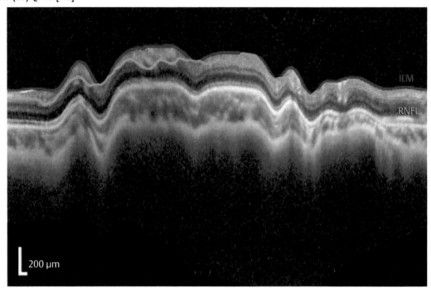

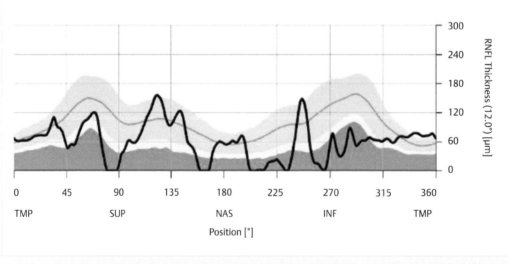

Fig. 8.3 Motion artifact. This is a retinal nerve fiber layer (RNFL) optical coherence tomography (OCT) of the left eye. Patient movement caused the retinal layers to have a wavy appearance (*top right panel*). This prevented segmentation inferiorly and temporally, leading to a lack of data in those quadrants (*bottom panels*) (Spectralis OCT, Heidelberg Engineering, Heidelberg, Germany).

blurred, wavy images that move outside the boundary of the rectangular display box and preclude accurate segmentation.

Today, different OCT machines employ different methods of motion correction. Some machines have a second laser beam to detect eye movement. Other machines include the use of additional B-scans obtained during the examination as a framework for realigning individual B-scans.[9]

So what can be done when there are wavy retinal layers or if the scan is cut off abnormally as a result of motion artifact? In the case of a tremor, an assistant can help to hold the patient's head against the bar during image acquisition to minimize movement. Have the technician describe the importance of minimizing movement to the patient, so that he or she knows it will affect his or her diagnosis and management. Finally, it may be necessary to be patient and take multiple images, which can be difficult in a busy clinic. Having a well-trained technician can be one of the most important ways to minimize motion artifact.

Missing Data

In certain instances, the RNFL OCT fails to acquire data in an area of the scan (▶ Fig. 8.4). If this area of missing data is along the scan circle, the RNFL thickness measurements will be affected.

Cut Edge

Cut edge (▶ Fig. 8.5) artifacts occur in 0.2% of RNFL circular peripapillary B-scans taken with the

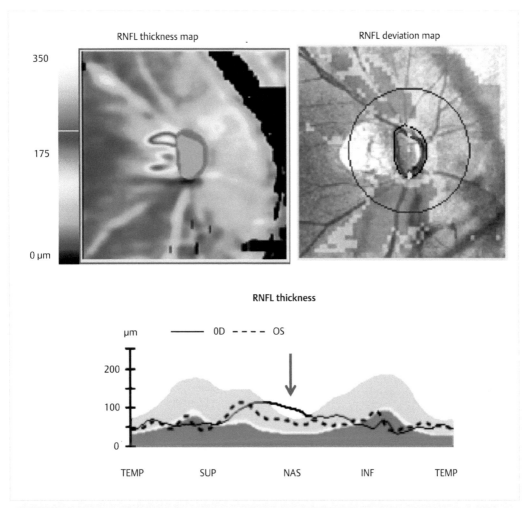

Fig. 8.4 Missing data. In this Cirrus optical coherence tomography (OCT) of the right eye, the top left panel has a black area nasally that indicates missing data (Cirrus OCT, Carl Zeiss Meditec, Inc., Dublin, California).

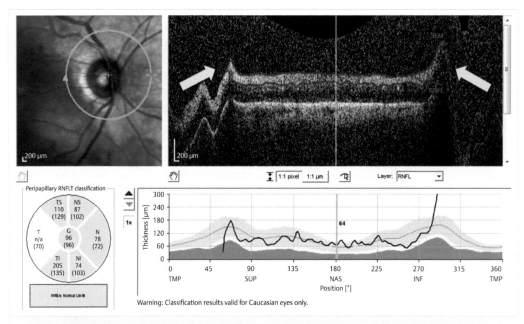

Fig. 8.5 Cut edge. The lateral edge of the retinal nerve fiber layer (RNFL) is abruptly truncated on both ends (yellow arrows), producing false measurements in the temporal region (Spectralis OCT, Heidelberg Engineering, Heidelberg, Germany). (Reproduced with permission from Liu Y, Simavli H, Que CJ, et al. Patient characteristics associated with artifacts in Spectralis optical coherence tomography imaging of the retinal nerve fiber layer in glaucoma. Am J Ophthalmol 2015;159(3):568.)

Spectralis SD-OCT machine (Heidelberg Engineering, Heidelberg, Germany).[2] A cut edge artifact refers to the abrupt truncation of the lateral edge of the RNFL. This may take place at one or both ends of the OCT scan and most likely results from patient movement.

8.2.2 Artifacts in Boundary Segmentation

The OCT instrument contains software that can identify specific layers of the retina, depending on the region and parameter of interest. In glaucoma patients, OCT is commonly used to measure and follow the thickness of the peripapillary RNFL over time. The OCT machine generates this measurement by first delineating the anterior and posterior borders of the RNFL and then calculating the distance between the two borders. These borders are marked by brightly colored (usually red, blue, or purple) lines. The anterior border represents the interface between the vitreous and the internal limiting membrane (ILM) of the retina, and the posterior border represents the interface between the ganglion cell nerve fibers and the ganglion cell bodies. OCT takes advantage of the higher reflectivity of the RNFL in order to locate these interfaces and

distinguish the RNFL from its surrounding layers. Therefore, anything that obscures the boundary between the RNFL and the vitreous anteriorly or the RNFL and the ganglion cell layer posteriorly will interfere with accurate segmentation.

Anterior Misidentification

Anterior RNFL misidentification (▶ Fig. 8.6) presents in 3.2% of peripapillary RNFL scans taken with the Spectralis SD-OCT machine (Heidelberg Engineering, Heidelberg, Germany).[2] These occur when the segmentation algorithm fails to correctly identify the anterior border of the RNFL. On the printout, the top red line drifts anteriorly (upward) into the vitreous, resulting in falsely increased or decreased thickness measurements, respectively.

A common cause of this type of artifact is the presence of an epiretinal membrane (ERM) or posterior vitreous detachment (PVD). In one study, ERMs were found in 47.3% (26 out of 55) of peripapillary scans with artifacts and tended to increase measurements of RNFL thickness.[10] If there is suspicion for an ERM, a basic clinical examination with or without a macular OCT would confirm the presence of this pathology. Similarly, certain features of the vitreous can confuse anterior

8

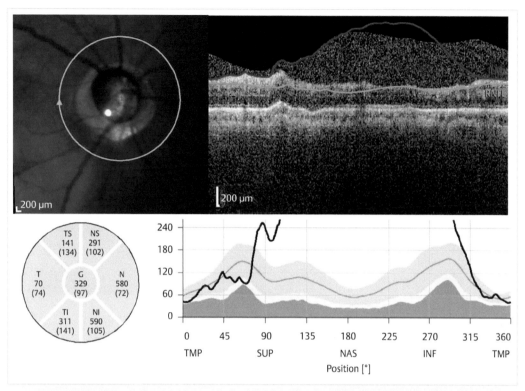

Fig. 8.6 Anterior segmentation artifact and poor signal. This is a retinal nerve fiber layer (RNFL) optical coherence tomography (OCT) of the right eye. The segmentation algorithm has misplaced the anterior boundary of the RNFL somewhere in the vitreous (*top right panel*) resulting in falsely thick measurements in the superior, nasal, and inferior quadrants (*bottom panels*). Note that the scan also has a grainy quality, which is the result of poor signal. This poor signal likely explains the inability of the OCT to accurately identify the anterior RNFL boundary (Spectralis OCT, Heidelberg Engineering, Heidelberg, Germany).

segmentation. Often in an area of vitreomacular traction (VMT), the hyaloid face appears as a hyperreflective line very near to the anterior boundary of the RNFL. In this case, the OCT may inaccurately segment the hyaloid face as the anterior RNFL. PVDs can induce other forms of artifact unrelated to segmentation errors, which is discussed further in the section *Artifacts Due to Ocular Pathology Unrelated to Glaucoma.*

Posterior Misidentification

Posterior RNFL misidentification (▶ Fig. 8.7) presents in 7.7% of peripapillary RNFL scans taken with the Spectralis SD-OCT machine (Heidelberg Engineering, Heidelberg, Germany).[2] These occur when the segmentation algorithm fails to correctly identify the posterior border of the RNFL, and this can lead to artifactually thick or thin RNFL measurements.

Glaucoma itself might contribute to this type of artifact, because glaucoma is associated with loss of RNFL reflectivity. Since OCT technology relies on differences in tissue reflectivity in order to construct the layers of the retina, loss of RNFL reflectivity means that the nerve fiber layer becomes less distinguishable from its surrounding layers. This change especially affects the interface between the RNFL and the less reflective deeper retinal layers. Theoretically, this would make glaucoma patients more prone to posterior misidentification artifact.

Incomplete Segmentation

Incomplete segmentation artifact (▶ Fig. 8.8) presents in 0.6% of peripapillary RNFL scans taken with the Spectralis SD-OCT machine (Heidelberg Engineering, Heidelberg, Germany).[2] The anterior and posterior segmentation lines should be present from the left-most side of the image to the right-most side of the image. However, if the software cannot trace part of the scan, this is referred

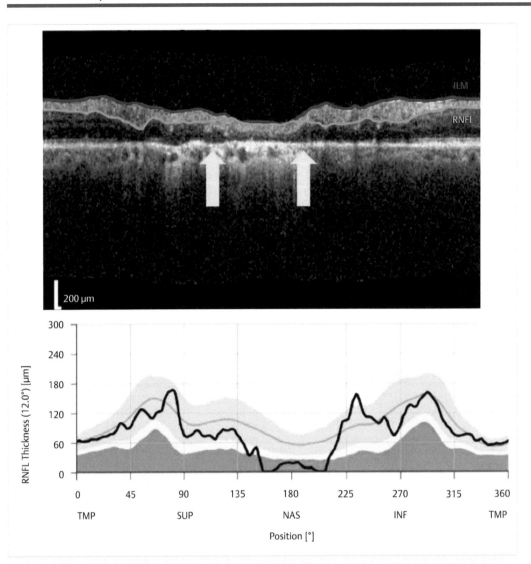

Fig. 8.7 Posterior segmentation artifact and going below the floor. This is a retinal nerve fiber layer (RNFL) optical coherence tomography (OCT) of the right eye. This patient appears to have thinning of the RNFL nasal quadrant, with RNFL thickness values of 0 μm. Due to a poor-quality scan, the segmentation algorithm has incorrectly identified the posterior boundary of the nasal RNFL (between *yellow arrows*) and displaced the posterior boundary anteriorly, resulting in falsely thin measurements. The floor effect refers to the fact that RNFL thickness measurements should not go below 50 μm, which is the thickness of nonneuronal components of the RNFL (Spectralis OCT, Heidelberg Engineering, Heidelberg, Germany).

to as incomplete segmentation. This should be an easy artifact for the clinician to spot, as long as he or she looks at the scan.

Floor Effect

Physiologically, the RNFL thickness can never be 0 μm. In fact, even in the most advanced glaucoma patient, RNFL thickness values cannot be less than around 50 μm, because the RNFL is partly comprised of nonneuronal tissue such as blood vessels and glial tissue. Despite this, the OCT machine will often report thickness values as low as 0 μm, which is below the floor of around 50 μm (▶ Fig. 8.7 and ▶ Fig. 8.10). This is an easy error to spot because the clinician can just look at the line graph and note that any points that drop to 0 μm are clearly artifacts. That being said, the RNFL may

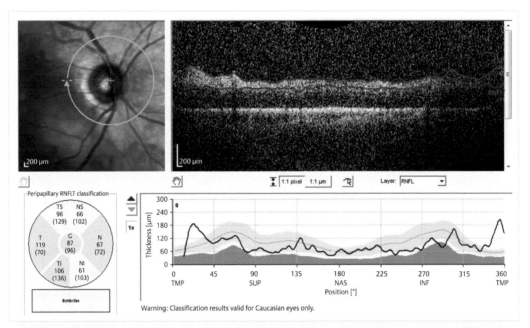

Fig. 8.8 Incomplete segmentation artifact. This is a retinal nerve fiber layer (RNFL) optical coherence tomography (OCT) of the right eye. At the left-most part of this image, you will see that the segmentation lines do not extend to the end of the scan. As a result, there is missing data and segmentation for the temporal quadrant. Incomplete segmentation occurs when there is failure to completely demarcate the RNFL borders along the entire 360-degree circumference of the scan (Spectralis OCT, Heidelberg Engineering, Heidelberg, Germany). (Reproduced with permission from Liu Y, Simavli H, Que CJ, et al. Patient characteristics associated with artifacts in Spectralis optical coherence tomography imaging of the retinal nerve fiber layer in glaucoma. Am J Ophthalmol. 2015;159(3):566.)

be very thin in that area, so physicians should refer back to the scan to understand why it was segmented incorrectly.

8.2.3 Artifacts due to Ocular Pathology Unrelated to Glaucoma

To be an expert in glaucoma, the clinician should also be able to identify nonglaucomatous pathology and know how it can affect measurements. To this end, abnormalities of the globe, retina, vitreous, and so on, can dramatically affect measurements and potentially render the scan unusable.

In a study at the Duke Eye Center in 2015 examining 277 patients in the glaucoma service, the most common ocular pathology causing artifacts in RNFL OCT scans included an ERM and VMT.[10] In a larger study by Massachusetts Eye and Ear in 2015 examining a total of 2,313 eyes, 14.4% of patients had artifact caused by PVD. Although less frequent, other ocular pathologies leading to artifacts included peripapillary atrophy (PPA), staphyloma, and myelinated nerve fiber layer (MNFL).[2]

Vitreomacular Traction/Posterior Vitreous Detachment

With normal aging, the vitreous may detach from the ILM. Initially, there may be a stage of VMT or partial PVD, which can progress to a complete PVD. The precise effects of PVD on RNFL artifact in the literature are varied. However, the rates of PVD-associated artifact is estimated to be approximately 14%. As the posterior hyaloid pulls off the ILM, some patients show focal artifactual thickening or "tenting" of the RNFL in the region of the VMT due to the physical pull from the vitreous (▶ Fig. 8.9a,b).[10] Subsequently, as the traction is released and as the PVD progresses from a partial to complete PVD, there can be relative RNFL thinning as the anterior RNFL surface may drop back more posteriorly. This is an important confounding factor for clinicians to be aware of in order to avoid incorrectly interpreting the decrease in RNFL thickness following the progression from partial PVD to complete PVD as a sign of glaucomatous changes to the RNFL.[11] It is important to know that the vitreous can create artifacts that can cause

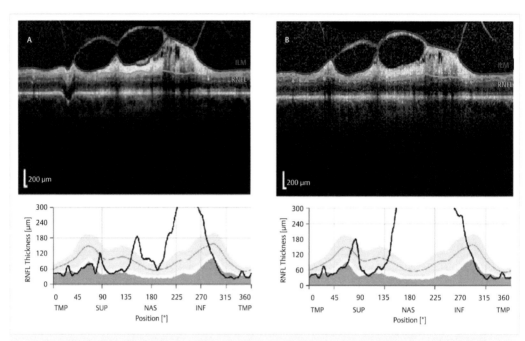

Fig. 8.9 Vitreous traction artifact. **(a)** Traction from the vitreous hyaloid face pulling on the retinal nerve fiber layer (RNFL) has caused artifactual thickening of the nerve fiber layer inferonasally. This can sometimes be seen in the setting of an impending posterior vitreous detachment (PVD). **(b)** After 2 years, the algorithm has additionally mistaken the hyaloid face nasally for the anterior border of the RNFL, leading to even greater thickness measurements. This leads to artefactual "growth" of RNFL thickness measurements between Panel A and Panel B (Spectralis OCT, Heidelberg Engineering, Heidelberg, Germany).

both falsely thickened and thinned RNFL. It is also important to know that this can change over time as the clinician follows a patient with sequential scans depending on the status of the vitreous traction. Another source of error during segmentation is if the detached or partially detached hyaloid face is misidentified as the anterior boundary of the RNFL (▶ Fig. 8.9b).[10,12] This is discussed further in the section *Artifacts in Boundary Segmentation*.

As an example, when monitoring a patient over time, if a focal decrease in RNFL thickness occurs at the same time as a newly diagnosed PVD, it would be prudent to carefully evaluate the scans and consider other diagnostic metrics prior to changing the patient's therapy, as this could be due to artifact.

Peripapillary Atrophy

Peripapillary atrophy (▶ Fig. 8.10) is a premature termination of the outer retinal layers near the ONH that is more common in patients with glaucoma. In a large study, 1.2% of glaucoma patients had PPA-associated error attributed both to poor scan quality and inaccurate thickness

measurements.[2] When imaging a patient with PPA, the scan circle diameter ideally should be large enough to encompass normal retinal tissue beyond the PPA. The Spectralis software (Glaucoma Module Premium Edition, GMPE) gives the option for different peripapillary RNFL circle scan sizes. When the scan circle crosses over an area of PPA, automatic segmentation can result in erroneously thin or thick measurements. To circumvent the problem of PPA, some physicians purposefully decenter the RNFL circle scan so that the scan circle does not cross over areas of PPA, and then that purposefully decentered scan is used as the baseline for subsequent similarly decentered scans. OCT can still prove useful in patients with PPA if the careful clinician, who notes this abnormality, adjusts the scan circle diameter and centration, and then correlates findings with other clinical metrics.

Myelinated Nerve Fiber Layer

MNFL occurs due to aberrant embryologic development whereby myelination extends past the lamina cribrosa. This anomaly results in thickening of the RNFL on OCT.[13] Despite the increased RNFL

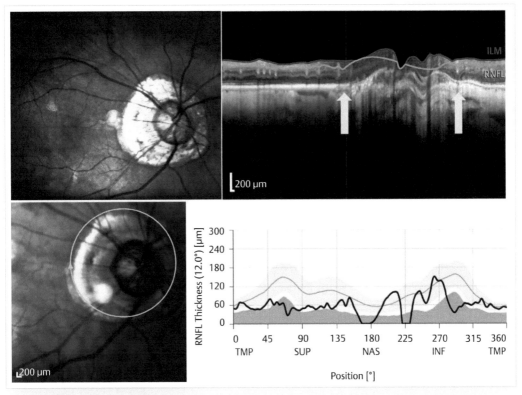

Fig. 8.10 Peripapillary atrophy-associated artifact and going below the floor. This is a retinal nerve fiber layer (RNFL) optical coherence tomography (OCT) of the right eye. Peripapillary atrophy (PPA) appears as a lighter colored crescent or halo around the optic nerve (*top left panel*). Most scan circles are large enough to capture normal retinal tissue beyond the PPA. In this case, the scan circle overlaps the PPA in the inferonasal quadrant (*bottom left panel*). As a result, there are absent outer retinal layers in this region (between *yellow arrows*), leading to inaccurate posterior RNFL segmentation and areas of artifactual thinning. In two areas, the incorrect segmentation leads to erroneous RNFL thickness measurements of 0 μm, which is below the floor of approximately 50 μm (*bottom right panel*) (Spectralis OCT, Heidelberg Engineering, Heidelberg, Germany).

thickness, some reports have shown that the automatic segmentation reports can be associated with artifactually thinned RNFL.[2] Care should be taken to evaluate patients with MNFL on a case-by-case basis, as this variant may lead to falsely thick measurements due to the additional myelin or thin measurements due to segmentation error. The clinician should be able to readily detect these abnormalities by paying attention to the segmentation and correlating with the clinical appearance of the optic nerve.

Staphyloma

A staphyloma is an outpouching of the ocular wall with a radius of curvature less than that of the surrounding ocular wall. These range in depth and can be present in the peripapillary region. The biggest issue is that staphylomas alter the imaging depth, and this affects the ability of the SD-OCT to resolve the retinal layers at greater depth. Newer swept-source OCT (SS-OCT) can allow for analysis of deeper tissues. However, its abilities have yet to be proven for glaucoma evaluation. Furthermore, SS-OCT is not used in most ophthalmology practices at this time. Given issues in resolution at this depth, the most common artifacts are poor signal quality and consequently inaccurate segmentation.[2] The clinician should carefully document a staphyloma on fundus examination and be highly skeptical of any OCT results obtained.

High Myopia

High myopia is an interesting pathology to consider. In a study by Massachusetts Eye and Ear, a large subgroup of 1,222 patients with documented high myopia and glaucoma did not show a significant difference in number of RNFL artifacts as compared to nonmyopic glaucoma patients.[2] A study by Duke Eye Center describes three patients with high myopia and OCT artifacts. One of these patients had retinoschisis affecting segmentation and another patient had poor signal artifact.[10] Even though patients with high myopia have higher incidence of other pathologies, such as retinoschisis and staphyloma, the relative infrequency of these events means that high myopia is not an independently statistically significant cause of OCT artifact.

That being said, the clinician must be aware of the presence of high myopia, which is a common cause of red disease (see section on *OCT Diseases*). Patients with high myopia but without glaucoma have been noted to have thinner RNFL values in all four quadrants. It is important to know that this is pathologic thinning, and not artifactual thinning. Differentiating myopic RNFL thinning from glaucomatous thinning requires evaluating the OCT scan in the context of other clinical testing as well as the clinical examination. For the purposes of this section on artifacts, know that high myopia does not significantly increase the rate of RNFL OCT artifacts seen. However, the clinician should be cautious if faced with related pathologies such as staphyloma or retinoschisis, as these can cause artifact.

Epiretinal Membrane

ERM can lead to errors in anterior segmentation, and is discussed further in the section *Artifacts in Boundary Segmentation*.

Anterior Segment Pathology

Corneal or lens abnormality can affect image quality and therefore induce artifact. This is discussed further in the section *Poor Signal*.

8.2.4 Artifacts due to Differences in OCT Machines

The OCT instruments that are commercially available today differ in key areas, which make their measurements noninterchangeable (see Chapter 7 on "Comparison of Common Devices"). For this reason, if a patient is scanned with one device and the following year is scanned with a different device, you cannot accurately follow disease progression.

First, different machines possess different reference databases (▶ Table 8.2). The reference database (or "normative database") is a collection of measurements taken from a population of normal subjects. When the OCT machine takes a measurement, it interprets the measured value based on the normal curve described by the reference database and color-codes them for easy interpretation. A color-coding of green ("within normal limits") suggests that the patient is normal and has nerve tissue values similar to age-matched normal subjects in the reference database. Yellow ("borderline") is a warning and suggests that the patient's values may be outside 95% of normal limits. Red ("outside normal limits") indicates that the patient may have glaucoma, due to nerve tissue that is abnormally thin and outside the 99% normal limits. Since different manufacturers built the reference databases using data from different subjects and ethnicities, the OCT machines may vary in their color categorizations for the same patient.

Second, measurements can vary among machines. This is evidenced by the different mean RNFL thicknesses for a healthy population who were all scanned on four different machines on the same day (Stratus 110.1 ± 12.8 μm, Cirrus 98.7 ± 10.9 μm, Spectralis 106.6 ± 12.8 μm, RTVue 112.8 ± 13.2 μm).[14]

8.3 Etiologies of ONH and Macula Artifacts

Artifacts can occur in ONH and macular scans as well. Different OCT machines have different scan protocols and different segmentation algorithms, as described in ▶ Table 8.1 of a review of SD-OCT by Chen et al.[15] For example, the Spectralis GMPE software (Heidelberg Engineering Inc., Heidelberg, Germany) measures neuroretinal rim thickness (i.e., Bruch's membrane opening–minimum rim width [BMO-MRW]) and evaluates for asymmetry in retinal thickness at the macula (i.e., posterior pole asymmetry analysis). In contrast, the Cirrus HD-OCT (Carl Zeiss Meditec, Inc., Dublin, CA) measures neuroretinal rim thickness and macular parameters from a 200-line cube scan over the optic nerve and macula. The RTVue-100 (Optovue Inc., Fremont, CA) measures disc parameters from a combination of 12 radial scans and a series of concentric circle scans centered over the ONH and measures macular parameters from a 15 horizontal lines (plus 1 vertical line) macular cube scan. The 3D OCT-2000 (Topcon Corporation, Tokyo, Japan) measures disc and macular parameters

Table 8.2 Characteristics of the reference databases of OCT instruments. Each brand of OCT uses a unique reference database for determining cutoffs for normal and abnormal parameters. This table lists the features of the reference database cohorts specific to each brand of OCT machine

Model	Carl Zeiss Meditec	Topcon Medical Systems	Heidelberg Engineering*	Optovue
Number of subjects	282	182	201	480
Age (years)	19 to 84	19 to 84	18 to 78	18 to 84
Gender (M/F)	133 M 149 F	Disc: 54 M / 92 F Macula: 112 F / 61 M	111 M 90 F	N/A
Ethnicity	43% Caucasian 24% Asian 18% African-American 12% Hispanic 1% Indian 6% Mixed ethnicity	64% Caucasian 21% African-American 15% Hispanic	Caucasian	33% Caucasian 22% Asian 20% African-American 12% Hispanic 12% Indian 1% Other
Anatomy evaluated	RNFL thickness Optic nerve parameters GCL + IPL thickness Macular thickness	Optic disc Macula	RNFL thickness	RNFL thickness Ganglion cell complex Macula thickness
Study locations	United States, China	United States	Germany	11 clinical sites worldwide

Abbreviations: GCL, ganglion cell layer; IPL, inner plexiform layer; OCT, optical coherence tomography; RNFL, retinal nerve fiber layer
Note: *Prior to Heidelberg 2016 update.

from a 512 × 128 volume scan over the optic nerve and macula.[15]

8.3.1 Bruch's Membrane Opening–Minimum Rim Width Artifacts

BMO-MRW is a measurement of the thickness of the neuroretinal rim, which is sensitive to early glaucomatous thinning. It is derived from a 24-line radial scan centered over the ONH. The printout shows 12 different B-scans per eye, each corresponding to a different clock hour of the nerve. In each of these, a red line marks the ILM and a green or yellow arrow marks the shortest distance from the BMO to the ILM. This distance represents the BMO-MRW and is averaged for global, quadrant, and sector values. Artifacts in BMO-MRW analysis can result from misidentification of Bruch's membrane (▶ Fig. 8.11) or the ILM or cup surface (▶ Fig. 8.12), which can lead to erroneously thick or thin measurements. If the margin of the optic nerve is incorrectly identified, Bruch's membrane may not even be present in the representative B-scan from that sector, leading to artifacts. In ▶ Fig. 8.11, the tilted nerves and PPA disrupt

identification of BMO in certain sectors. Theoretically, VMT and ERM could lead to misidentification of the ILM, similar to the artifacts they cause for RNFL segmentation. Poor signal, which was discussed previously, can also lead to segmentation errors of the BMO and the ILM.

8.3.2 Macular Asymmetry Analysis Artifacts

The posterior pole asymmetry analysis is used to identify asymmetry in retinal thickness at the macula between eyes (OD-OS asymmetry) and across hemispheres within each eye (hemisphere asymmetry). The 8 × 8 colored grid displays measurements of retinal thickness within each cell. Artifacts in these printouts commonly result when a patient blinks (▶ Fig. 8.13) or when a scan is not centered properly (▶ Fig. 8.14). During blinking or abrupt movement, the machine is unable to acquire data at that precise moment, and there is a dark band of missing signal on the grid. This can mislead the clinician to think that there is thinning. When inspecting the heat map grid of the macula, there is a well-demarcated dark horizontal stripe that is clearly not physiologic. Also, if the

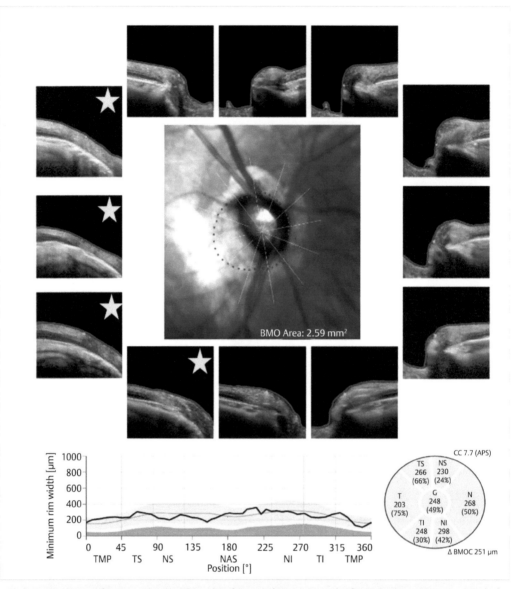

Fig. 8.11 Bruch's membrane opening (BMO) misidentification. This is an example of a Spectralis optic nerve scan, which determines Bruch's membrane opening–minimum rim width (BMO-MRW) or the neuroretinal rim thickness. In the center panel, the red dots incorrectly mark the disc margin or BMO border in the temporal and inferior regions. The reason the red dots are so far from the true temporal disc border is that the disc margin or BMO edge is incorrectly marked or segmented (see panels with *yellow stars*).

scan is not precisely centered at the fovea, thickness measurements will be inaccurate. There is usually a ring of thicker retina surrounding the fovea, which then thins beyond this ring. If the scan is decentered, there will be both erroneous thickening and thinning, depending on whether that quadrant has been shifted further from or closer to the true fovea. Look at the macular heat map (▶ Fig. 8.14, left eye); it should be readily apparent that the scan is decentered inferior to the fovea. Other errors in scan acquisition can lead to missing data (▶ Fig. 8.15) when parts of the temporal macula are entirely missing from the scan and associated analysis. In these instances, the image should be retaken. Other macular pathologies can also affect these results, including macular

8

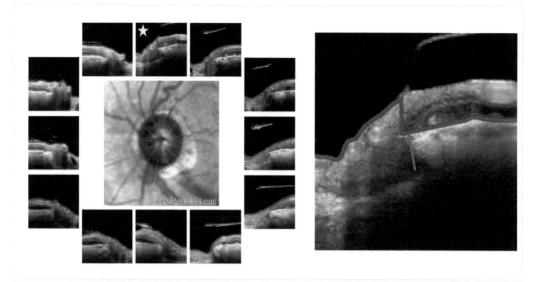

Fig. 8.12 Internal limiting membrane (ILM) misidentification. This is an example of a Spectralis optic nerve scan, which determines Bruch's membrane opening–minimum rim width (BMO-MRW) or the neuroretinal rim thickness. In this example, the algorithm failed to correctly identify the ILM or cup surface in one of the scans (see panel with the *yellow star*; same panel enlarged on the *right*). Note that the red line partly follows the retinal pigment epithelium instead of the ILM. Consequently, the BMO has also been incorrectly identified. Since the ILM and BMO were both misidentified, the green arrow, which is supposed to span the neuroretinal rim thickness, is incorrectly placed below the true neuroretinal rim.

atrophy, macular edema, VMT, and ERM; and changes in posterior pole asymmetry analysis measurements from these pathologies should be distinguished from changes due to glaucoma.

8.4 OCT Diseases

The OCT machine has attempted to simplify the job of the clinician by color-coding the results on the printout. An overall color classification of green appears to mean the patient is "normal," yellow that the patient is "borderline" or may have glaucoma, and red that the patient is "abnormal" and has glaucoma. The OCT machine's glaucoma software only has one disease in the differential diagnosis, which is glaucoma. This may suffice for glaucoma patients; however, strictly utilizing the color-coding system will inevitably result in misdiagnosis, especially in patients who have abnormal parameters from either an artifact or a nonglaucomatous disease process. These inaccurate OCT diagnoses are colloquially referred to as green, yellow, and red disease.

The green, yellow, and red RNFL cutoffs on the Cirrus™ OCT were derived from a reference database of which 43% were Caucasian, 24% were Asian, 18% were African-American, and 12% were Hispanic. Recent literature has shown that race affects baseline RNFL thickness. For example, blacks may have thinner temporal RNFLs, Asians may have thicker global, superior, and inferior RNFLs, and Hispanics may have thicker inferior RNFLs.[16] Since the OCT software does not adjust the final color classification for race, this could cause serious misinterpretation of outputs. For instance, since Asian patients have thicker RNFLs on average than white patients, the clinician may underestimate thinning. This is because the relative thinning is still within the normal (green) range as compared to the predominantly Caucasian cohort used as a reference by the Spectralis OCT software. This is an example of green disease, which is a "false negative" diagnosis of glaucoma and where the OCT indicates things are normal when in fact the RNFL is thinned from baseline. This example demonstrates that the clinician should not just trust the OCT interpretation, but rather utilize his or her own clinical judgment. There are many artifacts that cause red, yellow, and green disease, which we will go on to describe.

"OCT diseases" commonly affect clinical practice. For example, Mansberger et al looked at automated versus manual segmentation and the effect of manual correction on the final OCT color classification. This group found that 23.7% of patients with borderline (yellow) classifications on automated segmentation became normal (green) with manual

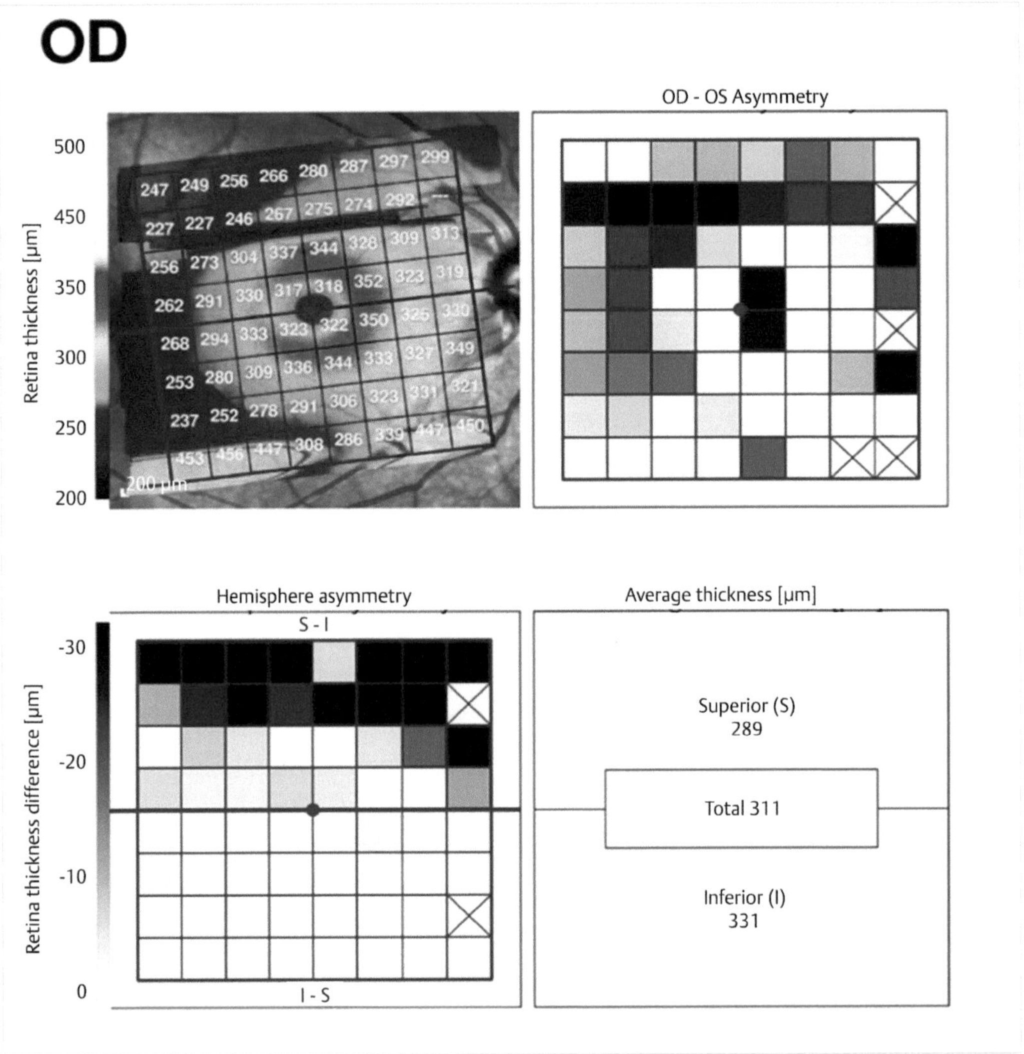

Fig. 8.13 Blink artifact. This is an example of a macular posterior pole asymmetry analysis scan from the Spectralis Glaucoma Module Premium Edition (GMPE) software. When a patient blinks or moves abruptly, the machine is unable to gather accurate information at that moment. This results in a horizontal rectangular area of abrupt color change that is readily seen in the color thickness map of the right eye. In this example, a dark gray horizontal line in the superior macula indicates that the patient had blinked (*top left panel*). Looking only at the hemisphere asymmetry analysis, the clinician would be misled to think there was true superior thinning, when in fact this is artifact.

segmentation.[17] This means that in a standard practice, approximately one quarter of patients being followed for borderline glaucoma or OCT thinning would in fact have no RNFL thinning at all.

8.4.1 Red Disease

Red disease is a "false positive" diagnosis of glaucoma, and this occurs when the OCT red color classification indicates glaucomatous thinning, when in fact the patient does not have glaucoma. Red disease may be due to artifactual thinning or due to real nonglaucomatous tissue thinning. In a busy clinic, it can be tempting to rely on the color map alone, but this can get the clinician into trouble.

Example 1

Consider this possible scenario: A patient presents to clinic for his or her glaucoma suspect follow-up. He or she has significant dry eyes requiring frequent artificial tears, but he or she did not use any

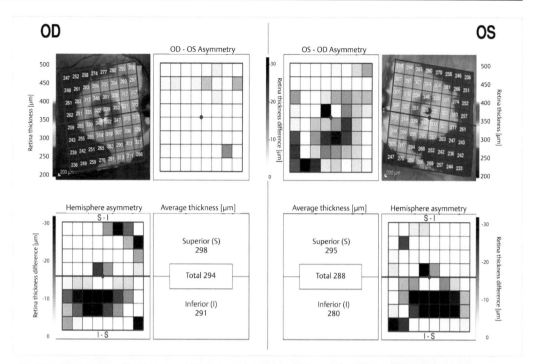

Fig. 8.14 Decentration. This is an example of a macular posterior pole asymmetry analysis scan from the Spectralis Glaucoma Module Premium Edition (GMPE) software. Normally, the grid should be centered precisely over fovea but it is tilted such that the horizontal gridlines are parallel to the fovea-to-disc (FoDi) axis. In this example, the grids for both eyes are decentered inferiorly (OS > OD). Since retinal thickness usually increases and then decreases moving away from the fovea in all directions, decentration can produce misleading results in the asymmetry maps between eyes (OD-OS asymmetry) and within the same eye (hemisphere asymmetry).

prior to the appointment. When the technician obtains the OCT, the patient is nervous about the test and does not blink. The printout shows areas of red on the thickness plot, which suggest to the clinician that the RNFL has thinned and the glaucoma may be progressing. Do you start topical pressure lowering drops given this change from his or her previous scan?

Start by looking at the actual OCT scan, not just the color analysis. This patient's OCT scan appears grainy due to poor signal from dry eyes. As discussed earlier in this chapter, dry eye can lead to falsely thinned RNFL values. Since the image quality was poor, the OCT inaccurately segmented the RNFL, and the data is unusable. Place artificial tears and repeat the scan for more accurate results. In this example, the OCT software diagnosed red disease, but the clinician astutely identified the inaccuracy.

Example 2

An established patient with a diagnosis of glaucoma suspect presents for yearly examination. His or her visual acuity and visual fields are unchanged. His or her thickness plot now reveals inferior thinning in the left eye. You worry that he or she is progressing to glaucomatous damage. What do you do?

First, look carefully at this patient's scan. Compared to the previous visit, the superior quadrant is thickened in addition to the thinning of the inferior quadrant. Additionally, the nerve looks slightly superiorly displaced in the scan circle. To recall, decentration of the nerve within the scan circle of even 10% can lead to significant changes in the thickness averages for those quadrants. Specifically, as you move farther from the nerve, the RNFL is thinner. Repeat this patient's scan with a well-centered scan circle and the color map will be green in all quadrants.

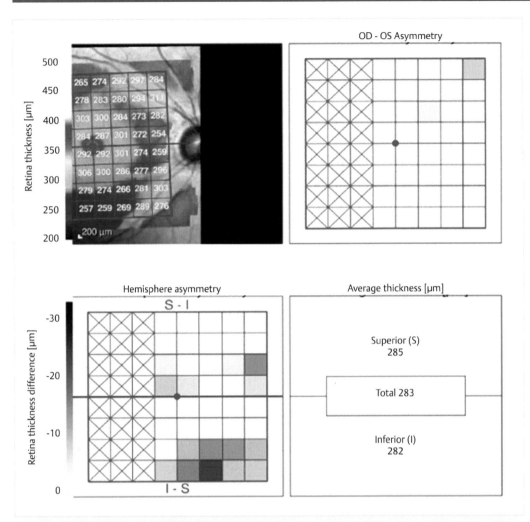

Fig. 8.15 Missing data. This is an example of a macular posterior pole asymmetry analysis scan from the Spectralis Glaucoma Module Premium Edition (GMPE) software. A large portion of the temporal macula is missing from this photo. The areas of the grid with "Xs" indicate the missing data. If a technician notices this problem, the scan should be repeated.

Example 3

A patient with advanced glaucoma on maximum medical therapy comes to clinic. The visual acuity is unchanged and the intraocular pressure is at goal. His or her visual field is reliable and unchanged from prior testing. Unfortunately, the OCT color map is now completely red in both eyes, where previously it still had a yellow temporal quadrant in both eyes. Should you start talking about surgical intervention?

This is a challenging case, but start by looking at the scan. In this example, the RNFL is difficult to identify due to reduced reflectivity. As a result, the posterior boundary of the segmentation is inaccurately placed in the middle of the RNFL. As was described previously in this chapter, glaucoma causes loss of reflectivity of the nerve fiber layer and makes it more difficult for the OCT to accurately segment. In some instances, the RNFL thickness may read as low as 0 μm, which we know is physiologically impossible as discussed in the earlier section *Floor Effect*. In this case, the OCT has diagnosed red disease of the temporal quadrants due to posterior boundary misidentification. However, manual resegmentation would reveal stable RNFL thickness as compared to the previous year's scan. Do not do surgery based on this finding alone because the OCT is stable on maximum medical therapy.

8.4.2 Green Disease

Green disease is dangerous due to the false reassurance it provides. It is comforting to point at a green thickness map and show the patient that the glaucoma is well controlled or that he or she does not have glaucoma at all. There are many artifacts that we have discussed that can lead to falsely thick measurements and cause the OCT to interpret things as normal when there is actually pathologic loss of the nerve fiber layer.

Example 1

A new patient comes in with a prior diagnosis of moderate glaucoma in the right eye and mild glaucoma in the left eye. The thickness plot of the right eye shows yellow superior and temporal quadrants and red inferior and nasal quadrants. The thickness plot of the left eye also shows yellow superior and temporal quadrants and a red inferior quadrant; however, the nasal quadrant is green. Here, the OCT confirms that his or her disease in the left eye is less severe, because of the reassuring green nasal quadrant. Do you agree that the left eye has less RNFL thinning than the right eye?

Carefully examine the OCT scan. In this case, the hyaloid face is tugging on the nasal peripapillary retina causing profound vitreous traction in the left eye. This traction is resulting in false thickening of the RNFL in the nasal quadrant, which the OCT labeled as green. In comparison, the right eye has no vitreous traction. The OCT has misleadingly reassured the clinician that the left eye has more mild glaucoma, when in fact this was only the result of an impending posterior vitreous detachment. A few months later, this patient has release of the vitreous traction and reports a new floater. A repeat OCT demonstrates that the previously green nasal quadrant in the left eye is now red since it is no longer being pulled anteriorly. This is an example of green disease falsely reassuring the clinician and leading to potential under treatment of disease.

Example 2

A patient with Parkinson's disease comes for a comprehensive eye examination. His or her intraocular pressures are 24 mmHg in both eyes. His or her RNFL OCT shows a completely green color map for both eyes. Is this ocular hypertension?

On his or her RNFL OCT scan, the retina appears to be a very wavy group of horizontal lines (retinal layers). This is the result of motion artifact due to the patient's Parkinson's disease. The OCT software cannot accurately segment this scan with motion artifact, and has arbitrarily assigned the anterior and posterior boundaries, making the calculated RNFL thickness above average. Instruct the technician to repeat the scan with an assistant gently holding the head still while the picture is being acquired. Now, the OCT demonstrates areas of pathologic RNFL thinning, and you start topical glaucoma therapy. If the clinician is rushed and fails to look at the scan, this green disease would result in misdiagnosis.

Example 3

A patient with mild glaucoma in both eyes returns to clinic for yearly follow-up. He or she reports that the vision in the right eye is more distorted than last year. His or her OCT is reassuring, and shows a green thickness map in the right eye, which was notably yellow last year. Could his or her glaucoma have improved in the right eye?

On dilated examination, there is a yellow sheen over the macula. Close examination of the OCT scan would reveal a thin white layer on the anterior surface of the retina consistent with an ERM. The OCT has misidentified this membrane as the anterior boundary for segmentation. The clinician should explain to the patient that his or her nerve fiber layer has not become thicker, but that he or she has an ERM that has resulted in segmentation artifact, causing the OCT to diagnose green disease.

8.5 A Relevant Summary of OCT Artifacts for Technicians

A good technician is invaluable. The technician is on the frontlines acquiring the data that is vital to how the clinician chooses to treat patients. Ultimately, the clinician is responsible for analyzing the scans and making clinical decisions; however, a well-trained technician can drastically improve clinical practice. Here, we detail a few points to share with your technicians so that they can also be on the watch for artifacts.

- Clean the lens. It sounds simple, but the "smudge artifact" can be a nuisance and make the scan unusable.

8

- Is the scan blurry or grainy appearing? Place artificial tears in the patient's eyes. This may not fix the problem, as the clinician may note another issue, like cataracts, but it is worth trying artificial tears first.
- Make sure the nerve is precisely in the center of the scan circle. If it is even 10% off the center, it may falsely look like the patient's glaucoma got worse, when it did not.
- Is the patient moving or do they have a tremor? The corresponding scan might make the retina look very wavy or part of it may be missing altogether. If the patient is unable to hold still, have someone else to help hold the patient's head against the bar so it does not move. It may be necessary to take multiple pictures and be patient despite a busy clinic.
- Is there a light-colored crescent or halo around the nerve? Make the scan circle diameter just large enough to encompass some of the retina beyond this area.
- Does the technician have other concerns about the scan quality? If so, he or she should notify the clinician. The technician devotes significant time to acquire a good image, and may be able to offer valuable insights.

8.6 Future Directions

8.6.1 Three-Dimensional Parameters

The use of three-dimensional OCT data has been proposed for evaluation of glaucoma. Three-dimensional RNFL volume has been shown to have the same or better diagnostic capability for glaucoma as compared to conventional two-dimensional RNFL thickness. If each individual B-scan used to create a three-dimensional volume scan is evaluated, the rate of artifact is approximately 21%. However, because the volume scan averages many B-scans to make this three-dimensional parameter, it is less subject to artifacts. Additionally, the algorithm used to generate three-dimensional RNFL volume scans automatically centers the ONH, therefore eliminating decentration artifact, which is the most common artifact affecting two-dimensional peripapillary thickness scans.

Another of these three-dimensional parameters is the ganglion cell complex (GCC) volume as derived from macular OCT scans. Data has shown that the GCC volume parameter has the same or better diagnostic capability as the conventional

two-dimensional peripapillary RNFL thickness parameter. Interestingly, 100% of the volume scans in this study had at least one B-scan with artifact. More importantly, manual deletion of the B-scans with artifact did not increase the diagnostic performance of these parameters. This is very interesting because even though artifacts are still present in this newer three-dimensional data analysis, they may not cause as much of an effect on the data output given the averaging effect over the depth of the scan.

8.6.2 OCT Angiography

Vascular dysfunction has been implicated in the pathogenesis of glaucoma. A study from 2014 demonstrated a significant 25% reduction in perfusion of the optic disc (disc flow index) in glaucoma versus normal eyes by using OCT angiography (OCTA).[18] Given such findings, OCTA may be used increasingly in the future to detect vascular changes as an early sign of glaucomatous progression. Unfortunately, OCTA is not without artifact. In fact, OCTA is a more technically challenging device for technicians and is subject to greater errors in image acquisition. In a study from 2019, the cumulative rate of any artifact in OCTA was 97%. Specifically, eye movement affected 93% of scans and defocus affected 75% of scans.[19] A well-trained technician could reduce both of these artifacts. We are likely to see OCTA play a greater role in the evaluation of glaucoma in the future, but given the high frequency of artifact clinicians will need to be highly attuned to the effects that artifacts can have on the diagnosis and management of glaucoma.

References

[1] Nakano N, Hangai M, Noma H, et al. Macular imaging in highly myopic eyes with and without glaucoma. Am J Ophthalmol. 2013; 156(3):511–523.e6

[2] Liu Y, Simavli H, Que CJ, et al. Patient characteristics associated with artifacts in Spectralis optical coherence tomography imaging of the retinal nerve fiber layer in glaucoma. Am J Ophthalmol. 2015; 159(3):565–76.e2

[3] Awadalla MS, Fitzgerald J, Andrew NH, et al. Prevalence and type of artefact with spectral domain optical coherence tomography macular ganglion cell imaging in glaucoma surveillance. PLoS One. 2018; 13(12):1–9

[4] Han IC, Jaffe GJ. Evaluation of artifacts associated with macular spectral-domain optical coherence tomography. Ophthalmology. 2010; 117(6):1177–1189.e4

[5] Ortega JdeL, Kakati B, Girkin CA. Artifacts on the optic nerve head analysis of the optical coherence tomography in glaucomatous and nonglaucomatous eyes. J Glaucoma. 2009; 18 (3):186–191

[6] Schrems-Hoesl LM, Schrems WA, Laemmer R, Kruse FE, Mardin CY. Precision of optic nerve head and retinal nerve fiber layer parameter measurements by spectral-domain optical coherence tomography. J Glaucoma. 2018; 27(5):407–414

[7] Stein DM, Wollstein G, Ishikawa H, Hertzmark E, Noecker RJ, Schuman JS. Effect of corneal drying on optical coherence tomography. Ophthalmology. 2006; 113(6):985–991

[8] Mwanza JC, Bhorade AM, Sekhon N, et al. Effect of cataract and its removal on signal strength and peripapillary retinal nerve fiber layer optical coherence tomography measurements. J Glaucoma. 2011; 20(1):37–43

[9] Baghaie A, Yu Z, D'Souza RM. Involuntary eye motion correction in retinal optical coherence tomography: hardware or software solution? Med Image Anal. 2017; 37:129–145

[10] Asrani S, Essaid L, Alder BD, Santiago-Turla C. Artifacts in spectral-domain optical coherence tomography measurements in glaucoma. JAMA Ophthalmol. 2014; 132(4):396–402

[11] Liu Y, Baniasadi N, Ratanawongphaibul K, Chen TC. Effect of partial posterior vitreous detachment on spectral-domain optical coherence tomography retinal nerve fibre layer thickness measurements. Br J Ophthalmol. 2020; 104(11):1524–1527

[12] Giani A, Cigada M, Esmaili DD, et al. Artifacts in automatic retinal segmentation using different optical coherence tomography instruments. Retina. 2010; 30(4):607–616

[13] Chen JJ, Kardon RH. Avoiding clinical misinterpretation and artifacts of optical coherence tomography analysis of the optic nerve, retinal nerve fiber layer, and ganglion cell layer. J Neuroophthalmol. 2016; 36(4):417–438

[14] Seibold LK, Mandava N, Kahook MY. Comparison of retinal nerve fiber layer thickness in normal eyes using time-domain and spectral-domain optical coherence tomography. Am J Ophthalmol. 2010; 150(6):807–814

[15] Chen TC, Hoguet A, Junk AK, et al. Spectral-domain OCT: helping the clinician diagnose glaucoma: a report by the American Academy of Ophthalmology. Ophthalmology. 2018; 125(11):1817–1827

[16] Poon LYC, Antar H, Tsikata E, et al. Effects of age, race, and ethnicity on the optic nerve and peripapillary region using spectral-domain OCT 3d volume scans. Transl Vis Sci Technol. 2018; 7(6):12

[17] Mansberger SL, Menda SA, Fortune BA, Gardiner SK, Demirel S. Automated segmentation errors when using optical coherence tomography to measure retinal nerve fiber layer thickness in glaucoma. Am J Ophthalmol. 2017; 174:1–8

[18] Jia Y, Wei E, Wang X, et al. Optical coherence tomography angiography of optic disc perfusion in glaucoma. Ophthalmology. 2014; 121(7):1322–1332

[19] Holmen IC, Konda MS, Pak JW, et al. Prevalence and severity of artifacts in optical coherence tomographic angiograms. JAMA Ophthalmol. 2020; 138(2):119–126

[20] Park EA, Budenz DL, Lee RK, Chen TC. Red and Green Disease in Glaucoma. In: Budenz DL, ed. Atlas of Optical Coherence Tomography for Glaucoma. Springer; 2020: 127–174

8

9 Anterior Segment Optical Coherence Tomography in Glaucoma

Ying Han and Julius Oatts

Summary

Anterior segment optical coherence tomography provides noninvasive, high-resolution, cross-sectional images of anterior segment structures and serves as an effective adjuvant tool in the diagnosis and management of glaucomatous conditions, particularly primary angle closure disease.

Keywords: optical coherence tomography, anterior segment, primary angle closure suspect, primary angle closure glaucoma, plateau iris

9.1 Introduction to Anterior-Segment OCT

Optical coherence tomography (OCT) is a powerful diagnostic technology which produces high-resolution cross-sectional images of the internal microstructure of living tissues, first described in the posterior and anterior segments of the eye in the 1990s.[1] Prior to this technology, the main imaging modality for evaluating the anterior segment of the eye was ultrasound biomicroscopy (UBM). Imaging of the iridocorneal angle and anterior segment anatomy is of particular interest to those diagnosing and managing different forms of glaucoma. UBM use frequencies from 35 to 80 MHz while OCT uses low-coherence, near-infrared light, allowing for very high resolution images. Apart from the increased resolution of anterior segment OCT (AS-OCT), it also has the advantage of significant ease in obtaining images. AS-OCT is noncontact and can be performed with patients sitting upright, compared to UBM which requires an eyecup, coupling medium with direct contact to the eye, and supine positioning. Anatomically, UBM confers the advantage of being able to image structures posterior to the iris, which is a limitation of AS-OCT imaging. A direct comparison between AS-OCT and UBM found no significant differences in anterior chamber parameters measured with both devices and a more easily identifiable scleral spur with AS-OCT compared to UBM.[2]

OCT technology was first described in 1991,[1] and though simplified, has been described as the optical equivalent of ultrasound imaging. Light is projected onto a biologic structure, in this case the eye, and the system detects reflected, nonscattered, coherent light. The two categories are time-domain OCT and the newer Fourier-domain, or spectral-domain, OCT. The former measures time-of-flight delay from light reflected off the tissue to that reflected from an adjustable, moving reference mirror. The latter uses a spectrometer to detect differences in light reflection between the tissue and a fixed reference mirror, using mathematical transformations to confer information about depth. Due to these differences, spectral-domain OCT provides higher image resolution and faster image acquisition. Swept-source OCT is an iteration of spectral-domain OCT and can be used for the anterior segment.

Image acquisition is similar to posterior segment imaging in that the patient is upright and no topical anesthesia is required. A wide palpebral fissure is required to fully image the anterior segment, and closed eyelids can affect image quality, particularly in the vertical meridian. This can be alleviated by manually opening the eyelids or using an eyelid speculum. The eye is aligned, the distance refraction is entered, and the patient is asked to focus on the internal fixation target at which point the images are obtained. Once images are acquired, geometric computational processes convert the optical distances from the images to physical distances taking refraction index variations from air, cornea, and aqueous humor into account. Since its initial application to the anterior segment in 1991, numerous advances have been made to AS-OCT.

9.2 Different AS-OCT Modalities and Systems

Compared to posterior segment OCT, AS-OCT typically uses a longer wavelength (1,310 nm compared to 830 nm). This longer wavelength further decreases scan acquisition time as well as decreases posterior segment exposure. This also allows improved penetration through structures that highly scatter light including the scleral and limbus.

▶ Table 9.1 is a list of specifications of historical and currently available AS-OCT imaging systems, a few of which are discussed in more depth below.[3]

Table 9.1 Specifications of AS-OCT imaging systems

	Stratus	Visante	SL-OCT	RTVue	Cirrus	Spectralis AS Module	CASIA
Manufacturer	Carl Zeiss Meditec	Carl Zeiss Meditec	Heidelberg Engineering	Optovue	Carl Zeiss Meditec	Heidelberg Engineering	Tomey
Year available	2002	2005	2006	2006	2007	2012	2008
Light source	Diode 820 nm	Diode 1,310 nm	Diode 1,310 nm	Diode 840 nm	Diode 840 nm	Diode 830 nm	Swept-source laser 1,310 nm
Axial resolution	10 μm	18 μm	<25 μm	5 μm	5 μm	3.9 to 7 μm	<10 μm
Scan size	6×2 mm	16×6 mm	15×7 mm	6×2 mm	3×1 mm	8×2.8 mm	16×6 mm
Scan speed	400 A-scans/sec	2,000 A-scans/sec	200 A-scans/sec	26,000 A-scans/sec	27,000 A-scans/sec	40,000 A-scans/sec	30,000 A-scans/sec

Abbreviations: AS-OCT, anterior segment optical coherence tomography.

Visante, the first AS-OCT imaging system to employ a higher wavelength, provided higher resolution than its predecessors but not enough to accurately determine the location of the trabecular meshwork. For this reason, areas of angle closure are determined by contact between the iris and the angle anterior to the scleral spur, thus overestimating angle closure when compared to gonioscopy. Also, due to its time-domain technology, scan acquisition time is significantly longer than its spectral-domain equivalents. The slit lamp OCT was unique in its integration into the slit lamp biomicroscope, though it had the same time-domain related constraints and there was poor agreement between that and the Visante.[4]

An update to spectral-domain OCT in the Cirrus, Spectralis, and CASIA systems was associated with increased scan quality and decreased scan acquisition time with improved visualization of the anterior chamber angle and the ability to image smaller structures including the trabecular meshwork, scleral spur, and Schwalbe's line. The CASIA further has the advantage of being able to obtain a 360-degree image of the anterior chamber using 128 cross-sections obtained in less than 3 seconds. Increasing image quality has contributed to a growing body of literature identifying and studying specific structures and parameters.

9.3 AS-OCT Identification of Anterior Segment Structures and Parameters

Many different angle parameters have been described to standardize the measurements obtained for clinical and research purposes, though longitudinal studies are needed to validate the diagnostic significance of these parameters.[5] Compared to UBM, there is a high level of correlation between anterior chamber angle measurements taken with UBM or older AS-OCT, though UBM angle parameters have been reported to be smaller, potentially due to pressure from the eyecup during UBM image acquisition.

Generally, AS-OCT measurements can be obtained with excellent repeatability and reproducibility with regard to angle parameters. With regards to image segmentation and quantification, there is still quite a bit of variability, and automated algorithms are needed. The Zhongshan Angle Assessment Program provided a semiautomatic algorithm to calculate various parameters, though this, like other measurements of angle parameters, is based on the ability to manually identify the scleral spur and the angle recess. A proposed method for automatic AS-OCT structure segmentation, measurement, and screening is promising, but not currently commercially available.

Identification of the scleral spur may vary among different graders and lead to differences in manual and semiautomatic measurements of the same angle parameters. In most situations, the system-generated automatic marking of these two landmarks is not accurate and needs manual correction. Cues including high pixel reflectivity or a subtle change in the contour of the inner scleral margin can help identify the scleral spur on AS-OCT images, though poor image quality or anatomically narrow angles can affect these and prevent accurate identification of the scleral spur.[6] A study using the Visante reported being unable to identify the scleral spur in as high as 25% of scans.[6] A

Table 9.2 AS-OCT parameters

Anterior chamber depth (ACD)	The perpendicular distance from the corneal endothelium at the corneal apex to the anterior lens surface
Anterior chamber width (ACW)	The distance between the two scleral spurs as identified in the horizontal meridian
Anterior chamber area (ACA)	The cross-sectional area of the anterior segment bounded by the corneal endothelium, anterior iris, and anterior surface of the lens
Lens vault (LV)	The perpendicular distance between the anterior pole of the crystalline lens and the line drawn between the two scleral spurs in the horizontal meridian (the line used to define ACW)
Angle opening distance (AOD)	The distance from the corneal endothelium to the anterior iris perpendicular to a line drawn along the trabecular meshwork 250, 500, and 750 μm anterior to the scleral spur along the anterior iris surface (AOD250, AOD500, AOD750)
Angle recess area (ARA)	The enclosed triangular area demarcated by the anterior iris surface, trabecular meshwork, and corneal endothelium measured 250, 500, and 750 μm from the scleral spur (ARA250, ARA500, ARA750)
Trabecular–iris space area (TISA)	The trapezoidal area with four boundaries: the line segment of AOD; a line drawn from the scleral spur perpendicular to the plane of the inner scleral wall to the opposing iris; the corneoscleral wall; the anterior iris surface (TISA 250, TISA 500, TISA 750)
Trabecular–iris angle (TIA)	The angle measured with the apex in the angle recess and the arms of the angle passing through the two endpoints of AOD segment (TIA250, TIA500, TIA750)

Abbreviation: AS-OCT, anterior segment optical coherence tomography.

similar study using Visante found similar rates of scleral spur identification, though were able to further stratify that the rates of identification were even lower in the superior and inferior quadrants.[7] ▶ Table 9.2 is a list of commonly measured and reported anterior segment parameters (▶ Fig. 9.1).

9.4 AS-OCT in Different Glaucomatous Conditions

AS-OCT is most helpful for patients with glaucoma with its objective qualitative and quantitative assessment of the anterior chamber angle. This is important in many conditions, but most revelatory in primary angle closure disease (PACD), a spectrum of conditions which includes acute primary angle closure, primary angle closure, primary angle closure suspect (PACS), and primary angle closure glaucoma (PACG). In these conditions, there is apposition between the peripheral cornea and the iris, blocking the trabecular meshwork and causing a narrow drainage angle. Gonioscopy remains the gold standard for diagnosing and following these conditions, but AS-OCT can serve as a useful adjunct. Although anterior segment imaging provides useful information in assessing PACD, it should not be considered a substitute for gonioscopy.[5]

9.4.1 Primary Angle Closure Suspect (PACS) (▶ Fig. 9.2)

PACS is defined as at least 180 degrees of iridotrabecular contact with nonvisualization of the posterior trabecular meshwork on gonioscopy, absence of peripheral anterior synechiae (PAS), intraocular pressure (IOP) ≤ 21 mmHg, and absence of glaucomatous optic neuropathy. Iris area and iris volume are AS-OCT metrics which have been described as a potential differentiator between PACS and PACG, with patients with PACG having thicker irides. Lens vault (LV) is a similar metric seen more in PACG compared to PACS, representing anterior displacement of the lens, a surrogate for iridolenticular contact leading to angle crowding. There is also growing interest in using deep learning as a tool to screen for and diagnose patients with PACD and has promising implications for future diagnostics.

9.4.2 Primary Angle Closure Glaucoma (PACG)

PACG is either acute PACG or chronic PACG based on the clinical presentation. Chronic PACG is characterized by elevated IOP, PAS for more than 180 degrees, and signs of glaucomatous optic

9

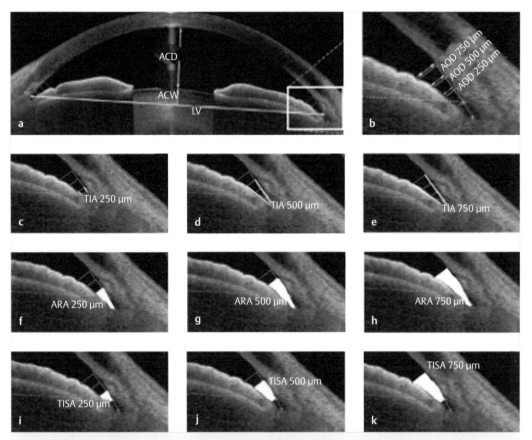

Fig. 9.1 Anterior chamber parameters in anterior segment optical coherence tomography (AS-OCT). Sample images show anterior chamber parameters for AS-OCT using the CASIA SS-1000 (Tomey, Japan). **(a)** Anterior chamber depth (ACD), anterior chamber width (ACW), and lens vault (LV). **(b)** Angle opening distance (AOD) at 250, 500, and 750 μm. **(c–e)** Trabecular–iris angle (TIA) at 250, 500, and 750 μm. **(f–h)** Angle recess area (ARA) at 250, 500, and 750 μm. **(i–k)** Trabecular–iris space area (TISA) at 250, 500, and 750 μm.

neuropathy (nerve head and visual field changes). In comparing AS-OCT to gonioscopy in this patient population, AS-OCT can detect more closed angles superiorly and inferiorly where gonioscopy detects more closed angles temporally and nasally.[8] This difference may represent the differences in acquisition between the dynamic, contact technique required for gonioscopy, and the noncontact light-based technology used by AS-OCT. AS-OCT has also been shown to detect more angle closure than gonioscopy, which could represent gonioscopy under-detection or AS-OCT over-detection, and further studies are required to determine the optimal clinical utility. Apart from anterior chamber angle measurements, eyes with PACG have thicker and more convex irides.[9] Subtle differences in anterior segment parameters could shed light on pathophysiology and subgroups within PACG.

9.4.3 AS-OCT Following Laser Peripheral Iridotomy (LPI) (▶ Fig. 9.3)

Successful LPI, a mainstay in the treatment of angle closure disease, inherently alters the anatomy of the anterior segment, something which can be measured quantitatively on AS-OCT. LPI widens the anterior chamber angle and increases the angle opening distance (AOD), angle recess area (ARA), and trabecular–iris space area (TISA).[5] There is some suggestion that AS-OCT parameters are affected differently following LPI in different subgroups of PACD. For example, patients with shallower pre-LPI anterior chamber depth (ACD) and higher LV may have a more robust anterior chamber deepening after LPI compared to those starting

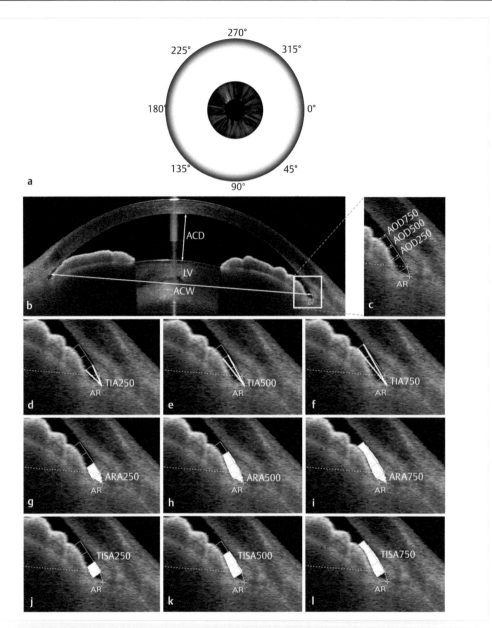

Fig. 9.2 Anterior segment optical coherence tomography (AS-OCT) images with anterior chamber parameters labeled, in a patient with primary angle closure suspect (PACS). **(a)** Schematic representation of the eight axes measured. **(b–i)** Sample images show anterior chamber parameters in SS-OCT. **(b)** Anterior chamber depth (ACD): the axial distance between the corneal endothelium and the anterior lens surface; anterior chamber width (ACW): the distance between the two scleral spurs; and lens vault (LV): the perpendicular distance from the anterior pole of the lens to the horizontal line between the scleral spurs. **(c)** Angle opening distance at 250, 500, and 750 μm (AOD250, AOD500, and AOD750): the distance between the posterior corneal surface and the anterior iris surface on a line perpendicular to the trabecular meshwork 250, 500, and 750 μm from the scleral spur. **(d–f)** Trabecular–iris angle at 250, 500, and 750 μm (TIA250, TIA500, and TIA750): an angle measured with the apex in the iris recess and the arms of the angle passing through a point on the trabecular meshwork 250, 500, and 750 μm from the scleral spur and the point on the iris perpendicularly. **(g–i)** Angle recess area at 250, 500, and 750 μm (ARA250, ARA500, and ARA750): the area of the angle recess bounded anteriorly by the AOD250, AOD500, and AOD750. **(j–l)** Trabecular–iris space area at 250, 500, and 750 μm (TISA250, TISA500, and TISA750): the area bounded anteriorly by AOD250, AOD500, and AOD750 as determined, posteriorly by a line drawn from the scleral spur perpendicular to the plane of the inner scleral wall to the iris, superiorly by the inner corneoscleral wall, and inferiorly by the iris surface.

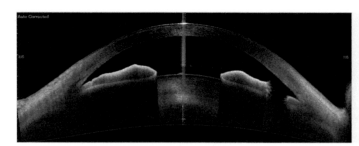

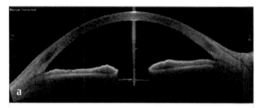

Fig. 9.3 Anterior segment optical coherence tomography (AS-OCT) after laser peripheral iridotomy (LPI). This example shows a cross-section image at the location of the LPI.

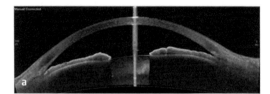

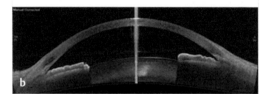

Fig. 9.4 Anterior segment optical coherence tomography (AS-OCT) before and after pupil dilation. Images were acquired **(a)** prior to dilation and **(b)** after pharmacologic dilation of the pupil.

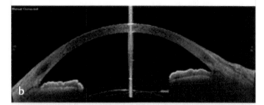

Fig. 9.5 Anterior segment optical coherence tomography (AS-OCT) after cataract surgery. These images were acquired from the same patient shown in ▶ Fig. 9.4 after subsequent cataract surgery, **(a)** prior to dilation and **(b)** after pharmacologic dilation of the pupil.

with deeper ACD.[10] This has implications for peri-LPI assessment with AS-OCT to stratify risk of angle closure and counsel and treat patients accordingly. Similarly, there may be racial differences in response to LPI, though further studies are needed.

9.4.4 AS-OCT Following Dilation (▶ Fig. 9.4)

Both physiologic and pharmacologic pupillary dilation are known to cause changes in anterior segment structures. For example, iris thickening induced by changing from light to dark conditions decreases AOD and contributes to the mechanism of angle closure.[11] Dilation-induced increases in ACD and anterior chamber width (ACW) on AS-OCT in normal and PACS eyes have been described, while others have found no change in these parameters in a similar cohort. AOD has been shown to increase significantly after dilation in normal eyes but not in eyes with PACS. Discrepancies

between studies may be due to variation in imaging devices, differences in patient population, or measurement error.

9.4.5 AS-OCT Following Lens Extraction (▶ Fig. 9.5)

Lens extraction is associated with anterior chamber deepening and widening of the anterior chamber angle,[12] a fact which has led some to advocate for lens extraction as the primary treatment for angle closure disease. Additionally, in patients with persistent narrow angles after LPI, lens extraction has been shown to further deepen the anterior chamber. In patients with narrow angles who undergo cataract or lens extraction, AS-OCT can serve as a helpful adjuvant to gonioscopy to demonstrate objective postsurgical changes in ACD and anterior chamber angle opening.

9.4.6 Other Glaucomatous Conditions

Plateau iris configuration refers to an anterior displacement of the ciliary body and iris root decreasing the iridocorneal angle. This can be treated with LPI, though these patients can have persistently narrow angles despite a patent LPI in which case laser iridoplasty is often performed. AS-OCT can effectively demonstrate increases in AOD and TISA after iridoplasty in those who did not show AS-OCT changes following LPI.[13] Additionally, AS-OCT allows for objective measurement of PAS, a useful addition to gonioscopic findings in equivocal cases or when attempting to stratify risk for angle closure.

Interestingly, AS-OCT has demonstrated angle deepening with Yttrium-Aluminum-Garnet (YAG) laser capsulotomy in pseudophakic patients with posterior capsule opacification and open angles. Anterior chamber depth and width both increased following YAG laser capsulotomy, suggesting a backward movement of the intraocular lens contributing to increased AOD, ACD, and ACW.

Finally, AS-OCT findings in pigment dispersion glaucoma have been described including significantly greater anterior chamber volume and higher degrees of iridolenticular contact when compared to control eyes. Additionally, the iris volume was lower in eyes with pigment dispersion, suggesting a mechanism that a weakly resistant iris may be more susceptible to iridolenticular contact and cause IOP elevation.

9.5 AS-OCT in Postoperative Care

In addition to its diagnostic value, AS-OCT can provide detailed postoperative information which could potentially improve postoperative care. The success of a trabeculectomy, a procedure which creates a connection between the anterior chamber and the subconjunctival space to lower IOP, relies on a well-filtering bleb. Postoperative trabeculectomy bleb morphology has been extensively reported. Blebs can be described by their appearance: diffuse, cystic, encapsulated, or flattened; or by the appearance of the fluid in the bleb: a single large fluid collection or multiple small communicating collections. Low reflectivity, diffuse, and cystic blebs on AS-OCT are thought to reflect aqueous humor, not fibrotic scar tissue, and signal good bleb morphology. Indeed, bleb wall reflectivity, a feature not assessable by slit lamp examination, may be the most useful parameter correlating with bleb functionality, with hyperreflective blebs associated with higher rates of failure.[14] Additionally, being able to identify a filtration opening on AS-OCT a few weeks following trabeculectomy correlated with IOP control 1 year after the procedure, suggesting another opportunity to use AS-OCT to improve surgical outcomes.[15] This can also be used serially before and after laser-suture lysis to demonstrate changes in bleb height and wall thickness.

AS-OCT can also be used to assess bleb morphology over glaucoma drainage devices. In patients with glaucoma who underwent Ahmed glaucoma valve implantation, a thin maximum bleb wall was associated with higher levels of surgical success.[16] AS-OCT can also be used in conjunction with specular microscopy to evaluate the health of the corneal endothelium following glaucoma drainage device surgery. Images obtained postoperatively can provide measures of the intracameral length of the tube, cornea-tube, and iris-tube distances as well as assessing tube patency (▶ Fig. 9.6 and ▶ Fig. 9.7).

With the increasing popularity of minimally invasive glaucoma surgery (MIGS), we can expect to see more data forthcoming regarding the AS-OCT findings in these procedures. One example showed successful bleb monitoring following Xen implantation, with hyperreflective blebs associated with higher rates of failure.[17]

Other postoperative conditions which may benefit from AS-OCT imaging include pupillary block, malignant glaucoma, and iris chafing secondary to intraocular lens placement.

9.6 AS-OCT in Additional Glaucoma-Related Situations

AS-OCT has been described in a few other contexts related to glaucoma. First, this technology has been used to measure central corneal thickness (CCT). CCT is an integral piece of data in patients with glaucoma, as it is known to cause artifacts in IOP readings, and thin CCT has been associated with increased glaucoma risk. Corneal thickness can be measured using optical pachymetry, Scheimpflug imaging, or ultrasound pachymetry which relies on the density and compressibility of the cornea to measure the amount of time needed for an ultrasound pulse to pass from and return to the transducer. Ultrasound pachymetry has

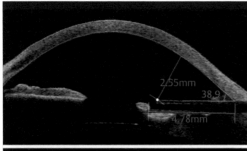

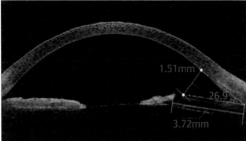

Fig. 9.6 Anterior segment optical coherence tomography (AS-OCT) of anterior chamber tube placement. The top image shows a glaucoma tube in the anterior chamber, and the bottom image shows a glaucoma tube in the sulcus entering the anterior chamber through the iris. Measurements of the AS-OCT parameters are shown.

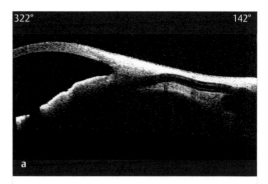

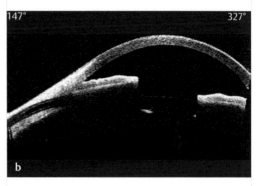

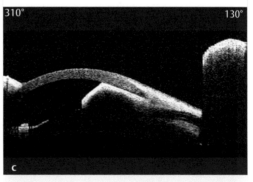

Fig. 9.7 Anterior segment optical coherence tomography (AS-OCT) of examples of sulcus tube placements, with and without peripheral anterior synechiae (PAS). Images from three different eyes are shown. **(a)** A typical example of a well-positioned sulcus tube. **(b)** An example where the sulcus tube is pushing the iris forward toward the cornea. **(c)** An example of significant PAS in a patient with traumatic glaucoma.

become more popular than optical pachymetry due to ease of use. Though there is some contradiction in the literature, generally compared to measurements taken with ultrasound pachymetry, CCT measured by AS-OCT measures 16 to 26 μm lower.[18,19] Some have reported no difference between the two modalities[64] and some have described thicker measurements with AS-OCT.

Lastly, AS-OCT can prove useful in following glaucoma in patients who have undergone Boston type I keratoprosthesis. In addition to providing information about the graft–host interface, AS-OCT can assess for the formation of PAS and angle closure. There is a high incidence of glaucoma in patients who have undergone this procedure, and often no view, gonioscopically or otherwise, to the anterior chamber angle. A prospective study of patients who had undergone this procedure found that 75% of patients with progression of anatomic angle narrowing on AS-OCT had no signs on clinical examination, emphasizing the potential value of this adjuvant imaging in these challenging patients.[20]

9.7 Conclusions

AS-OCT provides noncontact, quick, easy-to-obtain, detailed, high-resolution images of the anterior segment. This technology has led to improved understanding of the anatomical correlates of many glaucomatous conditions including PACD. In addition, AS-OCT can play a valuable role in the diagnosis and management of glaucoma through detailed qualitative and quantitative analysis of the anterior segment and anterior segment angle, though it is not an absolute substitute for gonioscopy. Although there are limitations to this technology including the inability to image beyond the posterior iris, it has a clear and evolving role in the management of glaucoma.

References

[1] Huang D, Swanson EA, Lin CP, et al. Optical coherence tomography. Science. 1991; 254(5035):1178–1181

[2] Dada T, Sihota R, Gadia R, Aggarwal A, Mandal S, Gupta V. Comparison of anterior segment optical coherence tomography and ultrasound biomicroscopy for assessment of the anterior segment. J Cataract Refract Surg. 2007; 33(5):837–840

[3] Leung CK, Weinreb RN. Anterior chamber angle imaging with optical coherence tomography. Eye (Lond). 2011; 25(3):261–267

[4] Leung CK, Li H, Weinreb RN, et al. Anterior chamber angle measurement with anterior segment optical coherence tomography: a comparison between slit lamp OCT and Visante OCT. Invest Ophthalmol Vis Sci. 2008; 49(8):3469–3474

[5] Smith SD, Singh K, Lin SC, et al. Evaluation of the anterior chamber angle in glaucoma: a report by the American Academy of Ophthalmology. Ophthalmology. 2013; 120 (10):1985–1997

[6] Narayanaswamy A, Sakata LM, He MG, et al. Diagnostic performance of anterior chamber angle measurements for detecting eyes with narrow angles: an anterior segment OCT study. Arch Ophthalmol. 2010; 128(10):1321–1327

[7] Sakata LM, Lavanya R, Friedman DS, et al. Assessment of the scleral spur in anterior segment optical coherence tomography images. Arch Ophthalmol. 2008; 126(2):181–185

[8] Sakata LM, Lavanya R, Friedman DS, et al. Comparison of gonioscopy and anterior segment ocular coherence tomography in detecting angle closure in different quadrants of the anterior chamber angle. Ophthalmology. 2008; 115(5):769–774

[9] Matsuki T, Hirose F, Ito S, Hata M, Hirami Y, Kurimoto Y. Influence of anterior segment biometric parameters on the anterior chamber angle width in eyes with angle closure. J Glaucoma. 2015; 24(2):144–148

[10] Han S, Sung KR, Lee KS, Hong JW. Outcomes of laser peripheral iridotomy in angle closure subgroups according to anterior segment optical coherence tomography parameters. Invest Ophthalmol Vis Sci. 2014; 55(10):6795–6801

[11] Hirose F, Hata M, Ito S, Matsuki T, Kurimoto Y. Light-dark changes in iris thickness and anterior chamber angle width in eyes with occludable angles. Graefes Arch Clin Exp Ophthalmol. 2013; 251(10):2395–2402

[12] Nonaka A, Kondo T, Kikuchi M, et al. Angle widening and alteration of ciliary process configuration after cataract surgery for primary angle closure. Ophthalmology. 2006; 113 (3):437–441

[13] Ramakrishnan R, Mitra A, Abdul Kader M, Das S. To study the efficacy of laser peripheral iridoplasty in the treatment of eyes with primary angle closure and plateau iris syndrome, unresponsive to laser peripheral iridotomy, using anterior-segment OCT as a tool. J Glaucoma. 2016; 25(5):440–446

[14] Ciancaglini M, Carpineto P, Agnifili L, et al. Filtering bleb functionality: a clinical, anterior segment optical coherence tomography and in vivo confocal microscopy study. J Glaucoma. 2008; 17(4):308–317

[15] Kojima S, Inoue T, Nakashima K, Fukushima A, Tanihara H. Filtering blebs using 3-dimensional anterior-segment optical coherence tomography: a prospective investigation. JAMA Ophthalmol. 2015; 133(2):148–156

[16] Jung KI, Lim SA, Park HY, Park CK. Visualization of blebs using anterior-segment optical coherence tomography after glaucoma drainage implant surgery. Ophthalmology. 2013; 120 (5):978–983

[17] Fea AM, Spinetta R, Cannizzo PML, et al. Evaluation of bleb morphology and reduction in IOP and glaucoma medication following implantation of a novel gel stent. J Ophthalmol. 2017; 2017:9364910

[18] Kim HY, Budenz DL, Lee PS, Feuer WJ, Barton K. Comparison of central corneal thickness using anterior segment optical coherence tomography vs ultrasound pachymetry. Am J Ophthalmol. 2008; 145(2):228–232

[19] Zhao PS, Wong TY, Wong WL, Saw SM, Aung T. Comparison of central corneal thickness measurements by visante anterior segment optical coherence tomography with ultrasound pachymetry. Am J Ophthalmol. 2007; 143(6):1047–1049

[20] Qian CX, Hassanaly S, Harissi-Dagher M. Anterior segment optical coherence tomography in the long-term follow-up and detection of glaucoma in Boston type I keratoprosthesis. Ophthalmology. 2015; 122(2):317–325

9

10 Special Considerations: OCT in Childhood Glaucoma

Tanya S. Glaser, Michael P. Kelly, Mays A. El-Dairi, and Sharon F. Freedman

Summary

Optical coherence tomography (OCT) is an important tool for managing glaucoma in children, particularly as children with glaucoma, especially younger children, are not able to perform visual field testing. Special considerations when performing OCT imaging in children with glaucoma include how to optimize and maximize the child's attention and cooperation for image acquisition, as well as how to interpret the OCT results in light of normal ocular development and ocular variations among children. This chapter provides a summary of how OCT can be performed in pediatric patients and also clinical pearls for image acquisition. Suggestions for OCT image interpretation for children and pitfalls to avoid are also discussed.

Keywords: pediatric glaucoma, congenital glaucoma, juvenile, infant, handheld OCT, portable OCT

10.1 Introduction

Glaucoma, being a progressive optic neuropathy, should ideally be monitored via objective functional and structural testing. Children with glaucoma should be monitored similarly to adults with glaucoma; however, the gold standard functional test (visual field testing) is almost impossible to obtain in the younger children. Of the available structural tests, optical coherence tomography (OCT), specifically spectral-domain OCT (SD-OCT), has become an important tool in managing glaucoma due to its ease of use and interpretation, high reproducibility, and sensitivity for progression.[1] For older, cooperative children, tabletop OCT can be used as in adults to aid in screening for and diagnosing of glaucoma, as well as for monitoring known glaucoma cases for progression. In infants and young children, handheld OCT devices are becoming more widely available, allowing for earlier analysis of optic nerve head and peripapillary retinal nerve fiber layer (pRNFL) features.

As we learn more about childhood glaucoma and its pathophysiology, we are discovering that there are special considerations for OCT in these children, including acquisition, anatomic and behavioral challenges, and interpretation. Although there are no published guidelines as to frequency and timing of OCT studies, we will describe what we do in our pediatric glaucoma practice.

10.2 Handheld and Portable OCT Imaging Modalities

The development of SD-OCT, with faster acquisition times and improved resolution compared to older OCT technology, has made imaging of children easier. The design of overhead mounted or handheld systems has allowed for supine imaging of awake neonates and infants, as well as anesthetized children undergoing examination or surgery. One common commercially used handheld OCT device is the Envisu C-class (previously Bioptigen, now Leica Microsystems, Wetzlar, Germany/NC, USA). This device has been used to successfully image infants in the office without anesthesia, as well as those in the operating room. The device is noncontact, can be performed through an undilated pupil, and can image both the anterior and posterior segments. Unfortunately, the Envisu C-class lacks automatic registration and automated analysis of the pRNFL or retinal layers, which are useful in the evaluation of glaucoma. We find this device to be most useful for qualitative information about the optic nerve, but less helpful for following changes in the ganglion cell and nerve fiber layers over time and identifying subtle changes.

The Spectralis (Heidelberg Engineering, Germany) tabletop model that has been converted for off-label handheld supine use,[2] and the OCT Spectralis with FLEX module (Heidelberg Engineering, Germany) are currently being used as research devices while awaiting FDA approval. The benefit of the Spectralis with FLEX module is the integrated software that allows for automated segmentation of retinal layers and familiar optic nerve head analysis, which is the same as the tabletop device used for older children and adults. The device also has eye-tracking and automated registration, which are necessary for obtaining aligned follow-up imaging and recognizing subtle changes among serial scans.

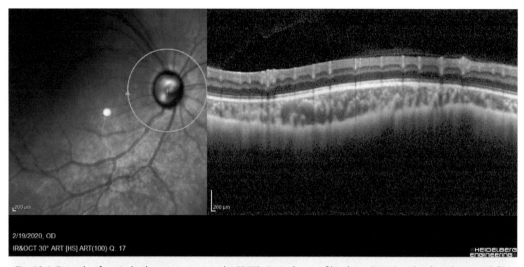

Fig. 10.1 Example of optical coherence tomography (OCT). Retinal nerve fiber layer (RNFL) with infrared image (*left*) circle scan (*right*) of a child with advanced glaucoma and nystagmus. OCT imaging was only possible under anesthesia with cessation of nystagmus.

10.3 Image Acquisition

10.3.1 How OCT Can be Used during Examination Under Anesthesia

For children too young to cooperate with tabletop OCT, handheld or overhead-mounted OCT imaging can be completed during examination under anesthesia or during anesthesia for ocular surgery. We generally perform this step after intraocular pressure (IOP) has been measured and the child's airway stabilized with either a laryngeal mask or endotracheal tube (as appropriate for the situation), but before B-scan ultrasound or photographic imaging, as the gel applied for these modalities can be hard to clear and may degrade the subsequent OCT images. We use an eyelid speculum during imaging. Anesthetic depth may need to be increased if the eyes are rotated upward or downward, as midline eyes are needed for optimal OCT imaging. Frequent topical lubricant drops are used as the ocular surface can dry quickly, which will degrade the OCT image. Knowledge of the patient's refractive error helps to focus the camera. Lastly, the imager must be adept at monitoring the proximity of the OCT device to the patient's cornea while simultaneously adjusting the direction and focus of the unit to capture the area of interest. In our institution, for clinical care we use the handheld Envisu (formally Bioptigen) OCT and for research we use the FLEX OCT.

We have found OCT performed during anesthesia to be helpful for infants, uncooperative children, or children with intellectual disability, as well as patients with poor visual fixation due to poor vision or nystagmus (which resolves under general anesthesia) (▶ Fig. 10.1).

10.3.2 Tabletop OCT for Children

Children over the age of 5 years are generally able to cooperate with tabletop OCT, though it is reasonable to attempt imaging on children as young as 3 years old, provided you have an experienced photographer, visual fixation is intact with minimal nystagmus, and there is a clear visual axis. To perform OCT imaging the child is seated in front of the imaging device. Depending on the child's height it might be easier for them to kneel on the chair or stand with their head resting on the chin rest, similarly to how they would be examined at the slit lamp. Smaller children can sit on a parent's or guardian's lap. For glaucoma evaluation, we like to have the following protocols: a peripapillary RNFL scan (or circle scan), a 61-line volume scan over macula, as well as attempting a Glaucoma

Lastly, the Optovue (Fremont, CA, USA) offers as a tabletop OCT and can be configured and used off-label as handheld device. Similar to the Spectralis, this device offers retinal tracking and automated analysis of the optic nerve and retina.

10

Table 10.1 Tips and tricks for acquiring OCT images in children

Pupil dilation is helpful in capturing an image, but imaging can be performed on the undilated or undilatable pupil, provided the visual axis is clear and fixation steady. Dilation is helpful for patients with nystagmus or poor fixation as it can make image acquisition easier and improve image quality.

Identify for the imager which eye and what specifically are the **areas of most interest**, as well as the fixation capability of each eye.

Plan and **prioritize in advance** which OCT scans are to be obtained, to facilitate efficiency and ensure complete OCT documentation.

Ready the device prior to bringing the child into the imaging room. Enter the demographic information into the imaging device, set the scan parameters and activate the first scan to be captured before bringing in the child and parent/guardian.

Turn the monitor away from and out of view of the child as it can be distracting.

In order to build trust, greet the parent/guardian and the child warmly by name. **Start with the room lights on** and provide a brief description of the imaging while adjusting the device to the height of the child.

Use the foot pedal for image capture, freeing both hands to manage the device and patient.

Start with the area of greatest interest when beginning to scan the eye. For example, if the RNFL is critical, scan the RNFL in both eyes first to ensure capture, then attempt macular scanning.

If the child refuses, **offer to scan the parent/guardian** or an available older sibling to reduce anxiety and provide assurance.

Consider an animated fixation target, such as cartoons on a portable screen, positioned behind the examiner (a parent's cell phone can often do the trick).

If fixation is drifting or if there are other difficulties with capture, **be prepared to reduce image averaging** (ART level), density and/or size of volume scan, or length of scan line, in order to speed up the testing time and achieve capture. And, as a last resort, turn off eye tracking, but know that the scan quality will be reduced and follow-up eye-tracked scanning will not be possible. (Eye tracking eliminates blink artifacts and allows for the follow-up scans to be in the exact same location.)

If fixation is achieved but drifts by a small amount, engage eye tracking and then **move the scan pattern on screen** with the mouse over the desired location.

It can sometimes be useful to **patch one eye when scanning the other** if the patient is struggling with fixation but able to see well enough to fixate with the eye being imaged.

Consider using a wide field OCT lens if both macula and optic nerve imaging is desired, as one scan can then capture both fully.

For high myopes, vertical line scanning can sometimes provide better volume scan alignment and coverage compared to horizontal line scanning for the macula.

Abbreviations: ART, automatic real time; OCT, optical coherence tomography; RNFL, retinal nerve fiber layer.

Module Premium Edition (GMPE, specific to Spectralis). ▶ Table 10.1 summarizes practical strategies for successful image acquisition.

10.3.3 Structural Considerations for Image Acquisition

Any type of media opacity can make OCT imaging difficult. Corneal scarring, clouding or Haab striae, especially if in the central cornea, can preclude imaging. Anterior segment dysgenesis, iris irregularities, and cataract can also make imaging challenging (▶ Fig. 10.2). In glaucoma following cataract surgery, it can be very challenging to focus the camera in aphakic eyes with large refractive errors. We often find that the en-face view and the OCT image cannot be focused at the same time. In severe glaucoma, the long axial length and the high myopia that are often present can also make OCT device focus challenging. It is critical in these cases to review the imaging quality and assess for any segmentation failures before interpreting the study.

10.4 Interpreting OCT Images in Pediatric Glaucoma

10.4.1 Optical and Anatomic Considerations for Image Acquisition and Interpretation

There are several anatomic changes that impact refraction and optics in very young eyes and must

10

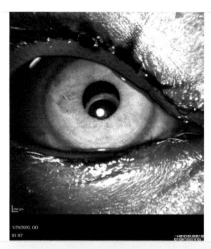 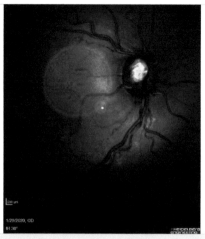

Fig. 10.2 Example of successful optical coherence tomography (OCT) imaging through a poorly dilated pupil with the visual axis limited by the small opening in the anterior capsule with Soemmering ring in this aphakic eye. External view demonstrating pupil size (*left*) and infrared image (*right*). We have been successful in imaging the optic nerve and fundus in some eyes where the size of the pupil precludes an indirect fundoscopic examination.

be considered when obtaining and interpreting OCT images. The greatest increase in axial length occurs after birth until about age 2 to 3 years, with an increase of about 2 mm every year. After age 5 or 6 years, the axial length increases by only about 1 mm more to reach its adult length.[3] There is minimal increase in axial length after age 10 to 15 years, in normal eyes. Corneal curvature also undergoes the largest change in the first few months of life. The neonatal cornea is steeper, with a mean keratometry value of 51.2 diopters at birth and 44.9 diopters by age 1 to 2 years. There is no significant change in corneal curvature after the age of 6 months.[3] Refraction and astigmatism also vary with age.

Due to the shorter axial length of the infant eye, the OCT image of the infant eye is magnified compared to that of an adult. In other words, there is an inverse relationship between axial length and retinal image size.[4] To summarize, due to these optical differences, the scan length in an infant is proportionally less (depending on age) than the scan length that is presumed for an adult. Work from Maldonado et al suggests age-specific imaging protocols to account for these optical changes[5,6] when using the handheld Bioptigen Envisu C-class. For the Spectralis FLEX, only the corneal curvature measurement can be adjusted.

There are small, but reproducible OCT measurement changes that occur with changing eye dimensions. Cross-sectional studies have suggested that the normative OCT values for pRNFL

vary with axial length for white children, with the average pRNFL thickness decreasing by about 2.6 μm with every 1-mm increase in axial length.[7] Similarly, in very young children (ages 0 to 5 years) mean pRNFL was inversely related to axial length.[8] It is possible that the inverse relationship between axial length and pRNFL thickness may be, at least in part, be due to a magnification artifact of OCT imaging, the result of a relative increase in the diameter of the projected circle scan and smaller size of the optic disc image with increasing axial length.[4,9,10] Practically, however, a 1.0 mm change in axial length (less than what is expected as a change in axial length from age 3 to 18 years) engenders a 2 to 3 μm change in pRNFL, which is less than the inter-test reproducibility of the OCT machine.

The relationship between age and pRNFL thickness seems to vary by study, with some studies suggesting a positive linear correlation of the average RNFL thickness with age[11] and others finding no relationship,[7] especially after controlling for variables such as refractive error.[8,12] Age, especially in very young children (less than 3 years), does seem to correlate with retinal layer thickness, especially near the fovea.[8] Specifically, the ganglion cell layer (GCL), inner nuclear layer (INL), and ganglion cell complex (GCC, which is the combined volumes of the macular nerve fiber layer, the GCL, and the inner plexiform layer) volumes showed an inverse relationship with age, while the photoreceptor layer's volume (calculated by combining the

Table 10.2 Summary of mean peripapillary retinal nerve fiber layers thickness across multiple studies of normal eyes of children using SD-OCT

Study	OCT	Age (mean, range, years)	n	Mean (µm)	SD (µm)
Rotruck et al[8]	Spectralis	2.3 (0–5)	56	107.6	10.3
Turk et al[14]	Spectralis	10.5 (6–16)	107	106.5	9.4
Yanni et al[13]	Spectralis	8.9 (5–15)	85	107.6	1.2
Al-Haddad et al[15,†]	Cirrus	10.7 (6–17)	108	95.6	8.7
Elía et al[17]	Cirrus	9.2 (6–13)	344	98.5	10.8
Barrio-Barrio et al[16,††]	Cirrus	9.6 (4–17)	283	97.4	9.0
El-Dairi et al[7,†††]	Stratus (OCT3)	8.5 (3–17)	286	108.3	9.8
Salchow et al[12,††††]	Stratus (OCT3)	9.7 (4–17)	92	107	11.1
Qian et al[11,†††††]	Stratus (OCT3)	10.4 (5–18)	398	112.4	9.2

Abbreviations: RNFL, retinal nerve fiber layer; SD, standard deviation; SD-OCT, spectral-domain optical coherence tomography.
Notes: Study population racial background predominantly white unless otherwise stated.
† Study population 100% white Middle Eastern children.
†† Study population race not specified, enrolled from Spanish hospitals.
††† Study population 40% black and 54% white, when analyzed by race, black children had statistically larger RNFL thicknesses compared to white children (110.7 ± 8.84 µm vs. 105.9 ± 10.18 µm).
†††† Study population 92% Hispanic.
††††† Study population 100% Chinese.

volume of layers from the external limiting membrane to the Bruch's membrane), increased logarithmically until about 2 years of age.[8] This corresponds histologically to the maturation of the foveal pit and increasing density of cones in the postnatal period. The published mean central macular thickness for very young children (0–5 years) is lower than that of older children (5–16 years) and should be taken into consideration when considering macular changes related to glaucoma.[8]

In summary, we can safely assume that the average pRNFL should be reproducible for the normal eye of a healthy child over time. The pRNFL quadrants or clock hours are expected to change over time due to changes in the tilt of the optic nerve in the growing eye.

10.4.2 Comparing to a Normative Database

None of the available OCT machines and software has integrated a normalized pediatric database. Instead, these devices use adult normative data to set the measurement ranges and parameters. Since pRNFL measurements are expected to be thicker in children than in adults,[13] any results obtained must be interpreted against published normative OCT values for children. Normative pRNFL and macula values for very young children (ages 0 to 5

years) was recently published using the overhead-mounted Spectralis FLEX OCT device.[8] Across several studies the average pRNFL for older children was similar, though the measurements obtained by Cirrus, Spectralis, and Stratus OCT (OCT3, Carl Zeiss Meditec, Dublin, CA) devices are not interchangeable (▶ Table 10.1).[7,8,11,13,14,15,16,17] There are likely racial variations in pRNFL thickness, with one study showing that the pRNFL in black children is thicker than in white children of a similar age.[7] This difference, however, is smaller than the magnitude of thinning expected in pRNFL due to disease (such as glaucoma), especially when looking at the average values.

▶ Table 10.2 summarizes mean pRNFL thickness across multiple studies of normal eyes of children using SD-OCT.

10.4.3 OCT Changes in Childhood Glaucoma

The current classification system for childhood glaucoma is summarized in ▶ Table 10.3 and ▶ Table 10.4.[18,19]

Unfortunately, there is no universally agreed upon definition for what constitutes mild, moderate, and severe stage glaucoma for childhood glaucoma. Instead, definitions tend to be clinically derived, with more emphasis placed on relative

Table 10.3 Criteria/signs used to define childhood glaucoma

Children less than age 18 years (USA) with at least two of the following:
• IOP >21 mmHg
• Optic nerve cupping (increasing c/d, asymmetry ≥0.2, focal thinning)
• Haab striae or increased K diameter (corneal diameter >11 mm in newborns, >12 mm in children younger than 1 year old, and >13 mm in children >1 year old)
• Progressive myopia, myopic shift, or increased axial length
• Visual field defect (glaucomatous)

Abbreviation: IOP, intraocular pressure.

Table 10.4 Types of childhood glaucoma and definitions

Type of childhood glaucoma	Definition
Glaucoma following cataract surgery	Meets glaucoma definition and glaucoma diagnosed only after cataract surgery
Glaucoma associated with nonacquired primarily ocular and/or systemic disease or syndrome	Meets glaucoma definition and congenital eye anomalies or systemic syndrome
Glaucoma associated with acquired conditions	Meets glaucoma definition with history of trauma, uveitis, steroid use, tumor, ROP, etc.
Primary congenital glaucoma (PCG)	Meets glaucoma definition with buphthalmos. Defined as neonatal onset if ≤1 month old, infantile onset if between ages 1 to 24 months, and late onset if older than 2 years of age.
Juvenile open angle glaucoma (JOAG)	Meets glaucoma definition with open angle, no buphthalmos, or other acquired or nonacquired ocular or systemic conditions and usually older than 4 years of age.
Childhood glaucoma suspect	Defined as having at least one of the following signs: intraocular pressure >21 mmHg on two separate occasions, suspicious visual field defect for glaucoma, increased axial length in the setting of normal IOP, increased corneal diameter in the setting of normal IOP, or suspicious optic disc appearance for glaucoma.[18]

Abbreviations: IOP, intraocular pressure; ROP, retinopathy of prematurity.

changes and clinical signs of glaucoma progression. Adding complexity to the situation, optic nerve and visual field damage may occur very early on (as in primary congenital and other forms of infancy-onset glaucoma, ▶ Fig. 10.3), compounded by visual dysfunction from anatomic changes such as corneal opacity and distortion, and amblyopia in unilateral or asymmetric bilateral disease. There may therefore be children with poor vision whose glaucoma is nonetheless controlled, and those (especially in older-onset cases such as juvenile open-angle glaucoma [JOAG]), where good vision persists despite severe glaucomatous optic neuropathy and visual field loss. Unlike adult patients, where glaucoma severity is based mainly on visual field loss, reliable visual fields are often challenging in the pediatric population. OCT, therefore, provides clinicians with a powerful objective tool to document baseline optic nerve health, and to monitor for glaucomatous progression, especially in milder cases or early in the disease course. As in adults with advanced glaucoma, OCT is a less sensitive tool for diagnosing disease progression in children with advanced disease and severe RNFL thinning, since further changes in pRNFL are difficult to detect once the measurement floor is reached.[20]

The role of OCT in pediatric glaucoma is a growing field; however, there are limited studies to date. Ghasia et al looked at pediatric eyes without glaucoma, with physiologic cupping, with mild glaucoma, and with moderate-to-severe glaucoma (defined as optic nerve head damage or poor control, cup-to-disc ratio > 0.5, and IOP > 21 mmHg) and found that there was no difference in the average pRNFL between normal eyes (104 ± 9 μm), physiologic cupping (99 ± 6 μm), and mild glaucoma (98 ± 9 μm). However, eyes with moderate-to-severe glaucoma had significantly thinner pRNFL (62 ± 18 μm) compared to the three other groups.[21] A limitation of this study was the small number of patients, with only 13 eyes in the moderate-to-severe glaucoma group. El-Dairi et al found that compared to healthy eyes of normal

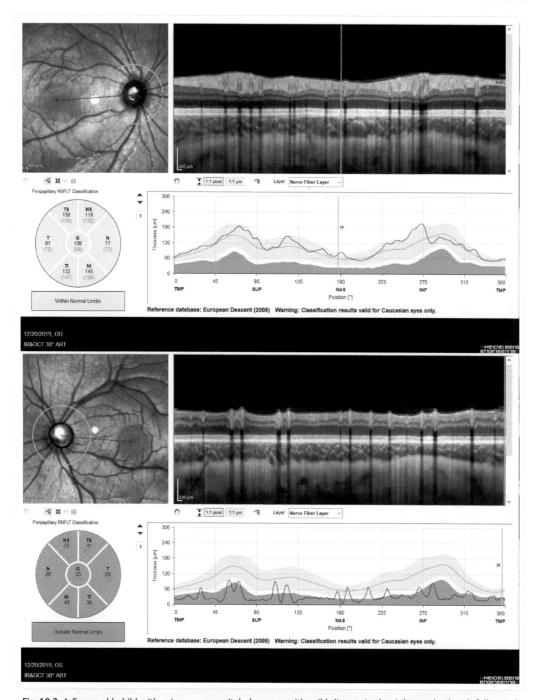

Fig. 10.3 A 5-year-old child with primary congenital glaucoma with mild disease in the right eye (*top*) with full retinal nerve fiber layer (RNFL) and advanced disease in the left eye with very thin RNFL (*bottom*). This patient was too young for reliable visual fields.

Table 10.5 Interpreting OCT of peripapillary RNFL in childhood glaucoma

Summary of RNFL findings

- Average pRNFL in advanced glaucoma (defined as optic nerve head damage or poor control, cup-to-disc ratio > 0.5, and IOP > 21 mmHg) was 62 ± 18 μm*
- Degree of pRNFL thinning inversely related to grade of glaucomatous damage determined by stereo photographs
- Degree of pRNFL thinning inversely related to cup-to-disc ratio
- The pattern of pRNFL loss in children can be diffuse instead of starting in the inferior and superior quadrants

Abbreviations: IOP, intraocular pressure; OCT, optical coherence tomography; pRNFL, peripapillary RNFL; RNFL, retinal nerve fiber layer.

Note: *Limited by small numbers, n = 13 eyes included in the moderate-to-severe glaucoma group

Table 10.6 Interpreting OCT of the macula in childhood glaucoma

Summary of OCT macular findings

- Macular volume is decreased in children with glaucoma
- GCC thickness is decreased in children with glaucoma
- The degree of GCC thinning corresponds to the cup-to-disc ratio

Abbreviations: GCC, ganglion cell complex; OCT, optical coherence tomography.

children, those with glaucoma had decreased average pRNFL thickness, with the degree of thinning increasing with increasing grade of glaucomatous damage as determined by review of stereo photographs.[22] Similarly, Srinivasan et al showed that older children who had undergone surgical treatment for primary congenital glaucoma (PCG) as infants had significantly thinner pRNFL when compared to healthy controls (86.4 ± 2.5 μm versus 113.6 ± 2.2 μm, respectively) and that pRNFL thickness correlated with the cup-to-disc ratio.[23] Morales-Fernandez et al also demonstrated thinner pRNFL in eyes diagnosed with PCG compared to healthy eyes (74.3 ± 26.3 μm versus 101.8 ± 9.9 μm, respectively).[24] Although adults typically exhibit initial pRNFL loss in the inferior and superior quadrants, several studies have suggested that pRNFL loss in children can be more diffuse, likely due to the severity of the disease at presentation.[22,23]

▶ Table 10.5 summarizes how to interpret OCT of pRNFL in childhood glaucoma.

Srinivasan et al also highlighted the importance of segmented macular volume scans in the evaluation of glaucoma. They showed that the GCC was decreased in children treated for PCG as infants. Furthermore, similar to pRNFL measures, the degree of GCC thinning correlated with the cup-to-disc ratio.[23] Similar results were published by Silverstein et al, who showed that eyes with glaucoma (PCG and JOAG) had significantly thinner mean macular nerve fiber layers, GCLs, and inner plexiform layers (the layers that make up the GCC).[25] In addition to GCC thinning, global macular volume was thinner in children with glaucoma compared to healthy controls.[25,26]

▶ Table 10.6 summarizes how to interpret OCT of the macula in childhood glaucoma.

Due to the observed changes in the retinal layers and macular volume associated with glaucomatous damage, we suggest that macular OCT scans, in addition to optic nerve scans, are important in the evaluation of children suspected of having, or known to have, glaucoma (▶ Fig. 10.4). When obtaining macular scans for pediatric glaucoma, remember that there may be abnormal but expected macular pathology in certain types of glaucoma associated with nonacquired system disease such as fovea plana in aniridia and choroidal hemangioma(s) in Sturge-Weber syndrome.

10.4.4 Postoperative Changes in OCT

Optic nerve head cupping reversal following IOP lowering in pediatric glaucoma is a well-known phenomenon, and thought to be an indicator of treatment success. However, despite the improved appearance of the optic nerve head on funduscopic examination, pRNFL thinning persists on OCT. Ely et al showed that the preoperative cup-to-disc ratio better predicted the postoperative pRNFL than the postoperative smaller "reversed" cup.[27] In other words, the appearance of the optic nerve head on funduscopic examination can be misleading in children treated for glaucoma and OCT may, in fact, be a better and more reliable indicator of optic nerve health.

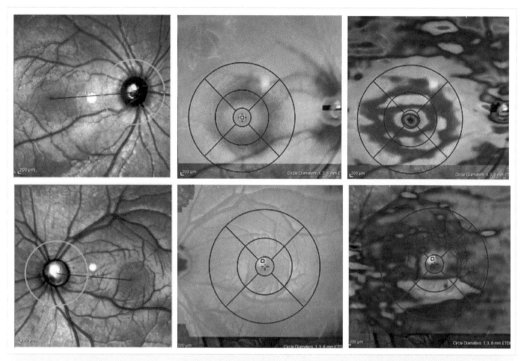

Fig. 10.4 A child with mild primary congenital glaucoma (PCG) (*top*) and advanced PCG (*bottom*). Note the advanced cupping on the infrared image (*bottom, left*). When comparing the top images to the bottom images, note that the eye with advanced glaucomatous optic atrophy shows corresponding macular thinning (*bottom, center*), most pronounced in the ganglion cell layer (*bottom, right*).

10

10.5 Pitfalls and Masqueraders of Pediatric Glaucoma

When using OCT to help evaluate for the presence of pediatric glaucoma, it is important also to consider masqueraders of glaucomatous optic neuropathy, especially if the other signs of glaucoma (elevated IOP, increasing axial length, myopic shift, or an enlarged cornea or Haab striae) are not present. Subtle optic nerve hypoplasia can present without the typical "double ring" sign, but with OCT showing diffuse thinning of the pRNFL that can mimic glaucoma. Patients with optic nerve hypoplasia should have smaller discs and cups, and many will also have associated hypoplastic fovea; the IOP should also be normal in these children.[28]

Any lesion that compresses the optic chiasm or optic nerve, such as a craniopharyngioma, pituitary adenoma, or optic pathway glioma, can lead to progressive pRNFL thinning over time and also nonglaucomatous cupping (▶ Fig. 10.5). Similarly, children with history of central nervous system disease, such as prior ventricular hemorrhage in premature infants, will likely later develop retrograde

pRNFL loss and cupping. These changes can mimic glaucomatous damage. As always, changes on OCT should be interpreted within the context of the entire clinical picture and medical history.

Other conditions with an anomalous optic nerve, such as optic nerve coloboma or optic disc pit, typically show chorioretinal–scleral excavation and a defect in the lamina cribrosa, respectively.[29] They may have associated maculopathy, retinoschisis, neovascularization, or herniation of retina into the optic nerve defect. OCT imaging of the macula can show subretinal fluid in these conditions.

Macular pathology on OCT can help differentiate glaucomatous and nonglaucomatous optic atrophy.[30] Specifically, changes to the outer retina should not be seen in glaucomatous optic atrophy in the absence of a history of uveitis or intraocular surgery. Inner-nuclear layer cysts are also much less common in glaucomatous optic atrophy compared to nonglaucomatous optic atrophy. Findings of outer retinal changes or inner-nuclear cysts should prompt an evaluation for causes of nonglaucomatous optic atrophy.

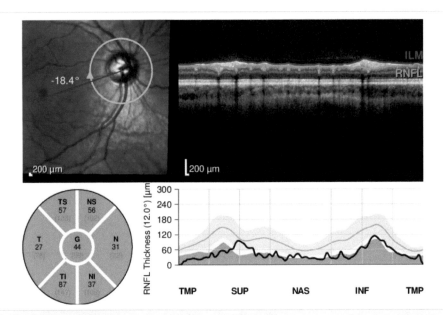

Fig. 10.5 Diffuse optic atrophy in a child with a history of a suprasellar pilocytic astrocytoma. Note the presence of nonglaucomatous cupping of the optic nerve in the infrared image (*top left*) reported as a 0.7 cup-to-disc ratio on fundoscopic examination.

Table 10.7 Examples of clinical scenarios and OCT imaging frequency

Clinical scenario	Suggested OCT imaging frequency
A child with elevated IOP but no other evidence of glaucoma	Recommend repeating imaging annually to watch for early evidence of OCT damage that would prompt more strict IOP control, etc.
A child with known glaucoma	The usual interval for OCT is annually, unless there is a period of very elevated IOP or an OCT showing loss that prompts a change in treatment such as a surgical intervention. In that case we usually repeat the OCT within several months, and continue at least every 6 months until the situation stabilizes and a new baseline is established.

Abbreviations: IOP, intraocular pressure; OCT, optical coherence tomography.

10.6 Imaging Guidelines and Recommended Frequency of Imaging

Tabletop OCT imaging of the optic nerve and macula is very useful to perform for any cooperative child with a relatively clear visual axis and central fixation (severe nystagmus can make it difficult to capture quality OCT images), who presents with known or suspected glaucoma, or even an abnormal finding such as an unusual-appearing optic nerve, macula, or isolated elevated IOP. If the OCT is normal, and the indication was an abnormal-appearing optic nerve head with normal IOP and vision, then it is reasonable to repeat in 1 year to verify the stability of the findings, and then only if something should change on the clinical examination. Alternatively, if one has a child with an abnormality, the frequency and number of times the OCT should be repeated depends upon the degree of suspicion for a true problem or the risk that it will develop.

▶ Table 10.7 summarizes OCT imaging frequency based on clinical scenarios in children.

For the general ophthalmologist or adult glaucoma specialist following now adult patients with a history of pediatric glaucoma we recommend following, treating, and managing as one would for adult-onset glaucoma.

References

[1] Xu L, Freedman SF, Silverstein E, Muir K, El-Dairi M. Longitudinal reproducibility of spectral domain optical coherence tomography in children with physiologic cupping and stable glaucoma. J AAPOS. 2019; 23(5):262.e1–262.e6

10

[2] Vinekar A, Sivakumar M, Shetty R, et al. A novel technique using spectral-domain optical coherence tomography (Spectralis, SD-OCT + HRA) to image supine non-anaesthetized infants: utility demonstrated in aggressive posterior retinopathy of prematurity. Eye (Lond). 2010; 24(2):379–382

[3] Gordon RA, Donzis PB. Refractive development of the human eye. Arch Ophthalmol. 1985; 103(6):785–789

[4] Sanchez-Cano A, Baraibar B, Pablo LE, Honrubia FM. Magnification characteristics of the Optical Coherence Tomograph STRATUS OCT 3000. Ophthalmic Physiol Opt. 2008; 28 (1):21–28

[5] Maldonado RS, Izatt JA, Sarin N, et al. Optimizing hand-held spectral domain optical coherence tomography imaging for neonates, infants, and children. Invest Ophthalmol Vis Sci. 2010; 51(5):2678–2685

[6] Vinekar A, Mangalesh S, Jayadev C, Maldonado RS, Bauer N, Toth CA. Retinal imaging of infants on spectral domain optical coherence tomography. BioMed Res Int. 2015; 2015:782420

[7] El-Dairi MA, Asrani SG, Enyedi LB, Freedman SF. Optical coherence tomography in the eyes of normal children. Arch Ophthalmol. 2009; 127(1):50–58

[8] Rotruck JC, House RJ, Freedman SF, et al. Optical coherence tomography normative peripapillary retinal nerve fiber layer and macular data in children 0–5 years of age. Am J Ophthalmol. 2019; 208:323–330

[9] Bayraktar S, Bayraktar Z, Yilmaz OF. Influence of scan radius correction for ocular magnification and relationship between scan radius with retinal nerve fiber layer thickness measured by optical coherence tomography. J Glaucoma. 2001; 10 (3):163–169

[10] Aykut V, Öner V, Taş M, Işcan Y, Ağaçhan A. Influence of axial length on peripapillary retinal nerve fiber layer thickness in children: a study by RTVue spectral-domain optical coherence tomography. Curr Eye Res. 2013; 38(12):1241–1247

[11] Qian J, Wang W, Zhang X, et al. Optical coherence tomography measurements of retinal nerve fiber layer thickness in Chinese children and teenagers. J Glaucoma. 2011; 20 (8):509–513

[12] Salchow DJ, Oleynikov YS, Chiang MF, et al. Retinal nerve fiber layer thickness in normal children measured with optical coherence tomography. Ophthalmology. 2006; 113 (5):786–791

[13] Yanni SE, Wang J, Cheng CS, et al. Normative reference ranges for the retinal nerve fiber layer, macula, and retinal layer thicknesses in children. Am J Ophthalmol. 2013; 155(2):354–360.e1

[14] Turk A, Ceylan OM, Arici C, et al. Evaluation of the nerve fiber layer and macula in the eyes of healthy children using spectral-domain optical coherence tomography. Am J Ophthalmol. 2012; 153(3):552–559.e1

[15] Al-Haddad C, Barikian A, Jaroudi M, Massoud V, Tamim H, Noureddin B. Spectral domain optical coherence tomography in children: normative data and biometric correlations. BMC Ophthalmol. 2014; 14:53

[16] Barrio-Barrio J, Noval S, Galdós M, et al. Multicenter Spanish study of spectral-domain optical coherence tomography in normal children. Acta Ophthalmol. 2013; 91(1):e56–e63

[17] Elía N, Pueyo V, Altemir I, Oros D, Pablo LE. Normal reference ranges of optical coherence tomography parameters in childhood. Br J Ophthalmol. 2012; 96(5):665–670

[18] Thau A, Lloyd M, Freedman S, Beck A, Grajewski A, Levin AV. New classification system for pediatric glaucoma: implications for clinical care and a research registry. Curr Opin Ophthalmol. 2018; 29(5):385–394

[19] Weinreb RN, Grajewski AL, Papadopoulos M, Grigg J, Freedman S, World Glaucoma Association. Childhood glaucoma: the 9th consensus report of the World Glaucoma Association. In: Consensus Series 9. Amsterdam, The Netherlands: Kugler Publications; 2013. https://wga.one/wga/consensus-9/

[20] Mwanza JC, Budenz DL, Warren JL, et al. Retinal nerve fibre layer thickness floor and corresponding functional loss in glaucoma. Br J Ophthalmol. 2015; 99(6):732–737

[21] Ghasia FF, Freedman SF, Rajani A, Holgado S, Asrani S, El-Dairi M. Optical coherence tomography in paediatric glaucoma: time domain versus spectral domain. Br J Ophthalmol. 2013; 97(7):837–842

[22] El-Dairi MA, Holgado S, Asrani SG, Enyedi LB, Freedman SF. Correlation between optical coherence tomography and glaucomatous optic nerve head damage in children. Br J Ophthalmol. 2009; 93(10):1325–1330

[23] Srinivasan S, Addepalli UK, Rao HL, Garudadri CS, Mandal AK. Spectral domain optical coherence tomography in children operated for primary congenital glaucoma. Br J Ophthalmol. 2014; 98(2):162–165

[24] Morales-Fernandez L, Jimenez-Santos M, Martinez-de-la-Casa JM, et al. Diagnostic capacity of SD-OCT segmented ganglion cell complex versus retinal nerve fiber layer analysis for congenital glaucoma. Eye (Lond). 2018; 32(8):1338–1344

[25] Silverstein E, Freedman S, Zéhil GP, Jiramongkolchai K, El-Dairi M. The macula in pediatric glaucoma: quantifying the inner and outer layers via optical coherence tomography automatic segmentation. J AAPOS. 2016; 20(4):332–336

[26] Hess DB, Asrani SG, Bhide MG, Enyedi LB, Stinnett SS, Freedman SF. Macular and retinal nerve fiber layer analysis of normal and glaucomatous eyes in children using optical coherence tomography. Am J Ophthalmol. 2005; 139(3):509–517

[27] Ely AL, El-Dairi MA, Freedman SF. Cupping reversal in pediatric glaucoma—evaluation of the retinal nerve fiber layer and visual field. Am J Ophthalmol. 2014; 158(5):905–915

[28] Pilat A, Sibley D, McLean RJ, Proudlock FA, Gottlob I. High-resolution imaging of the optic nerve and retina in optic nerve hypoplasia. Ophthalmology. 2015; 122(7):1330–1339

[29] Jeng-Miller KW, Cestari DM, Gaier ED. Congenital anomalies of the optic disc: insights from optical coherence tomography imaging. Curr Opin Ophthalmol. 2017; 28(6):579–586

[30] Jiramongkolchai K, Freedman SF, El-Dairi MA. Retinal changes in pediatric glaucoma and nonglaucomatous optic atrophy. Am J Ophthalmol. 2016; 161:188–95.e1

10

11 Special Considerations: High Refractive Errors

Ki Ho Park and Yong Woo Kim

Summary

As optical coherence tomography (OCT) uses optical principles to evaluate the retinal and optic nerve head (ONH) structures, special care must be taken when interpreting the OCT scans of eyes with high refractive errors. The prevalence of myopia is dramatically increasing in younger generations, especially in East and Southeast Asian countries. Given that myopia is an important risk factor for development of glaucoma, clinicians have to face challenging OCT cases in distinguishing glaucomatous changes in eyes with high myopia. The structural deformation common in highly myopic eyes, such as tilted disc, peripapillary atrophy, or posterior staphyloma, makes it difficult not only to obtain a clear image of an OCT scan but also to specify glaucomatous change from physiologically healthy status. The first half of this chapter describes the causes of OCT scan errors (i.e., ocular magnification errors, scan-circle diameter and location, insufficiency of normative database population, segmentation errors) that are incurred due to the anatomical characteristics of high myopia. The second half of this chapter introduces the new parameters additional to peripapillary retinal nerve fiber layer (RNFL) thickness (i.e., macular ganglion cell structure, Bruch's membrane opening (BMO)-based neuroretinal rim thickness) that are used for improved accuracy of glaucoma diagnosis in highly myopic eyes.

Keywords: high myopia, ocular magnification error, red disease, temporal raphe sign, Bruch's membrane opening-based minimum rim width, three-dimensional neuroretinal rim thickness, three-dimensional wide-field map

11.1 Introduction

Refractive errors, including myopia and hyperopia, prevent light from reaching the retina with precision focus. This affects visual acuity, certainly, but it can also impact the results of optical coherence tomography (OCT) imaging, which uses optical principles to observe the structure of the retina and optic nerve head (ONH). Changes in the ocular structure associated with refractive errors can influence the risk of developing glaucoma.

Hyperopic eyes are associated with a narrow angle, which increases the risk of primary angle-closure glaucoma (PACG). On the other hand, myopia is one of the major risk factors for development of primary open-angle glaucoma (POAG). When interpreting OCT images of eyes with high refractive error for diagnosis and monitoring of glaucoma, differing attention for myopic and hyperopic eyes is needed, in the following aspects: (1) careful anterior segment examination is more meaningful for PACG risk assessment in hyperopic eyes (discussed in Chapter 9); (2) structural anomalies of the posterior segment common to highly myopic eyes, such as tilted disc, chorioretinal and peripapillary atrophy, or posterior staphyloma, not only mimic glaucomatous change but also affect OCT scan characteristics.

Half of the world's population (approximately 5 billion people) is projected to be myopic by 2050, with as much as 10% highly myopic.[1] In developed countries in East and Southeast Asia, there is currently a myopia epidemic, the prevalence of myopia increasing more markedly at younger ages, reaching 80 to 90%. In the future, given that the risk of glaucoma increases as these generations age, clinicians will be challenged to interpret those eyes' OCT scans to distinguish glaucoma from myopia. This chapter summarizes the considerations for interpreting OCT scans in highly myopic eyes and provides practical tips for using OCT scans to improve the accuracy of glaucoma diagnosis in such eyes. The first half of this chapter discusses the causes of OCT scan errors due to the anatomical characteristics of high myopia as well as the cautions to be heeded in interpreting them; the second half introduces the new parameters for improved diagnosis of glaucoma in highly myopic eyes.

11.2 Technical Issues of OCT that Need to be Considered in High Myopia

11.2.1 Scan-Circle Size: Ocular Magnification Error

The commercially available OCT devices provide peripapillary retinal nerve fiber layer (RNFL)

thickness data as measured at a certain distance from the center of the optic disc. In order to derive the true size of an object on the fundus, it is necessary to take into account the curvature of the cornea, the anterior chamber depth, and the axial length, all of which contribute to the characteristics of the reflected image on the fundus. The relationship between the measurement of the OCT image and the actual fundus size can be expressed as $t = p \times q \times s$, where t is the actual fundus size, p is the magnification factor related to the camera of the OCT imaging system (known as 3.382 in the Cirrus HD-OCT system), q is the magnification factor related to the eye, and s is the measurement on OCT.[2] The ocular magnification factor q (in millimeters per degree) can be determined with the formula $q = 0.01306 \times (x - 1.82)$, where x is the axial length. In the case of Cirrus HD-OCT (Carl Zeiss Meditec, Dublin, CA, USA), the default axial length is 24.46 mm, and the scanning radius for the peripapillary RNFL scanning protocol is set to 1.73 mm. If the axial length of the eye is greater than the default (24.46 mm), which is a common condition in highly myopic eyes, the scanning radius is magnified (greater than 1.73 mm), and this effect, the so-called "magnification error," can skew the measurement of RNFL thickness.

The actual average RNFL thickness at the 1.73-mm-radius circle can be estimated according to the assumptions that (1) all of the retinal nerve fibers emerging from the retinal ganglion cells (RGCs) exit the eyeball through the ONH; (2) if the same number of retinal nerve fibers cross the different-sized circles with the same center, the larger scan circle will have a lower average RNFL thickness; and (3) the total cross-sectional areas of the retinal nerve fibers under the different circles will be equal, because the same number of retinal nerve fibers cross the circles.

The total cross-sectional area of the RNFL and the magnified radius of the scan circle can be estimated in the following equations:

Equation 1.

Total cross-sectional area of RNFL
$$= \text{(observed average RNFL thickness)} \times 2\pi \times \text{(magnified radius)}$$
$$= \text{(actual average RNFL thickness at 1.73 mm radius circle)} \times 2\pi \times 1.73 \; mm$$

Equation 2.

$$\text{Magnified radius} = 1.73 \times 3.382 \times 0.01306 \times \text{(axial length} - 1.82)$$

From Equations 1 and 2, the actual average RNFL thickness can be estimated as follows:
Equation 3.

Actual average RNFL thickness at 1.73 mm radius circle
$$= 3.382 \times 0.01306 \times \text{(axial length} - 1.82) \times \text{observed average RNFL thickness}$$

In the case of an eye with an axial length of 26.0 mm and an observed average RNFL thickness of 76 µm, the actual average RNFL thickness at the 1.73-mm-radius circle can be estimated as $3.382 \times 0.01306 \times (26.0 - 1.82) \times 76 = 81.17$ µm.

Spectralis OCT (Heidelberg Engineering, Heidelberg, Germany) uses a 3.5-mm-diameter scan circle and adjusts for ocular magnification error by entering the keratometry values of the subject. However, adjustment for ocular magnification error is not always ideal; that is, due to the fact that the optic disc size can also increase with myopia, even if the actual scanning radius is greater than 1.73 mm, it may not always indicate that the RNFL is being measured farther from the disc margin.[3] In this sense, the axial length and the optic disc size should be considered together when interpreting the RNFL thickness data from OCT scans in highly myopic eyes.

11.2.2 Scan-Circle Size: Pathologies Influencing the Scan Circle

Peripapillary pathologies, such as peripapillary atrophy (PPA), myelinated nerve fiber layers, or even vitreous floaters can invade the scanning circle area and affect RNFL thickness measurements. ▶ Fig. 11.1 shows a representative case of large PPA in highly myopic eyes invading the scanning circle. This can cause segmentation errors in the area of PPA and result in false-positive red signs on the color-coded map.

Spectralis OCT provides three peripapillary circle scans with diameters of 3.5, 4.1, and 4.7 mm. All of the circle scans are aligned to the individual fovea-to-BMO-center axis (BMO: Bruch's membrane opening). ▶ Fig. 11.2 shows the Spectralis OCT scan result for the same subject as in ▶ Fig. 11.1, demonstrating that the outer circle enables better measurement of the RNFL thickness. ▶ Fig. 11.3 shows another case with vitreous floater invading the scan circle, causing segmentation error and, newly in this case, false-positive

11

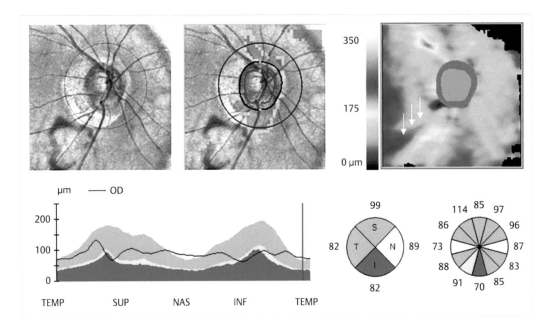

Fig. 11.1 Artifacts invading scan circle: large peripapillary atrophy. Cirrus HD-OCT scan of right eye of a 59-year-old male with high myopia. His refraction was –5.25 D, and the axial length was 26.66 mm. Retinal nerve fiber layer (RNFL) defect on red-free RNFL photography was hard to identify. Humphrey visual field (HVF) test revealed a within-normal-range visual field. A Cirrus HD-OCT optic disc cube scan reported the red sign in the inferior sector. The deviation map showed defects in the superior and inferior regions, and the thickness map revealed a slit-like defect in the inferotemporal area (*white arrows*). Note the large peripapillary atrophy (PPA) invading the scan circle and the vitreous floater in the inferotemporal area. These artifacts limit the ability to confirm OCT scan results.

red sign. Taken together, it should be kept in mind that any pathologies invading the scan circle can affect the segmentation outcome of RNFL and, in turn, the resulting thickness measurements.

11.2.3 Scan-Circle Location: Effect of Major Vessels in Tilted Discs

In myopic eyes, the process of emmetropization occurs by axial elongation and induces stretching of the peripapillary structure, usually in the temporal direction. The BMO enlarges with the development of gamma-zone PPA, and the optic disc changes to a more oval and tilted shape. At the same time, the major arcade vessels converge into the macular area, reducing the angle between the major superotemporal and inferotemporal blood vessels. Since the RNFL is distributed along the major blood vessels, the temporalization of those vessels as induced by axial elongation can alter the peak distribution of the RNFL (temporal deviation of RNFL humps, ▶ Fig. 11.4). The altered distribution of the peripapillary RNFL can lead to false-positive red signs in the superior and inferior

sectors and to relatively thickened RNFL in the temporal sector.

In Cirrus HD-OCT, these phenomena can be reduced by correcting the scan-circle location according to the center of the BMO rather than the center of the scleral canal opening.[4] This method of scan-circle correction originates from the idea that the temporal edge of the temporal PPA (approximately coincides with the BMO) and nasal scleral lip might be the original optic disc margin and the appropriate landmark for OCT RNFL thickness measurement. By manually moving the scan circle in a more temporal direction, the location of the superior and inferior peaks can be widened, thereby reducing false-positive errors (▶ Fig. 11.5).

11.2.4 Normative Database

The commercially available OCT devices compare their measurement values with the internal normative database and provide color codes as green (normal range), yellow (outside 95% normal limit), red (outside 99% normal limit), or white (thicker than normal range), accordingly. For Cirrus HD-

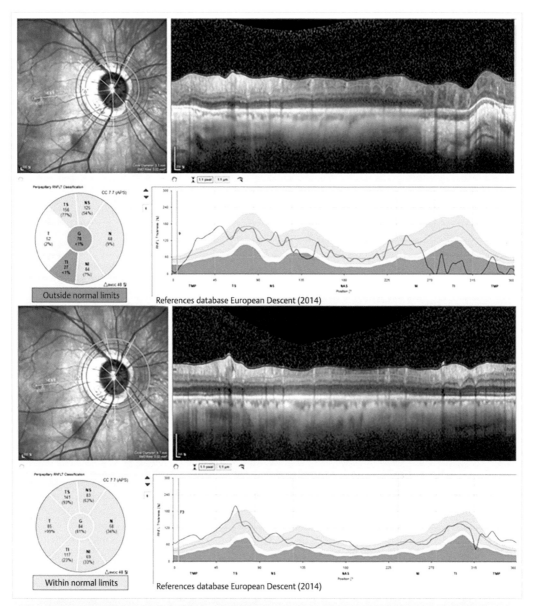

Fig. 11.2 Scan-circle diameter adjustment by Spectralis optical coherence tomography (OCT). Spectralis OCT scan of the same eye as in ▶ Fig. 11.1. The Glaucoma Module Premium Edition (GMPE) software provides three peripapillary circle scans with diameters of 3.5, 4.1, and 4.7 mm. All of the circle scans are aligned to the individual fovea-to-Bruch's membrane opening (BMO)-center axis. Note the segmentation error with the 3.5-mm scan circle in the inferotemporal area due to peripapillary atrophy (PPA). The larger scan-circle diameter (4.7 mm) enabled better evaluation and measurement of the retinal nerve fiber layer (RNFL) thickness. Since averaging can hide focal axonal defects on the color-coded classification chart, it is strongly recommended to have a detailed view to the height profile. The focal defect in the inferotemporal region (*black arrow*), which may be related to the inferotemporal defect on the Cirrus HD-OCT thickness map, needs to be monitored closely.

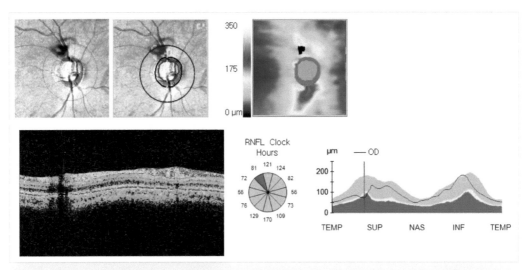

Fig. 11.3 Artifacts invading scan circle: vitreous floater. Cirrus HD-OCT scan of right eye of a 50-year-old female with myopia (axial length = 24.78 mm). Note the vitreous floater invading the scan circle in the superotemporal area and the resulting segmentation error in the same area. The retinal nerve fiber layer (RNFL) clock-hour map reported a false-positive red sign and a pseudo-defect on the temporal-superior-nasal-inferior-temporal (TSNIT) map at the site of the vitreous floater.

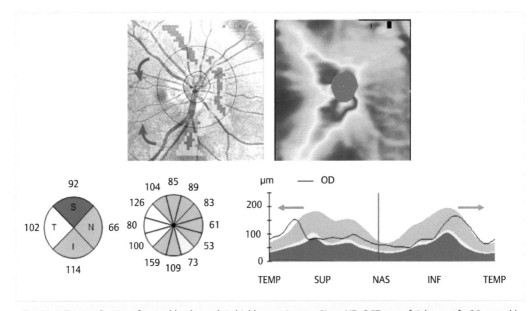

Fig. 11.4 Temporalization of major blood vessels in highly myopic eyes. Cirrus HD-OCT scan of right eye of a 26-year-old male with high myopia (refraction = –8.75 D, axial length = 26.31 mm). Note the temporally dragged major vessels at the superotemporal and inferotemporal arcades, which results in temporal migration of the retinal nerve fiber layer (RNFL) peaks on the temporal-superior-nasal-inferior-temporal (TSNIT) map. This made the RNFL relatively thicker in the temporal quadrant and thinner in the superior quadrant.

11

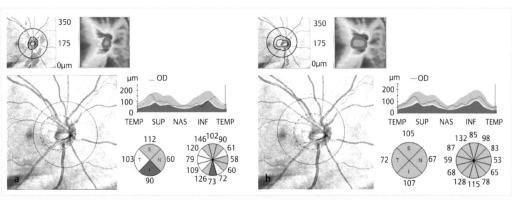

Fig. 11.5 Normalization of peak retinal nerve fiber layer (RNFL) distribution after scan-circle location correction. Cirrus HD-OCT scan of right eye of a 21-year-old male with high myopia (axial length = 25.38 mm). **(a)** Default optic disc cube scan of Cirrus HD-OCT. The device automatically detects the center of the optic disc based on Bruch's membrane opening (BMO), but it is often not distinguishable, especially in eyes with tilted optic disc and temporal peripapillary atrophy. Because of the reflectivity similarity, the device automatically detects the scleral opening as an optic disc margin. The actual border of the BMO is indicated by the red-dotted circle. In this case, the scan circle is relatively skewed to the nasal side of the BMO center, resulting in temporal migration of RNFL peaks, thickening of temporal RNFL, and thinning of inferior RNFL. **(b)** Manual correction of scan-circle location to center of BMO normalized RNFL peak distribution and demonstrated green signs for RNFL thickness.

OCT, the normative database for peripapillary RNFL thickness consists of 284 healthy subjects of various races (European, Chinese, African, and Hispanic). However, subjects with high refractive errors who fell outside the –12.00 to + 8.00 diopter range were excluded from this population. The mean spherical equivalent and axial length among the races ranged from –1.77 to + 0.22 diopters and from 23.6 to 24.2 mm, respectively. The normative database for ganglion cell–inner plexiform layer (GCIPL) thickness consists of 282 healthy subjects with a mean spherical equivalent of –1.00 ± 2.1 diopters and an average axial length of 23.94 ± 1.06 mm. Spectralis OCT references the age-adjusted data from 201 healthy subjects of European descent (age range: 18–78 years). Their refractive errors ranged from –7 to + 5 diopters, but the myopic population proportion has not been disclosed.

In myopic eyes, as the eyeball elongates without a change in the volume of the RGCs, there is a significant negative correlation between the degree of myopia and the thickness of peripapillary RNFL or macular GCIPL. Magnification errors of OCT also underestimate actual measurements. As the normative database for commercially available OCT devices does not contain enough healthy, highly myopic eyes, false-positive red signs for these eyes are common (so-called "red disease"). Building a new normative database containing myopic or highly myopic eyes significantly improved the specificity of RNFL defect detection as well as the diagnostic accuracy for glaucoma compared with the built-in normative database.[5,6] In this regard, clinicians should be aware of the coverage of the normative database and should not rely only on the color codes of the reported OCT data when monitoring a subject with high refractive errors.

11.2.5 Segmentation Errors

Highly myopic eyes are associated with macular pathology including myopic traction maculopathy, myopic choroidal neovascularization, and chorioretinal atrophy as well as ONH deformation manifesting as tilted disc, peripapillary atrophy, or posterior staphyloma. In addition, extremely elongated eyes are difficult to focus on, or obtain clear images of, by OCT scanning. These structural changes can limit the automated segmentation algorithms and affect RNFL and macular ganglion cell layer measurements (▶ Fig. 11.6). Clinicians should confirm the segmentation quality before referencing the color-coded reports from an OCT device. Some commercially available OCT devices provide a segmentation correction function by which more accurate information from highly myopic eyes is obtainable.

11

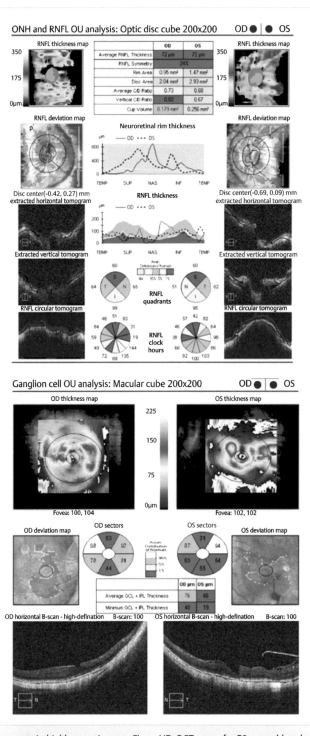

Fig. 11.6 Segmentation errors in highly myopic eyes. Cirrus HD-OCT scan of a 59-year-old male with high myopia. His refractions were −7.5 diopters in both eyes, and the axial lengths were 30.10 and 30.21 mm, respectively. Both eyes had posterior staphyloma with temporally stretched peripapillary scleral flange as well as tractional membranes at the macula. These pathologies limited the clear image scan of optical coherence tomography (OCT), resulting in segmentation errors and reporting of diffuse red signs.

11

11.3 Glaucoma Diagnosis in High Myopia

11.3.1 Macular Parameters for Glaucoma Diagnosis

Highly myopic eyes show variable sizes and shapes of optic disc as well as variations in peripapillary structures such as PPA. These features make RNFL thickness measurements inaccurate and alter the normal range, making glaucoma difficult to diagnose. Given that glaucoma is characterized by progressive degeneration of RGCs, the macula can be an alternative option for glaucoma diagnosis, as it contains more than 50% of the RGC. Current OCT devices provide macular parameters, but their definitions are slightly different from each other. The most commonly used macular parameters are measurements of inner retinal layer thickness in the macular area including the RNFL, ganglion cell layer (GCL), and inner plexiform layer (IPL). Cirrus HD-OCT reports the GCIPL thickness (the sum of the thicknesses of the GCL and IPL) and RTVue OCT (Optovue, Fremont, CA, USA) measures ganglion cell complex (GCC) thickness (the sum of the thicknesses of the RNFL, GCL, and IPL), both of which are representative macular measurements from OCT. GCIPL thickness is known to be less affected by the effect of optic disc rotation in myopic eyes than is peripapillary RNFL thickness or vertical cup-to-disc ratio. In this sense, both GCIPL and GCC thicknesses have shown, compared with peripapillary RNFL thickness, good and comparable diagnostic accuracy for glaucoma in highly myopic eyes.[7] However, caution is still needed, as these parameters do report false-positive signs for glaucoma (one study from Korea reported a prevalence of 40.4% from 104 healthy eyes), especially in eyes of longer axial length and larger fovea-disc angle.[8] In addition, macular pathologies common in extremely highly myopic eyes, including myopic macular degeneration or myopic traction maculopathy, can cause abnormalities in macular ganglion cell layers as well as segmentation errors.

Temporal Raphe Sign

The current OCT devices provide a thickness map for the macular parameters so that ganglion cell defects can be well detected in glaucomatous eyes. They often appear in an arcuate-to-crescent shape and are usually located in the temporal macular region along the horizontal raphe. The asymmetry of GCIPL thickness across the horizontal raphe in the temporal macula can be a good sign of early (or manifest) glaucomatous change. This is analogous to the glaucoma hemifield test of Humphrey visual field (HVF) for identification of glaucomatous visual field defect. Temporal raphe sign is defined as an identifiable horizontal straight line longer than one-half of the inner-to-outer-annulus distance on the macular GCIPL thickness map of Cirrus HD-OCT (▶ Fig. 11.7 and ▶ Fig. 11.8). According to a study from Korea including 195 highly myopic eyes (93 glaucomatous and 102 nonglaucomatous eyes), the temporal raphe sign showed better diagnostic ability (area under curve: 0.938) for glaucoma compared with any other OCT parameters.[9] This sign was also useful for discriminating glaucoma from nonglaucomatous optic neuropathies such as compressive optic neuropathy or optic neuritis.[10]

11.3.2 Neuroretinal Rim Parameters for Glaucoma Diagnosis

In the OCT era, the BMO, delineating the termination of the Bruch's membrane (BM), is an easily identifiable anatomic landmark for neuroretinal rim analysis. As the axons composing the optic nerve must pass through the BMO to exit the eye, it is reasonable to measure the neuroretinal rim thickness from the plane of the BMO. The BMO-based neuroretinal rim approach for the diagnosis of glaucoma in highly myopic eyes is attractive for the following reasons: (1) neuroretinal rim analysis can be less affected by temporal convergence of major vessels and RNFL peaks; (2) BMO-based rim analysis can theoretically better evaluate the actual amount of neuroretinal rim in a tilted optic disc with oblique insertion. Current OCT devices provide two neuroretinal rim parameters, Bruch's membrane opening-based minimum rim width (BMO-MRW) from Spectralis OCT, and three-dimensional neuroretinal rim thickness (3D-NRT) from Cirrus HD-OCT.

BMO-MRW, defined as the minimal distance between the BMO and the internal limiting membrane, has shown higher sensitivity than peripapillary RNFL thickness in diagnosing early glaucoma (▶ Fig. 11.9). This parameter has been shown to be more sensitive than conventional optic disc margin-based assessment and of similar sensitivity to that of RNFL thickness for identification of glaucoma in myopic eyes.[11] Similar to BMO-MRW, 3D-NRT is defined as the distance between the BMO

11

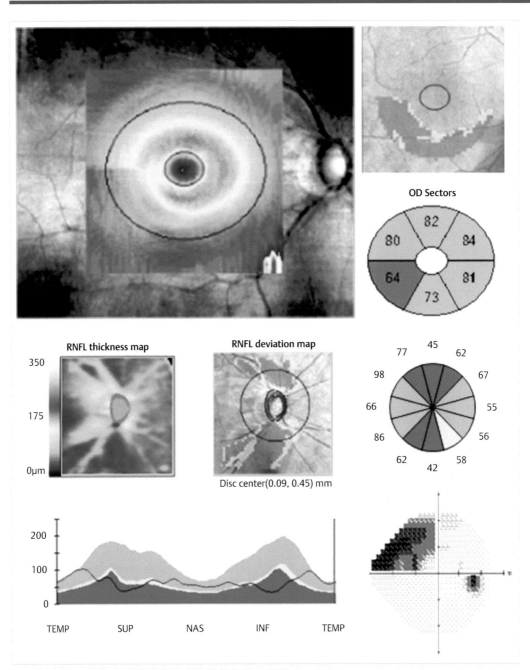

Fig. 11.7 Temporal raphe sign: positive. Cirrus HD-OCT scan of right eye of a 43-year-old male with primary open-angle glaucoma (POAG). His baseline intraocular pressure ranged from 16 to 20 mmHg, and the axial length was 26.16 mm. The temporal raphe sign is defined as positive when the horizontal straight line is confirmed to be longer than one-half of the inner-to-outer-annulus distance on the macular ganglion cell–inner plexiform layer (GCIPL) thickness map. The retinal nerve fiber layer (RNFL) maps demonstrated superior and inferior defects, and the GCIPL deviation map revealed arcuate-shaped inferotemporal defect. The automated Humphrey visual field (HVF) test showed superior arcuate visual field defect.

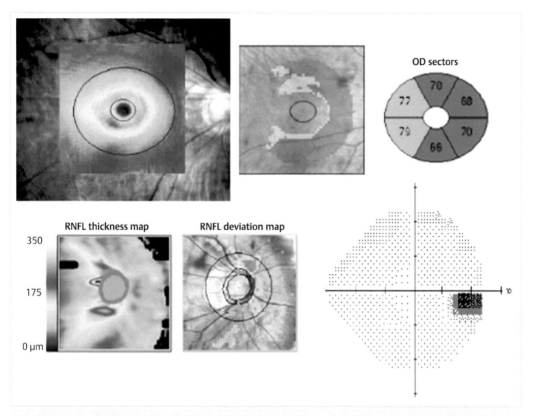

Fig. 11.8 Temporal raphe sign: negative. Cirrus HD-OCT scan of right eye of a 27-year-old male with high myopia (axial length = 30.47 mm). There was no identifiable asymmetrical ganglion cell–inner plexiform layer (GCIPL) thickness difference at the temporal macula; thus, the temporal raphe sign was deemed negative. Despite diffuse red signs on the GCIPL maps, the retinal nerve fiber layer (RNFL) maps revealed no definite defects, and the Humphrey visual field (HVF) test result was within the normal range.

and the vitreoretinal interface, which is associated with the minimum cross-sectional rim area in the given direction (▶ Fig. 11.10).[12] This parameter has shown a significantly lower false-positive rate than RNFL thickness (2.1 vs. 26.9%, $p < 0.001$) as well as a better diagnostic accuracy for diagnosis of glaucoma in myopic eyes.

However, the major limitation of the BMO-based neuroretinal rim approach is that the identification of the BMO can be indistinct in highly myopic eyes, especially in areas where glaucomatous neuroretinal rim loss is common. In addition, Cirrus OCT does not provide the normative database for 3D-NRT in eyes within an extreme range of disc area (< 1.3 or > 2.5 mm²), which renders discrimination of those eyes from glaucomatous eyes problematic.

11.3.3 All at One Glance: 3D Wide-Field Map in SS-OCT

Recent advances in swept-source OCT (SS-OCT) technology have made it possible to capture the macular and peripapillary area simultaneously from a single scan. DRI OCT Triton (Topcon, Tokyo, Japan) uses a wavelength-sweeping laser with a center wavelength of 1,050 nm to acquire 100,000 A-scans per second. DRI OCT Triton captures a 12 × 9 mm wide-field area including the macula and ONH in only 1.3 seconds. The built-in analysis software reports a wide-field thickness map, a thickness surface map, and a SuperPixel map for the RNFL, GCL++(equivalent to GCC) and GCL+ (equivalent to GCIPL) layers, respectively. Especially, the thickness surface map is displayed in three

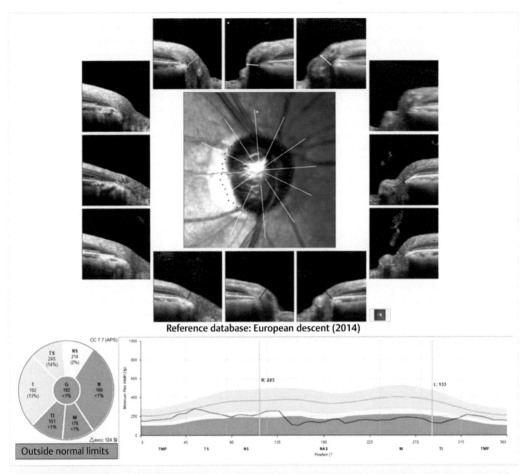

Reference database: European descent (2014)

Outside normal limits

Fig. 11.9 Diagnosis of primary open-angle glaucoma (POAG) by Bruch's membrane opening-based minimum rim width (BMO-MRW). Spectralis optical coherence tomography (OCT) scan of right eye of a 56-year-old male with POAG. The axial length was 25.56 mm, and the optic nerve head (ONH) had a combination of beta and gamma zones of temporal peripapillary atrophy. The outer edge of the hyper-reflective area in the infrared (IR) image corresponds to the retinal pigment epithelium (RPE) termination, and the Bruch's membrane (BM) goes further than the RPE does (*red dot*). The BMO-MRW is defined as the minimum distance between the Bruch's membrane opening (BMO) and the internal limiting membrane (ILM). The classification chart is color-coded according to percentile, as green (above the 5th percentile in the reference database), yellow (borderline, between the 1st and 5th percentiles), and red (outside normal limits, below the 1st percentile). In this case, the right eye had significant thinning of BMO-MRW in the inferior sector.

dimensions for the selected layers (RNFL, GCL++, or GCL+) and can be rotated or zoomed-in or -out by mouse operation (▶ Fig. 11.11). The 3D wide-field map in SS-OCT is expected to be advantageous to conventional spectral-domain OCT (SD-OCT) scans for the diagnosis of glaucoma in myopic eyes, for the following reasons.[13] First, the wide-field map enables three-dimensional evaluation of the

11

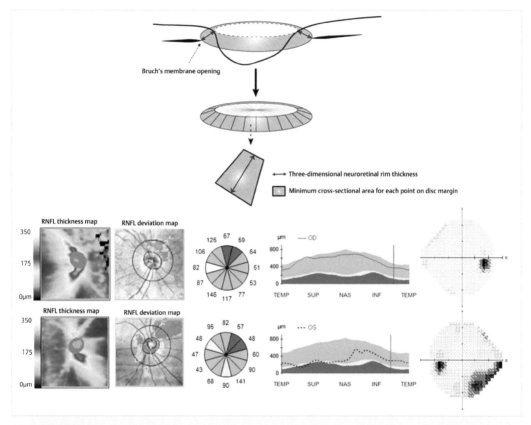

Fig. 11.10 Diagnosis of primary open-angle glaucoma (POAG) by 3D-NRT. Cirrus HD-OCT scan of a 37-year-old female with high myopia (axial lengths 26.14 and 26.06 mm, respectively) and POAG in left eye. The three-dimensional neuroretinal rim thickness (3D-NRT) is defined as the distance between the Bruch's membrane opening (BMO) and the vitreoretinal interface, which is associated with the minimum cross-sectional rim area in the given direction (trapezoid). In the right eye, despite red signs on the deviation map, the 3D-NRT was within the normal range in all quadrants, and the Humphrey visual field (HVF) test result was within the normal range. In the left eye, however, the 3D-NRT was reported to be thinned in the superonasal area, which was consistent with the thinning of the superotemporal retinal nerve fiber layer (RNFL) on the thickness and deviation maps and with the inferior arcuate visual field defect in the HVF test as well.

peripapillary and macular structure of myopic eyes, which may be more accurate than simply distinguishing by color differences on the two-dimensional thickness map from conventional SD-OCT. Second, SS-OCT provides a wider range of OCT scan compared with conventional SD-OCT. Conventional SD-OCT scans only a 6 × 6 mm² area of the peripapillary and macular regions, while SS-OCT scans a 12 × 9 mm² area at a time. Examining a wider range of RNFL structure at a glance will enable better understanding of glaucoma susceptibility in eyes with high refractive errors.

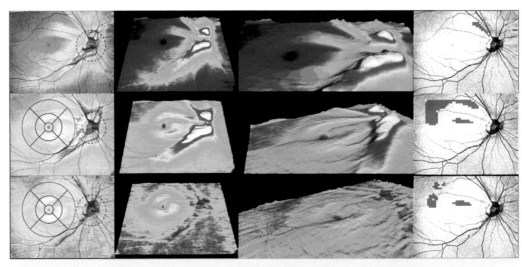

Fig. 11.11 Diagnosis of primary open-angle glaucoma (POAG) from 3D wide-field map. DRI OCT Triton scan of right eye of a 23-year-old male with POAG. He had a history of photorefractive keratectomy on both eyes. The intraocular pressure was 12 mmHg, and the axial length was 24.71 mm. He had inferonasal scotomas in the Humphrey visual field (HVF) test (mean deviation, –3.50 dB). DRI OCT Triton captures a 12 × 9 mm wide-field area including the macula and optic nerve head (ONH), and reports a wide-field thickness map (*left column*), a thickness surface map (*middle columns*), and a SuperPixel map (*right column*) for the retinal nerve fiber layer (RNFL, upper row), GCL + + (equivalent to ganglion cell complex [GCC], middle row), and GCL + (equivalent to ganglion cell–inner plexiform layer [GCIPL], lower row) layers, respectively. Especially, the thickness surface map is displayed in three dimensions for the selected layers (RNFL, GCL + +, and GCL +) and can be rotated or zoomed-in or -out by mouse operation. The wide-field maps all demonstrated glaucomatous defects in the superotemporal area.

References

[1] Holden BA, Fricke TR, Wilson DA, et al. Global prevalence of myopia and high myopia and temporal trends from 2000 through 2050. Ophthalmology. 2016; 123(5):1036–1042

[2] Littmann H. Determination of the true size of an object on the fundus of the living eye. By H. Littmann from the original article, "Zur Bestimmung der wahren Grosse eines Objektes auf dem Hintergrund des lebenden Auges," which originally appeared in Klinisches Monatsblatter fur Augenheilkunde 1982; 180:286–9. Translated by TD Williams. Optom Vis Sci 1992;69(9):717–720

[3] Jonas JB. Optic disk size correlated with refractive error. Am J Ophthalmol. 2005; 139(2):346–348

[4] Chung JK, Yoo YC. Correct calculation circle location of optical coherence tomography in measuring retinal nerve fiber layer thickness in eyes with myopic tilted discs. Invest Ophthalmol Vis Sci. 2011; 52(11):7894–7900

[5] Biswas S, Lin C, Leung CK. Evaluation of a myopic normative database for analysis of retinal nerve fiber layer thickness. JAMA Ophthalmol. 2016; 134(9):1032–1039

[6] Seol BR, Kim DM, Park KH, Jeoung JW. Assessment of optical coherence tomography color probability codes in myopic glaucoma eyes after applying a myopic normative database. Am J Ophthalmol. 2017; 183:147–155

[7] Choi YJ, Jeoung JW, Park KH, Kim DM. Glaucoma detection ability of ganglion cell-inner plexiform layer thickness by spectral-domain optical coherence tomography in high myopia. Invest Ophthalmol Vis Sci. 2013; 54(3):2296–2304

[8] Kim KE, Jeoung JW, Park KH, Kim DM, Kim SH. Diagnostic classification of macular ganglion cell and retinal nerve fiber layer analysis: differentiation of false-positives from glaucoma. Ophthalmology. 2015; 122(3):502–510

[9] Kim YK, Yoo BW, Jeoung JW, Kim HC, Kim HJ, Park KH. Glaucoma-diagnostic ability of ganglion cell-inner plexiform layer thickness difference across temporal raphe in highly myopic eyes. Invest Ophthalmol Vis Sci. 2016; 57(14):5856–5863

[10] Lee J, Kim YK, Ha A et al. Temporal raphe sign for discrimination of glaucoma from optic neuropathy in eyes with macular ganglion cell-inner plexiform layer thinning. Ophthalmology. 2019; 126(8):1131–1139

[11] Malik R, Belliveau AC, Sharpe GP, Shuba LM, Chauhan BC, Nicolela MT. Diagnostic accuracy of optical coherence tomography and scanning laser tomography for identifying glaucoma in myopic eyes. Ophthalmology. 2016; 123(6):1181–1189

[12] Kim YW, Park KH. Diagnostic accuracy of three-dimensional neuroretinal rim thickness for differentiation of myopic glaucoma from myopia. Invest Ophthalmol Vis Sci. 2018; 59 (8):3655–3666

[13] Kim YW, Lee J, Kim JS, Park KH. Diagnostic Accuracy of Wide-Field Map from Swept-Source Optical Coherence Tomography for Primary Open-Angle Glaucoma in Myopic Eyes. Am J Ophthalmol. 2020;218:182-191.

12 Future Directions: Optical Coherence Tomography Angiography for Glaucoma

Darrell WuDunn

Summary

Optical coherence tomography angiography (OCTA) is an emerging technology that provides detailed images of the microvasculature of the optic nerve, peripapillary, and macular regions. OCTA of the optic nerve and peripapillary nerve fiber layer plexus shows good correlation with glaucomatous retinal nerve fiber loss and visual field defects. Both macular and peripapillary OCTA show changes consistent with changes in their corresponding structural optical coherence tomography (OCT) measures. Compared to structural OCT, macular OCTA demonstrates a deeper floor effect and thus may be useful in more severe glaucoma cases. Although this technology offers unprecedented details of the circulation, its role in the diagnosis and management of glaucoma is still unclear. Currently available commercial instruments lack the robust analytical output of its more mature structural OCT brethren, so interpreting the OCTA results in the clinical setting may be challenging. Nevertheless, OCTA can provide complementary information alongside standard structural OCT and visual field measures.

Keywords: microvasculature, superficial vascular plexus, vessel density, blood flow, angiography

12.1 Introduction

12.1.1 The Role of Ocular Blood Flow in Glaucoma

The circulation of the optic nerve has long been thought to play an important role in the development and progression of glaucoma. However, the precise mechanism of how blood flow to the optic nerve relates to glaucomatous optic neuropathy remains poorly understood. Epidemiologic evidence indicates a strong association between lower ocular diastolic perfusion pressure, the difference between diastolic blood pressure and intraocular pressure, and prevalence of glaucoma in multiple different ethnic and geographic populations.[1] Several studies have suggested that treatment of systemic hypertension is associated with increased optic disc cupping and is a significant predictor of the development of glaucoma.

Proponents of a vascular-associated pathogenesis of glaucoma optic neuropathy propose that optic nerve head ischemia results from decreased blood perfusion, which may be due to elevated intraocular pressure and/or decreased systemic blood pressure. The increased pressure gradient between intraocular pressure and blood pressure at the optic nerve head may impede blood flow into the eye because of the increased pressure the ocular arterial system must overcome. Numerous studies have shown that ocular blood flow to the optic nerve head is decreased in eyes with glaucomatous nerve damage.[1] However, it remains unclear if the decreased blood flow is the critical factor that leads to nerve fiber loss, or if the decreased metabolic demands of the glaucomatous optic nerve results in decreased blood flow to the optic nerve head.

Prior to the development of optical coherence tomography angiography (OCTA), studies of ocular blood flow relied on technology that could only visualize or measure flow through large vessels such as the central retinal artery or the posterior ciliary arteries and their primary tributaries.[1] Because OCTA can image the microvasculature, it has become a useful tool in investigating the ocular microvasculature in glaucomatous optic neuropathy.

12.1.2 Optical Coherence Tomography Angiography Technology

Basic Technology

OCTA is an emerging technology that enables noninvasive imaging of blood vessels within the retina, choroid, and optic nerve.[2] Advancements in the acquisition speed and the depth of tissue penetration of OCT technologies have enabled the development of commercially available OCTA devices. OCTA uses the same basic technology of OCT, whereby two superimposed beams of coherent light produce an interference pattern based on the structure of the tissue being imaged. OCTA images blood vessels by detecting changes in sequential B-scan images of

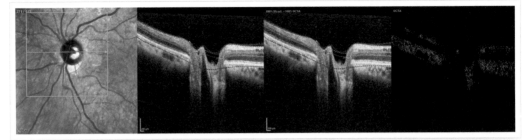

Fig. 12.1 Single B-scan of a peripapillary optical coherence tomography angiography (OCTA) scan. *Far left image:* Greyscale image of left optic nerve. The colored square shows the area of the OCTA scan and the colored arrow shows the B-scan depicted in the subsequent images. *Near left image:* Structural optical coherence tomography (OCT) image. *Near right image:* Combined structural OCT and OCTA image. *Far right image:* OCTA image in which the individual colored spots represent individual blood vessels.

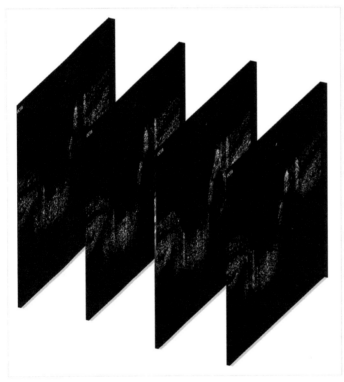

Fig. 12.2 Four adjacent raster B-scan images used to create a volumetric optical coherence tomography angiography (OCTA) image. OCTA identifies blood vessels by detecting change in the position of blood cells flowing through a vessel. By assembling consecutive B-scan slices, an image of a vessel coursing through the tissue can be created.

the same tissue. For the most part, the only difference between successive B-scans of the given tissue is the varying position of blood cells as they flow through vessels. This motion contrast is what the OCTA device interprets as blood vasculature at that particular location in the tissue (▶ Fig. 12.1). As with typical OCT scans, OCTA scans combine successively displaced raster B-scan data over an area of tissue to yield volumetric OCTA data (▶ Fig. 12.2). This enables three-dimensional representation of the microvasculature and allows segmentation of

the different retinal layers and their microvasculature, as is typically visualized in standard OCT. The OCTA device then projects en face views of the microvasculature, including for several segmentation layers.

Commercial OCTA Instruments

Although all the available commercial OCTA instruments image the microvasculature using the same basic principles, they use different

Table 12.1 Technical features of three commercial OCTA instruments

System	AngioVue	AngioPlex	Spectralis OCTA
OCT instrument	RTVue XR Avanti SD-OCT	Cirrus HD-OCT 5000 SD-OCT	Spectralis OCT2 SD-OCT
Manufacturer	Optovue Inc., Fremont, CA	Carl Zeiss Meditec, Inc., Dublin, CA	Heidelberg Engineering, Heidelberg, Germany
Algorithm	SSADA	OMAG	Probabilistic approach
Light source (nm): center/ bandwidth	840 50	840 90	870 50
A-scans/second	70,000	68,000	85,000
Axial resolution (microns)	5	5	5
Transverse resolution (microns)	15	15	6
A-scan count (HxV)	304×304, 400×400	245×245, 350×350	256×256, 512×512
Repeat B-scan count	2	2, 4	7
Scan duration per image (seconds)	2.7×2, 4.6×2 Scans in x and y direction	3.6 Scans in one direction only	5.4, 21.6 Scan in one direction only

Abbreviations: OCT, optical coherence tomography; OCTA, optical coherence tomography angiography; OMAG, optical microangiography; SSADA, split-spectrum amplitude decorrelation angiography.
Source: Data from Li et al.[3]

algorithms for signal processing and image generation.[3] Current Fourier-domain OCT systems generate signals that contain amplitude and phase information. To detect motion contrast (blood flow), algorithms are based on phase and/or amplitude information from the Fourier-transformed OCT signal, and include split-spectrum amplitude decorrelation angiography (AngioVue, Optovue, Fremont, CA), optical microangiography (AngioPlex, Carl Zeiss Meditec, Dublin, CA), and full-spectrum probabilistic approach (Spectralis OCTA, Heidelberg, Germany) (▶ Table 12.1).

The OCT RT XR Avanti with AngioVue detects motion contrast using split-spectrum amplitude decorrelation angiography (SSADA). The technique analyzes the amplitude of variation of the OCT signal over time for each location and calculates decorrelation. Stationary tissue will show low decorrelation (high correlation) since the signal will vary minimally over time, whereas flowing blood cells will show high decorrelation because the signal amplitude will shift widely over time as the blood cells shift in position. Blood flow through a vessel is detected if the decorrelation exceeds a threshold value.

Optical microangiography (OMAG) by AngioPlex uses both phase and amplitude information to generate motion contrast information. Phase information is extracted by measuring the phase change between adjacent B-scans, which depends on the incident angle between the direction of blood flow and the OCT beam. The Spectralis algorithm applies a probabilistic approach to detect motion contrast. The changes in OCT signal from static tissue and from flowing blood follow two distinct distributions and by analyzing multiple repeated scans (seven for the Spectralis), the algorithm determines the probability that the signal at that location corresponds to one of the two distributions.

The commercial instruments use the same optical source as their structural OCT protocols with the wavelength centered in the 840 to 880 nm range for SD-OCT or 1,050 nm for swept-source OCT.

OCTA instruments differ in the number of repeat B-scans they use to detect motion contrast, usually two or four, but seven for the Spectralis, as noted above. There is a tradeoff between acquisition speed and sensitivity when considering the optimal number of repeat B-scans. In addition, the longer acquisition times for OCTA scans make them more prone to artifacts due to bulk eye or head movement. To lessen these bulk motion signal artifacts, each manufacturer uses its own eye-tracking technology to register repeated B-scans to each other.

In addition to the modalities described above, differences among commercial OCTA devices also include time delay between repeat B-scans, algorithms to compensate for bulk motion and other artifacts, signal processing, noise reduction, and

12

image analysis. Because of these differences, OCTA images may not be directly comparable among different instruments.[3]

As with structural OCT, good signal quality is critical for proper interpretation of OCTA scan results. The commercial instruments generally use the same quality indices for OCTA scans as those used for structural OCT scans (e.g., signal strength index, signal quality).

Advantages of OCTA

Incorporated into standard OCT devices, OCTA can be performed in conjunction with standard (structural) OCT, which enables correlation between microvasculature and retinal nerve fiber layer results. Segmentation of the different retinal layers based on structural OCT enables en face visualization of different retinal capillary plexuses, including superficial or retinal nerve fiber layer plexus, deeper retinal capillary beds, and even the choriocapillaris. This is a major advantage over other vascular imaging technologies, such as fluorescein or indocyanine angiography, which presents the entire retinal vasculature en face. In addition, OCTA does not require intravenous injection of contrast dye.

Limitations of OCTA

OCTA images are prone to the same artifacts that can plague standard structural OCT images, such as decentration, segmentation error, defocus, tilt, and projection.[4] Segmentation is a particular problem because, in contrast to a structural OCT RNFL annular scan that is essentially a single B-scan cross section, the en face projection of a capillary plexus layer requires the proper segmentation across the entire scan volume of several hundred B-scans. This is particularly a problem in eyes with retinal pathology that disrupts an area of the normally organized stack of retinal layers. In addition, since OCTA requires multiple re-scanning of the same tissue plane to detect motion contrast, OCTA requires either faster imaging speeds or longer image acquisition times compared to structural OCT. Longer acquisition times leave OCTA more prone to bulk movement or blink artifacts. Overall, OCTA is more prone to artifacts than standard OCT.[4]

OCTA visualizes the vascular structure, but does not measure actual blood flow, although the intensity of the vessel image may reflect the flow speed up until saturation of the image pixel. It does not detect microvasculature containing blood that is stagnant or moving too slowly to detect a change during sequential scans. As in structural OCT, OCTA scan details tend to diminish in deep structures such as the choroid and the optic nerve head deep to the lamina cribrosa.

Care should be taken when interpreting OCTA results from different instrument manufacturers. OCTA image results may not be directly comparable among different OCT devices.[3] Each OCTA manufacturer uses its own scan protocols, signal processing, data analysis, and visualization methods to render the OCTA information. The output of results also varies tremendously among the different devices. The data analysis output for OCTA is not as mature as the output for structural OCT. At the time of this writing, normative databases were not yet available for most devices and the data outputs are mostly qualitative rather than quantitative, potentially leaving the clinician at a loss for how to interpret the OCTA results or how to apply them to clinical practice.

12.2 OCTA of the Optic Nerve Head and Peripapillary Microvasculature

12.2.1 OCTA of the Optic Nerve Head Microvasculature in Normal Eyes

Since the optic nerve is the principal structure affected by glaucoma and the optic nerve head is the primary site of damage, most OCTA studies in glaucoma focus on the optic nerve and peripapillary microvasculature. The optic nerve is perfused from several arterial plexuses depending on the section of the nerve within the eye, the lamina cribrosa, and the retrobulbar region.[1,2] The optic nerve head prelaminar region is supplied by the choroid consisting of the scleral short posterior ciliary arteries and the recurrent choroidal arteries. These vessels enter the sclera medially and laterally and act as end arteries, which leaves the optic nerve head susceptible to ischemia. The centripetal branches from the short posterior ciliary arteries form the circle of Zinn and Haller and supply the lamina cribrosa. The retrolaminar region of the optic nerve is supplied by a peripheral centripetal system from the pial network of vessels or from an axial centrifugal supply of the central retinal artery. The primary glaucomatous changes are

12

thought to occur in the deep optic nerve head region supplied by the posterior ciliary arteries.

Although major vessels obscure significant portions of the laminar capillaries, OCTA based on SD-OCT (840–880 nm source) can generally provide distinct images of the microvasculature within the lamina cribrosa.

The peripapillary retinal nerve fiber layer is supplied by the radial peripapillary capillary network, and this network can be well visualized by OCTA. Scan protocols of commercial OCTA instruments typically include 3 × 3 mm square en face images centered on the optic disc at three or four stacks or layers. The retinal nerve fiber layer microvasculature is usually segmented between the internal limiting membrane (ILM) and the inner plexiform layer (IPL).

12.2.2 OCTA of the Optic Nerve and Peripapillary Microvasculature in Glaucoma

Optic disc images of glaucomatous eyes by OCTA may show decreased capillary density compared to normal eyes (▶ Fig. 12.3).[5] The vessel density (the proportion of the area covered by white pixels representing vessels out of the whole area of measurement) generally correlates with the degree of glaucomatous nerve damage and is more easily discernible in more advanced disease, given the lack of quantitative output from most OCTA systems. Vessel density of the peripapillary superficial capillary plexus (between ILM and IPL) that supplies the nerve fiber layer also shows a strong correlation with glaucoma severity and may be easier to discern because of its close anatomic correspondence to the OCT RNFL annulus (▶ Fig. 12.4).

Decreased vessel density within a peripapillary sector or hemifield will typically reflect a corresponding decrease in OCT RNFL thickness in the same sector or hemifield (▶ Fig. 12.5).[6,7,8,9] This may be particularly the case for defects in the inferotemporal sector where glaucomatous damage most commonly occurs (▶ Fig. 12.6).[7,9]

Normative datasets and quantitative analysis of OCTA images are not readily available yet on some commercial instruments. Thus, the extent of microvascular defects may be difficult to ascertain on the en face images. In general, clinicians are better able to qualitatively assess thickness, as seen on structural OCT cross-sectional annular RNFL images, compared to pattern density, as seen on en face OCTA images. Changes in serial OCTA scan images may be easier to notice on visual inspection, as some vessels may fade out over time. However, the reproducibility of serial scans has not been firmly established. In addition, how the optic nerve and peripapillary microvasculature, as depicted by OCTA, evolve as individuals age has not been well described.

Some studies have detected subtle decreases in whole image optic disc and peripapillary vessel density in glaucoma suspects and preperimetric glaucoma eyes compared to normal eyes,[10] although such detection required statistical image analysis not currently available on commercial OCTA instruments. In the absence of meaningful quantitative analysis on commercial instruments, distinguishing glaucoma suspects from normal eyes is difficult.

12.3 OCTA of the Macular Microvasculature

12.3.1 OCTA of the Normal Macular Microvasculature

Patients with glaucoma often have thinning of their macular region, especially of the ganglion cell complex. Paracentral visual field defects are also

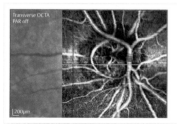
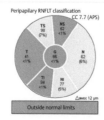
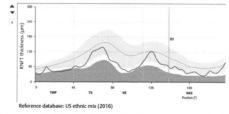

Fig. 12.3 Optic nerve optical coherence tomography angiography (OCTA) scan and optical coherence tomography (OCT) retinal nerve fiber layer (RNFL) scan, right eye, of a 53-year-old woman with moderate glaucoma. The OCTA scan includes the full retina and choroid slabs.

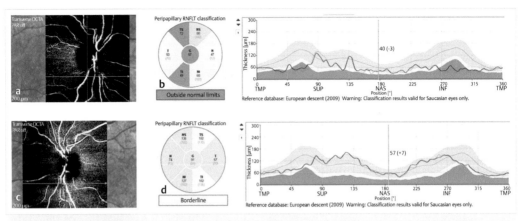

Fig. 12.4 Optic nerve optical coherence tomography angiography (OCTA) scans **(a, c)** and optical coherence tomography (OCT) retinal nerve fiber layer (RNFL) scans **(b, d)** of a 71-year-old woman with severe glaucoma in right eye and mild glaucoma in left eye. OCTA scans show the nerve fiber layer venous plexus. The right eye **(a, b)** shows much less microvasculature present than in the left eye **(c, d)**.

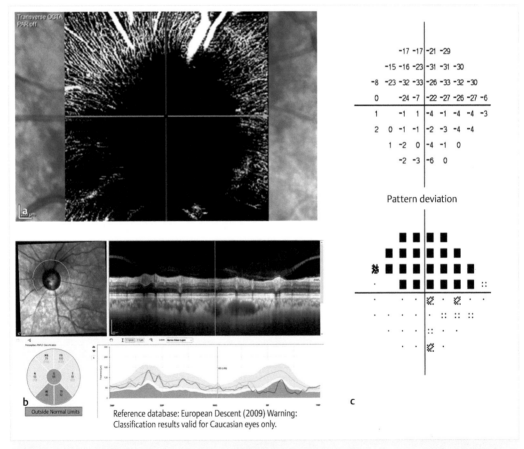

Fig. 12.5 Optic disc optical coherence tomography angiography (OCTA) and optical coherence tomography (OCT) retinal nerve fiber layer (RNFL) scans of left eye of a 59-year-old man with inferior neuroretinal rim loss and superior altitudinal loss in his visual field. Decreased vessel density within a peripapillary sector or hemifield will typically reflect a corresponding decrease in OCT RNFL thickness in the same sector or hemifield. In this case, he has severe loss of microvasculature within the inferior nerve fiber layer vascular plexus, **(a)** corresponding to the thinning inferiorly on OCT RNFL scan **(b)** and superior hemifield loss in his visual fields **(c)**.

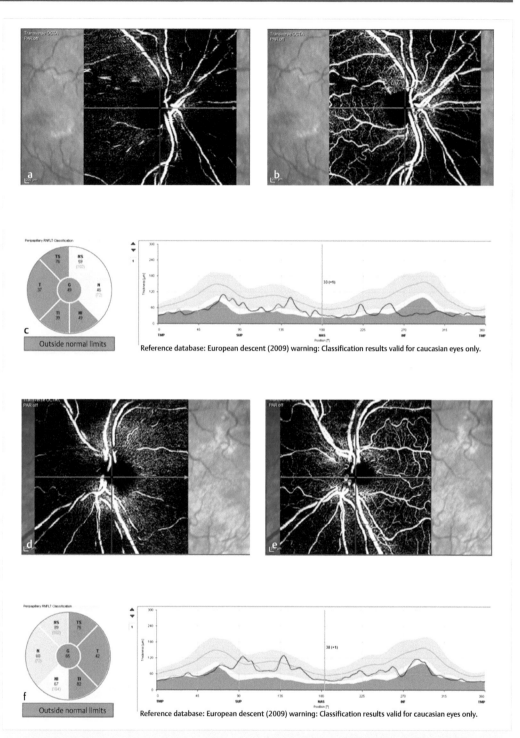

Fig. 12.6 Optic nerve optical coherence tomography angiography (OCTA) of a 62-year-old man with moderate glaucoma in both eyes, but worse in right eye (**a–c**) than left eye (**d–f**). His right eye has slightly more damage in the inferior retinal nerve fiber layer (RNFL) than in the superior RNLF (**c**). His retinal nerve fiber vascular plexus (**a**) and superficial vascular plexus (**b**) also show more microvasculature loss inferiorly compared to superiorly and more loss overall compared to the microvasculature of his left eye (**d, e**).

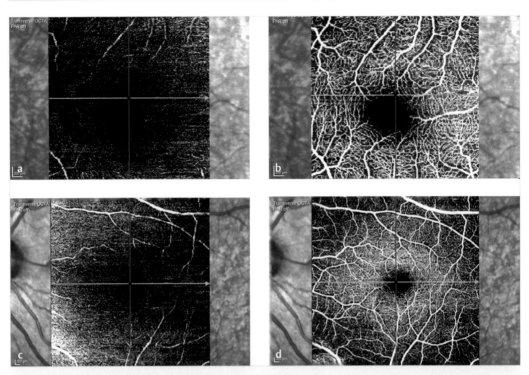

Fig. 12.7 Macula optical coherence tomography angiography (OCTA) scans of 40-year-old man without eye disease. OCTA of the macula is probably best directed at the superficial vascular plexus within the inner layers of the retina (internal limiting membrane [ILM] to inner plexiform layer [IPL]) and which supply the nerve fiber layer and ganglion cell complex layer. OCTA scans of the nerve fiber layer vascular plexus ([a] right eye; [c] left eye) show the microvasculature within the most superficial retinal layer and which includes the retinal nerve fiber layer. OCTA scans of the superficial vascular plexus ([b] right eye; [d] left eye) include the ganglion cell layer.

12

common in glaucoma patients, particularly those with normal tension glaucoma. The macular microvasculature supplies a major portion of the ganglion cells.[2] Hence, OCTA scans of the macular region may provide important insight into a patient's glaucoma.

The inner two-thirds of the retina is supplied by retinal capillaries via retinal arterioles that branch out from the central retinal artery.[1,2] Blood is drained via the retinal venules and veins to the central retina vein. The outer third of the retina is supplied by the choriocapillaris, which represents the terminal arterioles of the short posterior ciliary arteries. To provide optimal clarity of central vision, the foveal avascular zone (FAZ) contains no blood vessels, which would distort or impair light arriving at the fovea. The FAZ is bordered by a continuous capillary network. The nerve fiber layer is supplied by long capillaries that are arranged parallel to the nerve fibers as they radiate out from the peripapillary area (radial peripapillary capillary plexus). Just below this, the microvasculature

of the retinal ganglion cell layer forms a dense lattice pattern capillary network (superficial vascular plexus) that is supplied by successive branches of the arteries of the vascular arcade. The blood from the macular area drains via small venules that coalesce into successively larger venules and then into the arcade veins.

OCTA of the macula is probably best directed at the superficial vascular plexus within the inner layers of the retina (ILM to IPL) and which supply the nerve fiber layer and ganglion cell complex layer (▶ Fig. 12.7). Imaging of the deeper vascular plexus is prone to projection artifacts from overlying superficial vessels.

12.3.2 OCTA of Macular Microvasculature in Glaucoma

Glaucoma patients with paracentral scotomas and/or macular thinning on OCT are well suited for macular OCTA imaging. Studies have demonstrated significant correlation between macular

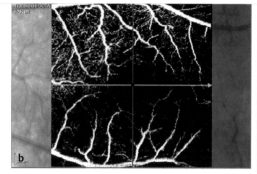
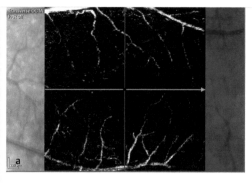
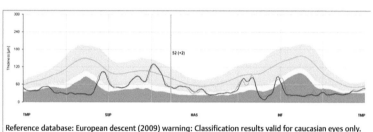
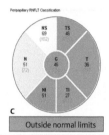

Fig. 12.8 Macula optical coherence tomography angiography (OCTA) scans of 69-year-old man with severe glaucoma in his left eye. His structural optical coherence tomography (OCT) retinal nerve fiber layer (RNLF) scan (c) shows more severe loss in the inferior hemifield. This is reflected in his nerve fiber layer vascular plexus (a) and superficial vascular plexus (b) which also show more severe microvascular loss inferiorly.

vessel density by OCTA and macular or ganglion cell complex thickness by OCT. Macular OCTA may show decreased vessel density in moderate and severe glaucoma, especially with more severe central vision loss (▶ Fig. 12.8).[8,11,12] Subtle vessel density loss may be seen in early glaucoma patients (even before visual field loss) and glaucoma suspects.[7,13,14] However, the paucity of quantitative analysis from commercial OCTA instruments makes detecting subtle changes in vessel density very difficult. In general, macular OCTA results parallel findings from structural OCT and visual field testing, in both severity and location.[14,15,16]

The size and shape of FAZ may also be useful for glaucoma diagnosis and monitoring. The FAZ may become larger and more irregularly shaped as glaucoma progresses, especially in eyes with central visual field defects. Since OCTA is extremely well suited for visualizing the FAZ, it should be quite informative in eyes with central defects.[11]

Macular OCTA may be particularly useful in severe glaucoma, when OCT of the macula and RNLF reach a measurement floor, at which the structural width measurement will no longer decrease despite further loss of visual field. The floor effect typically occurs when the visual field mean deviation (MD) falls below −15 to −17 dB. In

contrast, macular OCTA images may continue to show vessel density loss until the visual field MD reaches about −25 dB.[17] It should be realized, however, that subtle changes in OCTA macular vessel density are difficult to detect, especially without quantitative output from commercial OCTA instruments. Hence, although macular OCTA may have a broader dynamic range than structural OCT variables, it may be less sensitive for monitoring glaucoma progression.

12.4 OCTA of the Choroid

As described earlier, the peripapillary choroid is supplied primarily from the short posterior ciliary arteries, which also provide blood to optic nerve including the prelaminar and laminar regions.[1] Thus, the peripapillary choroid circulation may serve as a surrogate for the optic nerve head microvasculature in patients with glaucoma.

12.4.1 OCTA of the Normal Choroid

The short posterior ciliary arteries pass through the sclera near the optic nerve and branch out to form the arterioles of the choroid outer layer, which then terminate in the choriocapillaris. The choriocapillaris is a single layer anastomotic network of fenestrated capillaries, whose basement membrane form the outer layer of Bruch's membrane.

The choroid is often difficult to image due to its location beneath the retinal vasculature and retinal pigment epithelium. Enhanced depth imaging (EDI) and swept-source OCT are two modalities that improve imaging of the choroid. In addition, in areas of beta-zone peripapillary area, the choroidal vasculature can be better visualized due to the absence of overlying retinal pigment epithelia.

12.4.2 OCTA of the Choroid in Glaucoma

Patients with glaucoma may sometimes show areas of regional choroidal or deep-layer microvascular dropout, which is not typically seen in normal individuals.[18,19,20] Most areas of choroidal microvascular dropout occur in the inferior or inferotemporal sectors. Eyes with choroidal microvasculature dropout often have associated paracentral visual field defects, more advanced RNFL thinning on structural OCT, and worse mean deviation on visual fields. They may also show more rapid progression of visual field loss and RNFL thinning than eyes without choroidal microvasculature dropout.[18] Disc hemorrhages and focal laminar cribrosa defects are also associated with choroidal microvasculature dropout.[20]

12.5 OCTA in the Future

As manufacturers develop and refine their software for analyzing OCTA data, OCTA is expected to become more integrated into clinical practice for diagnosing and monitoring patients with, or suspected to have, glaucoma. It may prove useful in predicting subsequent visual field loss if microvasculature changes precede visual function changes. It may help assess the rate of visual field progression if repeatability is confirmed to be consistent. OCTA may become particularly helpful in severe glaucoma, when the floor effect diminishes the usefulness of structural OCT and of the probability plots of visual field analyzers.

References

[1] Harris A, Guidoboni G, Siesky B, et al. Ocular blood flow as a clinical observation: Value, limitations and data analysis. Prog Retin Eye Res. 2020:100841 (Online ahead of print)

[2] Spaide RF, Fujimoto JG, Waheed NK, Sadda SR, Staurenghi G. Optical coherence tomography angiography. Prog Retin Eye Res. 2018; 64:1–55

[3] Li XX, Wu W, Zhou H, et al. A quantitative comparison of five optical coherence tomography angiography systems in clinical performance. Int J Ophthalmol. 2018; 11(11):1784–1795

[4] Holmen IC, Konda MS, Pak JW, et al. Prevalence and severity of artifacts in optical coherence tomographic angiograms. JAMA Ophthalmol. 2020; 138(2):119–126

[5] Miguel AIM, Silva AB, Azevedo LF. Diagnostic performance of optical coherence tomography angiography in glaucoma: a systematic review and meta-analysis. Br J Ophthalmol. 2019; 103(11):1677–1684

[6] Chen CL, Bojikian KD, Wen JC, et al. Peripapillary retinal nerve fiber layer vascular microcirculation in eyes with glaucoma and single-hemifield visual field loss. JAMA Ophthalmol. 2017; 135(5):461–468

[7] Kurysheva NI, Maslova EV, Zolnikova IV, Fomin AV, Lagutin MB. A comparative study of structural, functional and circulatory parameters in glaucoma diagnostics. PLoS One. 2018; 13(8):e0201599

[8] Manalastas PIC, Zangwill LM, Daga FB, et al. The association between macula and ONH optical coherence tomography angiography (OCT-A) vessel densities in glaucoma, glaucoma suspect, and healthy eyes. J Glaucoma. 2018; 27(3):227–232

[9] Rao HL, Kadambi SV, Weinreb RN, et al. Diagnostic ability of peripapillary vessel density measurements of optical coherence tomography angiography in primary open-angle and angle-closure glaucoma. Br J Ophthalmol. 2017; 101 (8):1066–1070

[10] Hou H, Moghimi S, Zangwill LM, et al. Inter-eye asymmetry of optical coherence tomography angiography vessel density in bilateral glaucoma, glaucoma suspect, and healthy eyes. Am J Ophthalmol. 2018; 190:69–77

[11] Choi J, Kwon J, Shin JW, Lee J, Lee S, Kook MS. Quantitative optical coherence tomography angiography of macular vascular structure and foveal avascular zone in glaucoma. PLoS One. 2017; 12(9):e0184948

[12] Wan KH, Lam AKN, Leung CK. Optical coherence tomography angiography compared with optical coherence tomography macular measurements for detection of glaucoma. JAMA Ophthalmol. 2018; 136(8):866–874

[13] Hou H, Moghimi S, Zangwill LM, et al. Macula vessel density and thickness in early primary open-angle glaucoma. Am J Ophthalmol. 2019; 199:120–132

[14] Penteado RC, Zangwill LM, Daga FB, et al. Optical coherence tomography angiography macular vascular density measurements and the central 10–2 visual field in glaucoma. J Glaucoma. 2018; 27(6):481–489

[15] Wu J, Sebastian RT, Chu CJ, McGregor F, Dick AD, Liu L. Reduced macular vessel density and capillary perfusion in glaucoma detected using OCT angiography. Curr Eye Res. 2019; 44(5):533–540

[16] Yarmohammadi A, Zangwill LM, Diniz-Filho A, et al. Peripapillary and macular vessel density in patients with glaucoma and single-hemifield visual field defect. Ophthalmology. 2017; 124(5):709–719

[17] Moghimi S, Bowd C, Zangwill LM, et al. Measurement floors and dynamic ranges of OCT and OCT angiography in glaucoma. Ophthalmology. 2019; 126(7):980–988

[18] Kwon JM, Weinreb RN, Zangwill LM, Suh MH. Parapapillary deep-layer microvasculature dropout and visual field progression in glaucoma. Am J Ophthalmol. 2019; 200:65–75

[19] Lin S, Cheng H, Zhang S, et al. Parapapillary choroidal microvasculature dropout is associated with the decrease in retinal nerve fiber layer thickness: a prospective study. Invest Ophthalmol Vis Sci. 2019; 60(2):838–842

[20] Park HL, Kim JW, Park CK. Choroidal microvasculature dropout is associated with progressive retinal nerve fiber layer thinning in glaucoma with disc hemorrhage. Ophthalmology. 2018; 125(7):1003–1013

12

13 Future Directions: Swept-Source OCT for Glaucoma

Hana L. Takusagawa and Elizabeth Ann Zane Cretara

Summary

Swept-source optical coherence tomography (SS-OCT) is an emerging imaging modality used for the diagnosis and monitoring of patients with glaucoma. Compared to spectral domain OCT technology, SS-OCT uses a tunable, longer wavelength of light. This facilitates high resolution imaging of intraocular structure with improved range of depth and significantly increased scan speed. Current research is investigating the role of SS-OCT in imaging intraocular structures relevant to glaucoma, namely, the anterior segment, macula, choroid, and optic nerve including the lamina cribrosa. Future research is needed to establish the role of this new technology and determine how it fits into the larger framework of clinical glaucoma patient care.

Keywords: swept-source, optical coherence tomography, glaucoma, optic nerve, macula, choroid, lamina cribrosa

13.1 Introduction

Swept-source optical coherence tomography (SS-OCT) is an emerging ophthalmic imaging modality with many applications in the field of ophthalmology. We will concentrate on the role that SS-OCT may play in the diagnosis and monitoring of glaucoma. The technology represents an advancement compared to previous OCT platforms by replacing the fixed wavelength of spectral domain OCT with an ultra-high speed wavelength-tuned or "swept-source" laser, thereby improving range of depth, while shortening scan times.[1] Wide-field, 12 mm × 12 mm swept-source can image both the macula and optic nerve with a single scan.[2] Similarly, in the anterior segment, a single scan can simultaneously image the cornea, iris, and anterior lens.[2] In the United States, the Food and Drug Administration (FDA) approved the PLEX Elite 9000 Carl Zeiss Meditec (Jena, Germany) for research use in 2016 and in 2018 they approved the Triton Topcon SS-OCT system (Topcon, Tokyo, Japan) for clinical use.[3] Both of these can be used for imaging the posterior segment. The Tomey Casia SS-OCT (Tomey, Nagoya, Japan) is dedicated to imaging the anterior segment and is currently pending FDA approval but has been used in Asia since 2012 for both clinical and research purposes. Research continues to develop novel SS-OCT prototypes.

The commercially available SS-OCT devices scan the posterior pole at a rate of 100,000 A-scans/second at wavelengths centered at 1,050 nm with a range of approximately 100 nm, producing an axial resolution of 6.3 to 8 μm and a transverse resolution of 20 μm. Research prototypes have reported axial resolutions down to 5 μm.[2] By comparison, previous spectral domain OCT (SD-OCT) technology uses a fixed wavelength of 840 nm with scan speeds of 25,000 to 100,000 axial scans per second yielding axial resolution in the range of 2 to 7 μm and transverse resolution of 20 μm.[4] SD-OCT represented an improvement in speed and scan quality compared the previous time domain OCT (TD-OCT) technology by acquiring images at 50 × the speed of TD-OCT and applying a Fourier transform to the interference spectrum detected.[5]

Anterior segment OCT (AS-OCT) utilizes different wavelengths of light to optimize visualization of anterior ocular structures. SS-AS-OCT captures 30,000 A-scans per second, at 1,310 nm wavelength, yielding axial and transverse resolution of 10 and 30 μm, respectively, and permitting 360-degree scans in 2.4 seconds.[6] By comparison, SD-AS-OCT utilizes a central wavelength of 830 nm, with axial resolution of < 10 μm, and TD-AS-OCT utilizes 1,310 nm wavelength with axial resolution of 18 μm.[7] Research devices have demonstrated comparable imaging performance between enhanced depth imaging (EDI)-SD-OCT-AS and SS-OCT-AS.[8]

13.2 Imaging of Intraocular Structures Using SS-OCT in Glaucoma

Many intraocular structures are relevant to the study of glaucoma, namely, the anterior segment, macula, choroid, and optic disc including the lamina cribrosa. Since SS-OCT has become more widely used, research has focused on establishing its role in relationship to previous OCT imaging modalities in imaging intraocular structures. The majority of studies have focused on clinical applications in glaucoma diagnosis and monitoring

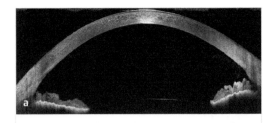

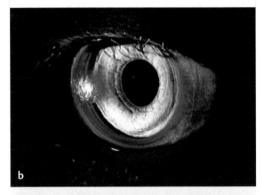

Fig. 13.1 Anterior segment swept-source optical coherence tomography (SS-OCT). **(a)** B-scan of anterior chamber (OS) of a healthy 38-year-old male. **(b)** SS-OCT volumetric rendering of anterior segment of a healthy 22-year-old woman. (Figure by Ryan McNabb, PhD, and Anthony Kuo, MD, of the Duke Eye Center.)

while others have focused on the potential of the technology to investigate the underlying pathophysiology.

13.2.1 Anterior Segment Application of SS-OCT in Glaucoma (▶ Fig. 13.1)

AS-OCT has been used to examine angle configuration for aid in diagnosis of angle anomalies relevant to glaucoma including narrow angle and plateau iris and has been used to monitor response to treatment, that is, laser peripheral iridotomy.[9] Research in the field of SS-AS-OCT has focused on comparing anterior segment measurements with those obtained with previous technologies including SD-AS-OCT and TD-AS-OCT.[10,11,12] One of these studies demonstrated that SS-AS-OCT was superior to SD-AS-OCT in visualizing deeper angle structures including the scleral spur.[11] In the area of angle closure, researchers have explored the role of SS-AS-OCT in visualizing peripheral anterior synechia (PAS) and studying changes in iris volume in response to pupillary dynamics and have found that PAS can be reproducibly imaged

and the findings are comparable to gonioscopy.[13,14] The specifics of these articles are discussed below.

Xu et al compared anterior segment parameters measured by SS-OCT and SD-OCT and found excellent inter-device reproducibility for measurements of angle opening distance (AOD), trabecular iris space area (TISA), and lens vault (LV).[10] However, anterior chamber width (ACW) showed low agreement. The authors hypothesized the difference might be due to variability in scan location between the two devices.[10] They concluded that although both the measurements are reliable, they should not be used interchangeably.

Qiao et al compared the ability of SS-OCT with SD-OCT to distinguish deeper angle structures including Schwalbe's line, Schlemm's canal, and scleral spur.[11] They compared scans from 67 healthy subjects obtained with SS-OCT versus SD-OCT, using anatomical markers (i.e., conjunctival blood vessel) to ensure equivalent positioning of both scans. Their results showed that SS-OCT had improved visualization of the scleral spur. They suggest that the improved depth of resolution possible with SS-OCT might be of particular benefit in visualizing angle structures in older patients with higher rates of pinguecula and pterygium.

Chansangpetch et al compared anterior segment parameters measured by SS-OCT and TD-OCT.[12] They found strong correlation between measurements of anterior chamber depth (ACD), LV, and ACW. However, AOD, TISA, and angle recess area (ARA) demonstrated variability, with SS-OCT tending to give larger numbers. They concluded that the measurements from different devices are reproducible but not interchangeable. They hypothesized that differences in measurements might be influenced by differences in speed, resolution, segmentation, or scan location.

Lai et al used SS-OCT to measure the area and degree of PAS.[13] They found good reproducibility of the PAS measurements by SS-OCT and found agreement with PAS assessment by gonioscopy. Synechial and appositional angle closure were demonstrated with dynamic dark-light OCT imaging. The authors propose this could be a new clinical tool for quantitative monitoring of PAS progression.

Mak et al compared iris volume in primary angle closure (PAC) or PAC suspect (PACS) with primary open-angle glaucoma (POAG) in response to light, dark, and pharmacologic dilation.[14] They found iris volume decreased after dilation in POAG and PAC and PACS and the degree of reduction was less in eyes with smaller anterior chamber volume. In

13

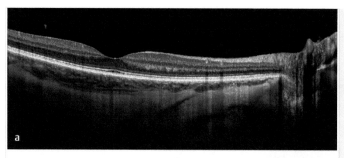

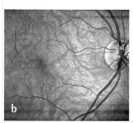

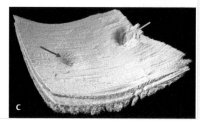

Fig. 13.2 Macular swept-source optical coherence tomography (SS-OCT). (a) Macular B-scan (OD) of a healthy 33-year-old woman. With SS-OCT, choroid is visible without enhanced depth imaging (EDI). (b) Summed volume projection provides *en face* view of retinal vessels and choroid below. (c) SS-OCT volumetric rendering of macula showing foveal pit (red arrow) and optic nerve head cup (yellow arrow). (Figure by Ryan McNabb, PhD, and Anthony Kuo, MD, of the Duke Eye Center.)

addition, they found larger iris volume was associated with a smaller angle width. The authors suggest SS-OCT may provide insights into the pathophysiology of angle closure.

13.2.2 Analysis of Macular and Peripapillary Retina by SS-OCT (▶ Fig. 13.2 and ▶ Fig. 13.3)

Several studies have explored the use of macular and peripapillary retina SS-OCT scans including their diagnostic value compared with SD-OCT scan for glaucoma.[15,16,17] In general, studies have shown SS-OCT obtains thinner measurements for most retinal layers compared to SD-OCT. However, the glaucoma discriminating ability overall was comparable.[15,17] Another study performed this same comparison using wide-field technology and found that specific layer measurements were more equivalent between SD-OCT and SS-OCT.[16] SS-OCT has also been used to assess asymmetry of the macula as a tool for glaucoma diagnosis.[18] The specifics of these articles are discussed below.

Yang et al compared macular thickness and diagnostic ability of macular ganglion cell layer plus inner plexiform layer (mGCIPL), macular ganglion cell complex (mGCC), and circumpapillary retinal nerve fiber layer (cpRNFL) between wide scan SS-OCT and standard macular SD-OCT. Although the diagnostic accuracy was equivalent between SS-OCT and SD-OCT scans, the measurements of specific layers were not. They found that mGCIPL and mGCC were thinner in both normal

and glaucomatous eyes using SS-OCT compared to SD-OCT, while the opposite trend was noted with the cpRNFL. Of the three layers, cpRNFL had the highest sensitivity and specificity for differentiating glaucoma for both SS-OCT and SD-OCT (area under the curve [AUC] = 0.83 and 0.85, respectively). The authors hypothesized differences in retinal subfield measurements might be due to different segmentation algorithms and scan quality.[15]

Lee et al compared macula scans by SD-OCT and SS-OCT including measurements of mGCIPL and macular RNFL (mRNFL) in glaucoma and evaluated their diagnostic ability.[17] They found the ability to distinguish glaucoma from normal was comparable; however, the specific layers and retinal subfield measurements were not. Although these differences varied by layer and retinal subfield and also between glaucoma and control, overall SS-OCT was noted to produce thinner measurements than SD-OCT, similar to findings of Yang et al. The highest AUC was noted to be SD-OCT mGCIPL in the outer temporal zone (AUC = 0.894).[17]

Hong et al compared glaucoma-discriminating abilities of SD-OCT macular and disc scans with SS-OCT wide scans which encompass both structures. They found that the AUC for standard macula and disc scans versus wide scans were not significantly different.[16] Unlike Yang et al and Lee et al, they found excellent agreement between retinal layer measurements performed by the two imaging modalities. The best individual parameter for differentiating glaucoma from normal was total cpRNFL using standard SD-OCT disc scans (AUC = 0.902).

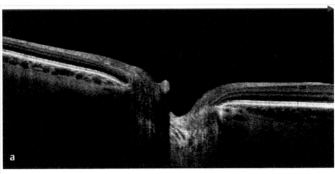

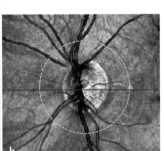

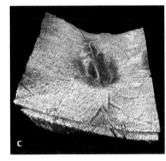

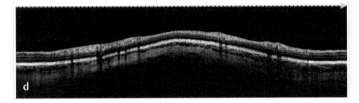

Fig. 13.3 Single volume acquisition optic nerve head swept-source optical coherence tomography (SS-OCT). **(a)** B-scan from optic nerve head volume (OS) of a healthy volunteer. **(b)** Summed volume projection provides *en face* view of retinal vessels and nerve head. Red line indicates location of B-scan in **(a)**. Gold dashed circle indicates location of peripapillary scan in **(d)**. **(c)** SS-OCT volumetric rendering of optic nerve head cup. **(d)** Peripapillary scan extracted from SS-OCT volume. (Figure by Ryan McNabb, PhD, and Anthony Kuo, MD, of the Duke Eye Center.)

Another study by Lee et al used SS-OCT technology to evaluate the glaucoma-differentiating ability of measurement asymmetry between macular layer thickness between fellow eyes. Their design was based on the premise that normal eyes tend to display a high degree of symmetry, which is disturbed by the glaucoma disease-state. They compared mRNFL, mGCIPL, mGCC, and total retina thickness between the two eyes. They found that overall glaucoma patients had thinner retinal layers and higher asymmetry. The AUCs of the average thickness differences ranged from 0.748 to 0.894. Authors reports their results were similar to previous studies using SD-OCT and might enhance diagnostic capabilities, although their study did not compare the OCT technologies.[18]

13.2.3 Choroidal Application of SS-OCT in Glaucoma

The choroid is thought to play a role in the vascular component of glaucoma. A recent paper used optical coherence tomography angiography (OCTA) to evaluate choroidal microvascular dropout in patients with POAG. They found the prevalence of choroidal microvascular dropout was significantly higher in POAG patients with disc hemorrhage, central visual field loss, and severe glaucomatous nerve damage.[19] Although choroidal imaging is not currently used in clinical evaluation of patients with glaucoma, research has explored the role of SS-OCT and SD-OCT in measuring macular and peripapillary choroidal thickness in glaucoma patients as a diagnostic tool.[20,21,22]

Hirooka et al used EDI SD-OCT to show choroidal thinning correlated to worsening glaucoma severity, particularly notable in the area nasal to the fovea in patients with normal-tension glaucoma (NTG).[20] Song et al compared peripapillary and macular choroidal thickness (PCT and MCT) between glaucoma and normal using SS-OCT and found both were thinner in glaucoma; however, only PCT was significantly thinner after controlling for confounding factors such as age, axial length,

13

and disc area.[21] They did not find any correlation with glaucoma severity, suggesting this technology might be helpful for diagnosis but not so for monitoring disease progression. They conclude their results are similar to previous EDI SD-OCT studies. However, they did not compare the performance of the modalities.

Zhang et al also measured choroidal thickness by SS-OCT in glaucomatous and normal eyes and found that it was thinner in the peripapillary and macular regions in glaucoma compared with control.[22] However, when they accounted for age and longer axial length, they found glaucoma was in fact not independently associated with choroidal thickness. An interesting secondary finding was that the relationship between older age and thinner choroid may be stronger in glaucoma compared with controls suggesting that glaucoma might modulate age-related changes to choroidal thickness.

13.2.4 Optic Nerve Head Application of SS-OCT in Glaucoma (▶ Fig. 13.3 and ▶ Fig. 13.4)

The optic nerve is the primary site of damage in glaucoma. Previous studies have described characteristic thinning in the ganglion cell layer which comprises the optic nerve cup.[23] Clinicians use OCT to monitor and track these changes over the course of treatment. Researchers have compared the ability of SS-OCT and SD-OCT to measure optic nerve head rim area and volume. They found their glaucoma-differentiating ability overall comparable.[24] Another study explored unique optic nerve head measurements obtained by SS-OCT and their ability to discriminate between glaucoma and myopia.[25] The specifics of these articles are discussed below.

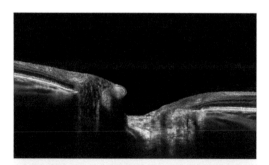

Fig. 13.4 High resolution B-scan of healthy (OS) nerve head. (Figure by Ryan McNabb, PhD, and Anthony Kuo, MD, of the Duke Eye Center.)

Kudsieh et al found that optic nerve measurements including cup-to-disc ratio and vertical cup-to-disc ratio showed excellent agreement between SS-OCT and SD-OCT imaging modalities.[24] In POAG patients, the rim area and volume were higher in SS-OCT compared with SD-OCT. For differentiating glaucoma from normal eyes the best parameter was cup-to-disc ratio by both SD-OCT and SS-OCT (AUC = 0.876 and AUC = 0.850, respectively).

Kim et al used optic nerve head measurements taken by SS-OCT to determine diagnostic power to differentiate between myopic normal and myopic NTG.[25] They found misalignment of optic disc angle (a novel marker used in this study indicating alignment between optic discs and posterior sclera) and horizontal tilt demonstrated best discrimination between myopic NTG and myopic normal (AUC = 0.696 and 0.682, respectively).

13.2.5 Lamina Cribrosa Application of SS-OCT in Glaucoma

The ability of SS-OCT to image deeper intraocular structures promises to improve our ability to image the lamina cribrosa, a structure deep within the optic nerve head, thought to be the primary site of axonal damage in glaucoma.[23] The following discussion benefits from the recent literature review by Takusagawa et al.[3]

Several studies report visibility of the anterior lamina cribrosa structures is generally more reliable than the posterior.[3]

SS-OCT scans of patients with glaucoma have demonstrated an increased lamina cribrosa depth, the distance from the plane of Bruch's membrane opening to the anterior surface of the lamina cribrosa. These findings have been shown to correlate with severity of glaucoma as well as younger age and higher untreated intraocular pressure and show dynamic reversal in response to glaucoma therapy. SS-OCT and SD-OCT measurements of the lamina cribrosa depth have been shown to be equivalent.[3]

SS-OCT scans of patients with glaucoma show more posteriorly located anterior lamina cribrosa insertion compared with normal, defined as the vertical distance between anterior laminar insertion to scleral wall and plane of Bruch's membrane opening. This finding appears to be more pronounced in patients with high-tension glaucoma compared with NTG.[3]

SS-OCT scan of patients with glaucoma demonstrate increased lamina cribrosa curvature index

13

(LCCI) compared with normal, defined as the difference between the mean lamina cribrosa depth and the anterior lamina cribrosa insertion depth. Likewise, this finding is more notable in high-tension glaucoma compared with NTG. Studies have shown that LCCI has good sensitivity and specificity for diagnosing glaucoma.[3]

SS-OCT scans of the lamina cribrosa thickness in glaucoma patients showed significant thinning compared with controls. Thinning appeared to correlate with glaucoma severity. This measurement has been shown to differentiate glaucoma from normal eyes with high degree of sensitivity and specificity.[3]

Anterior focal lamina cribrosa defects (FLCD) can be identified by SS-OCT and although this finding can also be seen in myopia, it is more specific for glaucoma. Studies have demonstrated its association with disc hemorrhages and corresponding visual field defects.[3]

SS-OCT has been used in an attempt to characterize the microarchitectural changes in glaucoma patients, such as the dimensions of the laminar pores and beams. Several studies found laminar pores are smaller with increased variability in size and tortuosity in glaucoma compared with normal. However, the results remain limited by overall poor visibility of the structures.[3]

SS-OCT is significantly better than unmodified SD-OCT at imaging the anterior and posterior lamina cribrosa and lamina cribrosa insertions. However, modified SD-OCT scans employing EDI and "adaptive compensation" (AC) performed equally well as SS-OCT.[3]

13.3 Future Research in SS-OCT for Evaluation of Glaucoma

Since SS-OCT is a relatively newly available technology in the United States, most of the studies to date have been performed in Asia. Given the variability in glaucoma subtypes based on ethnicity, such as higher rates of angle closure glaucoma and NTG in certain Asian populations, it will be interesting to see studies applying SS-OCT within the United States and comparing diagnostic properties in this context.

Another potential future direction for SS-OCT in glaucoma will be as an underlying platform for OCT-A (▶ Fig. 13.5). The advantages of SS-OCT— the ability to quickly obtain high-resolution images of large areas with deep penetration—also make it a favorable platform to study vascular

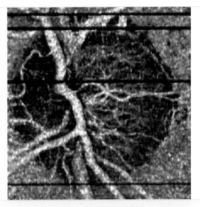

Fig. 13.5 Optical coherence tomography (OCT) angiography of optic nerve head. (Figure by Ryan McNabb, PhD, and Anthony Kuo, MD, of the Duke Eye Center.)

changes in glaucoma using OCT-A by decreasing artifacts and allowing imaging of deeper structures.

13.4 Conclusions

We have reviewed the current literature regarding use of SS-OCT in evaluation of glaucoma. This modality of OCT technology facilitates the imaging of intraocular structures with high resolution, range of depth, and increased scan speeds. Applications in glaucoma include improved imaging of the anterior chamber including visualization of deeper angle structures such as the scleral spur. Applications of SS-OCT in scanning of the retina include a single wide format scan which encompasses the macula and peripapillary area in a single scan which has been shown to be equivalent in differentiating glaucoma from normal as previous SD-OCT separates macula and peripapillary scans, which required longer time to acquire. Imaging of the optic disc and choroid with SS-OCT show noninferiority to the SD-OCT technology. Most studies have found that ocular measurements, whether involving the anterior segment or posterior segment, are well correlated between SD-OCT and SS-OCT, but the measurements are not interchangeable. Finally, SS-OCT shows potential advantages in imaging the deeper optic nerve structure of the lamina cribrosa; however, more evidence is required to differentiate its role from SD-OCT with enhanced depth imaging. We conclude SS-OCT is a promising new innovation in the realm of ophthalmic imaging with many applications in the field of glaucoma. Further research is needed to establish

13

its role among pre-existing imaging modalities and to also examine results among more diverse populations, including glaucoma patients in the United States.

References

[1] Lim H, Mujat M, Kerbage C, et al. High-speed imaging of human retina in vivo with swept-source optical coherence tomography. Opt Express. 2006; 14(26):12902–12908

[2] Potsaid B, Baumann B, Huang D, et al. Ultrahigh speed 1050 nm swept source/Fourier domain OCT retinal and anterior segment imaging at 100,000 to 400,000 axial scans per second. Opt Express. 2010; 18(19):20029–20048

[3] Takusagawa HL, Hoguet A, Junk AK, Nouri-Mahdavi K, Radhakrishnan S, Chen TC. Swept-source OCT for evaluating the lamina cribrosa: a report by the American Academy of Ophthalmology. Ophthalmology. 2019; 126(9):1315–1323

[4] Dong ZM, Wollstein G, Wang B, Schuman JS. Adaptive optics optical coherence tomography in glaucoma. Prog Retin Eye Res. 2017; 57:76–88

[5] Forte R, Cennamo GL, Finelli ML, de Crecchio G. Comparison of time domain Stratus OCT and spectral domain SLO/OCT for assessment of macular thickness and volume. Eye (Lond). 2009; 23(11):2071–2078

[6] Radhakrishnan S, Yarovoy D. Development in anterior segment imaging for glaucoma. Curr Opin Ophthalmol. 2014; 25 (2):98–103

[7] Li P, Johnstone M, Wang RK. Full anterior segment biometry with extended imaging range spectral domain optical coherence tomography at 1340 nm. J Biomed Opt. 2014; 19 (4):046013

[8] Li P, An L, Lan G, Johnstone M, Malchow D, Wang RK. Extended imaging depth to 12 mm for 1050-nm spectral domain optical coherence tomography for imaging the whole anterior segment of the human eye at 120-kHz A-scan rate. J Biomed Opt. 2013; 18(1):16012

[9] Shan J, DeBoer C, Xu BY. Anterior segment optical coherence tomography: applications for clinical care and scientific research. Asia Pac J Ophthalmol (Phila). 2019

[10] Xu BY, Mai DD, Penteado RC, Saunders L, Weinreb RN. Reproducibility and agreement of anterior segment parameter measurements obtained using the CASIA2 and Spectralis OCT2 optical coherence tomography devices. J Glaucoma. 2017; 26(11):974–979

[11] Qiao Y, Tan C, Zhang M, Sun X, Chen J. Comparison of spectral domain and swept source optical coherence tomography for angle assessment of Chinese elderly subjects. BMC Ophthalmol. 2019; 19(1):142

[12] Chansangpetch S, Nguyen A, Mora M, et al. Agreement of anterior segment parameters obtained from swept-source Fourier-domain and time-domain anterior segment optical coherence tomography. Invest Ophthalmol Vis Sci. 2018; 59 (3):1554–1561

[13] Lai I, Mak H, Lai G, Yu M, Lam DS, Leung CK. Anterior chamber angle imaging with swept-source optical coherence tomography: measuring peripheral anterior synechia in glaucoma. Ophthalmology. 2013; 120(6):1144–1149

[14] Mak H, Xu G, Leung CK. Imaging the iris with swept-source optical coherence tomography: relationship between iris volume and primary angle closure. Ophthalmology. 2013; 120 (12):2517–2524

[15] Yang Z, Tatham AJ, Weinreb RN, Medeiros FA, Liu T, Zangwill LM. Diagnostic ability of macular ganglion cell inner plexiform layer measurements in glaucoma using swept source and spectral domain optical coherence tomography. PLoS One. 2015; 10(5):e0125957

[16] Hong EH, Shin YU, Kang MH, Cho H, Seong M. Wide scan imaging with swept-source optical coherent tomography for glaucoma diagnosis. PLoS One. 2018; 13(4):e0195040

[17] Lee KM, Lee EJ, Kim TW, Kim H. Comparison of the abilities of SD-OCT and SS-OCT in evaluating the thickness of the macular inner layer for glaucoma diagnosis. PLoS One. 2016; 11(1):e0147964

[18] Lee SY, Lee EK, Park KH, Kim DM, Jeoung JW. Asymmetry analysis of macular inner retinal layers for glaucoma diagnosis: swept-source optical coherence tomography study. PLoS One. 2016; 11(10):e0164866

[19] Rao HL, Sreenivasaiah S, Dixit S, et al. Choroidal microvascular dropout in primary open-angle glaucoma eyes with disc hemorrhage. J Glaucoma. 2019; 28(3):181–187

[20] Hirooka K, Fujiwara A, Shiragami C, Baba T, Shiraga F. Relationship between progression of visual field damage and choroidal thickness in eyes with normal-tension glaucoma. Clin Exp Ophthalmol. 2012; 40(6):576–582

[21] Song YJ, Kim YK, Jeoung JW, Park KH. Assessment of open-angle glaucoma peripapillary and macular choroidal thickness using swept-source optical coherence tomography (SS-OCT). PLoS One. 2016; 11(6):e0157333

[22] Zhang C, Tatham AJ, Medeiros FA, Zangwill LM, Yang Z, Weinreb RN. Assessment of choroidal thickness in healthy and glaucomatous eyes using swept source optical coherence tomography. PLoS One. 2014; 9(10):e109683

[23] Quigley HA, Addicks EM, Green WR, Maumenee AE. Optic nerve damage in human glaucoma. II. The site of injury and susceptibility to damage. Arch Ophthalmol. 1981; 99(4):635–649

[24] Kudsieh B, Fernandez-Vigo JI, De-Pablo-Gómez-de-Liaño L, Fernández-Vigo C, Ruiz Moreno JM, Fernández-Vigo JÁ. Agreement between Fourier-domain and swept-source optical coherence tomography used for optic nerve head measurements. J Fr Ophtalmol. 2020; 43(1):25–30

[25] Kim YC, Cho BJ, Jung KI, Park CK. Comparison of diagnostic power of optic nerve head and posterior sclera configuration parameters on myopic normal tension glaucoma. J Glaucoma. 2019; 28(9):834–842

13

14 Future Directions: Artificial Intelligence Applications

Atalie Carina Thompson

Summary

Recent advances in the field of artificial intelligence, especially the development of deep learning algorithms, have spurred a surge of interest in their application for the detection of ophthalmic diseases such as glaucoma. As the leading cause of irreversible blindness worldwide, early and reliable diagnosis of glaucoma is critical so that appropriate treatment can be initiated. Optical coherence tomography (OCT) is the most commonly acquired imaging test to assess for early structural changes in the optic nerve head and macula due to glaucoma, but application of artificial intelligence (AI) may be able to glean additional information beyond current automated segmentation software. Several groups have demonstrated that deep learning algorithms can be trained to accurately distinguish between eyes with glaucomatous changes and healthy controls on OCT. Attention class activation maps, or heat maps, may point to additional structural changes from glaucoma that are not captured by the standard summary parameters provided by current OCT software. Deep learning (DL) models have also been developed to predict quantitative values from OCT, such as the retinal nerve fiber layer or Bruch's membrane opening–minimum rim width, from a color fundus photograph. Future studies will need to assess the performance of these different algorithms in real-world settings and explore whether novel algorithms can be built to detect glaucomatous progression on OCT.

Keywords: artificial intelligence, deep learning, machine learning classifiers, glaucoma, spectral domain optical coherence tomography

14.1 Introduction

Glaucoma is the leading cause of irreversible visual disability and blindness worldwide, with some studies estimating that nearly 112 million people will be impacted by the year 2040.[1]

However, the majority of patients with glaucoma are not aware they have this disease, which may be due to poor public awareness about glaucoma[2] and the fact that glaucoma remains relatively asymptomatic until the advanced stages. The concern that patients with glaucoma may not present until late in the disease has spurred interest in the development of affordable public health interventions to screen for and diagnose glaucoma so that effective treatments can be prescribed before the onset of substantial vision loss. However, prior efforts to screen for glaucoma using perimetry and tonometry have shown poor sensitivity and specificity at a population level.[3] Low-cost nonmydriatic fundus photographs are easy to acquire but require laborious subjective review by human graders. Moreover, studies have shown that human grades of color fundus photos have poor reproducibility[4] and poor sensitivity[5] for glaucoma in screening settings. The accuracy of these qualitative grades can be further limited in the cases of large physiologic cups, small optic nerve heads, or myopic tilted discs which can be challenging to evaluate.

Spectral domain optical coherence tomography (SD-OCT) has become the *de facto* standard for objective quantification of structural changes in the retinal nerve fiber layer (RNFL) and macula due to glaucoma because of its excellent reproducibility and accuracy.[6] SD-OCT can detect early structural glaucomatous changes before the onset of detectable visual field loss on standard automated perimetry. Although SD-OCT has been widely adopted in clinical practice, its high cost and the reliance on skilled operators for image acquisition have limited its utility in population-based screening.

Nevertheless, with recent advances in AI, especially the development of DL algorithms, there has been rising interest in building algorithms capable of diagnosing glaucoma on SD-OCT imaging. DL algorithms may be able not only to discriminate between eyes with and without glaucoma, but also to learn novel features on SD-OCT imaging that improve its discriminatory ability. By assessing the entire SD-OCT B-scan, DL algorithms may also obviate reliance on parameters derived from automated segmentation which can be prone to segmentation errors and artifacts. One group has also demonstrated a novel approach in which SD-OCT

14

data was used to develop DL algorithms that detected glaucomatous damage on color fundus photographs, thus improving the prospect of screening for glaucoma with low-cost photos. The purpose of this chapter is to provide a brief overview of AI with an emphasis on DL, and to then review select pivotal papers that have recently demonstrated how SD-OCT data can be used to develop DL algorithms capable of diagnosing glaucoma.

14.2 Artificial Intelligence

Artificial intelligence is a broad term that refers to the development of computer programs that can automate tasks in a way that mimics intelligent human behavior despite receiving minimal human input.[7] Broadly speaking, AI encompasses both machine learning classifiers (MLCs) and DL algorithms (▶ Fig. 14.1). MLCs are trained, rather than explicitly programmed, to find statistical patterns in datasets by being presented multiple relevant examples, and by this process they learn to automate the task. For traditional MLCs, the features need to have been already identified by humans using their domain knowledge. A distinct advantage of MLCs over traditional statistical programming is that MLCs can handle complex, large datasets that would not be practical to analyze using traditional statistical approaches. There are many types of MLCs including random forest (RF), logistic regression (LR), support vector machine (SVM),

independent component analysis (ICA), and Gaussian mixture model (GMM). Although research has been conducted using MLCs to classify glaucoma data, these previous studies were limited in the types of data that could be processed and often relied on the input of parameters from automated segmentation. This is because MLCs could only process data in one or two dimensions, and were not well suited for complex image processing.

The development of sophisticated convolutional neural networks (CNNs) has shifted the focus in AI in glaucoma to application of DL methods. DL refers to a relatively novel advance in machine learning in which a CNN autonomously learns features and tasks from a training dataset. Data is input, processed, and weighed through successive layers of these neural networks, which consist of series of interconnected nodes, until the algorithm develops a system of classifications capable of making a prediction (▶ Fig. 14.2). CNNs are substantially more complex and refined than MLCs. DL algorithms do not require that the specific features of interest in an image be identified a priori by the human programmer. Also, unlike MLCs which can only process data in a small number of dimensions, DL algorithms can process very complex data in multiple dimensions, and are thus better suited to the processing of ophthalmic imaging.

14.2.1 Development of a Deep Learning Algorithm

Training of a CNN goes through three basic stages: training, validation, and testing. There are also three approaches to training a CNN: supervised, unsupervised, and semi-supervised learning. In supervised learning, the DL algorithm is trained using a dataset where every image has a label, such as glaucoma or healthy. Unsupervised learning, on the other hand, exposes the algorithm to unlabeled data and allows it to extract novel patterns from the data. In semi-supervised learning the algorithm first trains on a large unlabeled dataset and then a much smaller labeled dataset in order to improve its performance. Next the DL algorithm must be validated to determine how well the model fits the training dataset. Finally, the performance is evaluated by applying the DL algorithm to a separate test dataset. It is important that the images from the same patient or same eye do not exist in both the testing dataset and the training/validation datasets because this can lead to biased overestimates of the algorithm's performance.

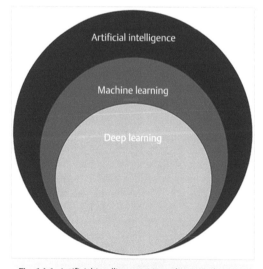

Fig. 14.1 Artificial intelligence. Venn diagram showing the relationship of deep learning and machine learning within the framework of artificial intelligence.

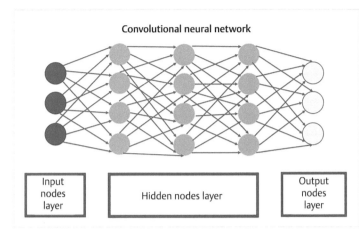

Convolutional neural network

Input nodes layer

Hidden nodes layer

Output nodes layer

Fig. 14.2 Convolutional neural network. Schematic diagram showing layers of nodes, including input, hidden, and output nodes.

Transfer Learning

Due to their complexity, DL algorithms require much larger datasets to train in the order of millions of ophthalmic images, which is not practical to obtain. Thus, transfer learning techniques are increasingly applied to improve the performance of DL algorithms in ophthalmology.[8] Transfer learning makes use of a CNN that has already been trained to be a general image classifier using a very large general image dataset such as ResNet34 or InceptionV3. Additional training is then conduced with a much smaller dataset of ophthalmic images to improve its performance for a specific task, such as discriminating between glaucomatous and healthy eyes. Application of transfer learning has enhanced the feasibility of developing high-performing DL algorithms for detecting glaucoma on SD-OCT and other ophthalmic imaging.

14.2.2 Deep Learning Algorithms to Diagnose Glaucoma on SD-OCT

Several groups have developed novel DL algorithms that can distinguish eyes with glaucoma from those without glaucoma when applied to SD-OCT images. CNNs can be developed to make predictions directly from the OCT imaging or can be combined in hybrid approaches that harness the CNN to extract the relevant features from OCT imaging so that machine learning techniques can be applied to classify the images. Muhammad and colleagues,[9] for example, generated a hybrid deep learning model (HDLM) for diagnosing glaucoma from OCT. They obtained 9 × 12 mm swept-source OCT images in 102 eyes (57 with glaucoma and 45 no glaucoma according to expert diagnosis using clinical information and imaging); and from these OCT scans

they generated six images to be input to the CNN: (1) three-color channel thickness map for the retinal ganglion cells (RGCs), (2) three-color channel thickness map for the RNFL, (3) RNFL probability map, (4) RGC probability map, (5) en face projection image, and (6) a combination image where the red channel was replaced with the RNFL probability values, the green channel with the RGC probability values, and the blue channel with normalized RNFL thickness values. Using AlexNet, a two-dimensional CNN pretrained on ImageNet, they performed feature extraction with the Caffe DL framework using each of the six aforementioned images as input to the CNN. The extracted features were then used as input to a RF model for classification of the images as glaucomatous or healthy, and the predictions were compared against traditional visual field and OCT metrics. In this study, the HDLM based on the RNFL probability map had the highest accuracy and lowest variability (93.1% +/- 0.57%), and was significantly better than conventional clinical metrics such as OCT quadrant analysis (accuracy 83.7%) or 24–2 Humphrey visual field mean deviation (80.4%) (all $p < 0.001$). However, other features did not perform well; for example, the en face projection showed the poorest accuracy and greatest variability (65.7% +/- 1.53%). One limitation of this study was the very small size of the training set. Transfer learning was performed using AlexNet but it is possible the accuracy of the algorithm would be higher if trained only on OCT images, especially given the small size of the OCT training set. Moreover, one can argue that outperforming isolated clinical metrics like OCT or perimetry parameters is not that difficult.

Asaoka et al[10] conducted a much larger, multi-institutional study to determine if a DL model would perform better than traditional MLCs for

14

distinguishing early glaucoma from normal eyes on OCT macular maps of the RNFL and ganglion cell layer complex. Pretraining was performed using a large OCT (RS 3000 OCT, Nidek Co., Gamagori, Japan) dataset from the Japanese Archives of Multicentral Images of Glaucomatous Optical Coherence Tomography database, and consisted of 4,073 OCT images from 1,371 eyes in 747 subjects with open angle glaucoma and 243 images from 193 healthy eyes in 113 subjects. Then additional training was conducted on a smaller separate dataset of images acquired with the Topcon OCT-1000 or OCT-2000 machine (Topcon Corporation, Tokyo, Japan) in 94 eyes/subjects with early open angle glaucoma (OAG) and mean deviation (MD)> −5 dB and 84 normal eyes/subjects. The 8×8 grid macular RNFL and ganglion cell complex layer thickness from SD-OCT was input to the DL model. Testing of the DL algorithm was performed on a separate dataset of 114 eyes/subjects with OAG and MD>−5 dB, and 82 normal eyes/subjects. The diagnostic accuracy of the DL model was significantly greater than that of two traditional MLCs, namely, RF and SVM (area under the receiver operating characteristic [AUC] curve = 93.7% vs. 82.0% or 67.4%, respectively, $p < 0.001$). However, a notable limitation of this model was the reliance on macular map data without any input of circumpapillary RNFL data, which is more commonly acquired in clinical practice and which may have been able to improve the model's performance.

Another drawback common to the two approaches just described is their reliance on OCT parameters and maps derived from the OCT machine's automated segmentation software. Thus, the accuracy of these DL algorithms relied on the accurate segmentation of the acquired OCT images. However, OCT segmentation can be prone to artifact and segmentation errors, especially in older patients or cases of advanced glaucoma. Studies have suggested that segmentation errors may be present on 20 to 40% of OCT scans, which can undermine the accuracy of segmented parameters. Moreover, in the aforementioned studies, the selected input was restricted to those structural features on OCT that are already known to be affected by glaucoma, such as the RNFL and ganglion cell complex, thus excluding the possibility of learning from other structural features on OCT. Application of DL algorithms directly to raw, unsegmented B-scans from the OCT can allow the DL algorithm to learn from the entire B-scan image, rather than preselected features or parameters, and thus may prove more accurate.

In a recently published work, Maetschke et al[11] developed a "feature agnostic" 3D CNN that could distinguish between healthy and glaucomatous eyes from raw, unsegmented OCT volumes of the optic nerve head. Their study consisted of 263 scans in 137 healthy patients and 847 scans in 432 primary open-angle glaucoma (POAG) patients. They compared this novel approach to the more traditional feature-based approach where various MLCs were trained using 22 segmented measurements from the Cirrus OCT (i.e., peripapillary RNFL thickness at 12 clock-hours, peripapillary RNFL thickness in four quadrants, average RNFL thickness, rim area, disc area, average cup-to-disc ratio, vertical cup-to-disc ratio, and cup volume). Logistic regression had the highest AUC among MLCs in the test dataset (0.89 ± 0.028) but this was significantly lower than the performance of the feature agnostic DL algorithm which achieved an AUC of 0.94 +/− 0.036 ($p < 0.05$). Also of note was the fact that the class activation maps of the volume scans highlighted additional regions important in the algorithm's classification, such as the lamina cribrosa, which may be a useful biomarker for glaucoma. Thus, this paper demonstrated that a DL model trained on a raw OCT volume scan outperformed MLCs that were trained using features derived from automated segmentation.

Another advantage of a DL model trained on unsegmented OCT B-scans is that it can produce a single probabilistic output for a diagnosis of glaucoma, which can be preferable to simultaneous interpretation of individual parameters. When faced with a high number of summary parameters, clinicians can find it difficult to determine which parameters are most important especially if they do not correspond with each other. Moreover, the more the number of parameters available the greater the likelihood of committing a type I error, or finding a false-positive test. This point was recently highlighted in a paper by Thompson et al.[12] In this study, a DL algorithm was trained to discriminate between glaucomatous and healthy eyes using the raw unsegmented peripapillary SD-OCT B-scan. The dataset consisted of 20,806 RNFL circle B-scans in 1,154 eyes of 635 participants. The ResNet34 architecture, which had been previously trained on ImageNet, was used for additional training of the DL algorithm. When analyzing the segmentation-free circle B-scan, the DL algorithm had a significantly greater AUC than conventional SD-OCT parameters like global RNFL thickness (0.96 vs. 0.87) or each of the RNFL sector values for discriminating between glaucomatous and control eyes (all $p < 0.001$). The sensitivity at both 80 and 95% specificity was also substantially greater for the DL algorithm than RNFL. Finally, when stratifying on glaucoma severity using the Hodapp-Parrish-Anderson criteria, the AUC was larger for the DL algorithm than for global RNFL at each level of severity, especially among those with preperimetric or mild glaucoma ($p < 0.001$). The application of this segmentation-free DL algorithm in clinical practice may improve the accuracy and sensitivity of SD-OCT for glaucoma diagnosis relative to the use of conventional RNFL from automated segmentation. Also, by providing a single probabilistic output rather than multiple SD-OCT summary parameters, use of the DL algorithm could decrease the risk of "red disease" or erroneously detecting glaucoma due to a false-positive test. Another advantage is that use of this algorithm obviates the reliance on potentially error-prone segmentation. Finally, class activation maps in this study highlighted areas on the SD-OCT B-scan beyond the RNFL, suggesting that other parts of the retinal architecture may also be important in detecting glaucoma.

14.2.3 Deep Learning Algorithms Trained to Assess Color Fundus Photos Using SD-OCT

The early success of DL algorithms trained on SD-OCT data to diagnose glaucoma on SD-OCT is not entirely surprising. However, the application of these algorithms is more likely to be in a clinical setting, as SD-OCT is not likely to be used in screening scenarios due to its high cost and operator requirements. Thus, numerous groups have focused on the development of DL algorithms that can diagnose glaucoma from color fundus imaging.[13,14,15] Although many of these landmark studies demonstrated excellent accuracy for detection of glaucoma, the approach had several notable limitations and underlying assumptions. The subjective label provided by human graders was used as the ground truth for these algorithms. However, human gradings of photos for glaucoma tend to have poor reproducibility,[4,16,17] low interrater reliability,[4,5,17] and decreased sensitivity particularly in a screening setting.[5,18,19,20] Clinicians tend to overdiagnose glaucoma in physiologically enlarged cups and underdiagnose it in small optic nerve heads.[14] The process of human grading is also laborious and time-consuming. Thus, human graders may not provide a suitable reference standard

for training a DL algorithm. Moreover, it is possible that DL algorithms trained to detect glaucoma based on subjective human grades will replicate common human errors.

In response to these challenges, Medeiros et al developed a novel approach of training a machine-to-machine (M2M) DL algorithm in which color fundus photographs were labeled with an objective reference standard, the corresponding global RNFL thickness measurement from SD-OCT.[21] Because the label was a quantitative number, the M2M algorithm learned to predict the global RNFL value when evaluating a color fundus photograph, thus estimating the amount of neuroretinal damage from glaucoma. The DL algorithm's predicted RNFL value from color fundus photo was strongly and significantly correlated with the actual RNFL value from the corresponding SD-OCT (Pearson $r = 0.832$, $p < 0.001$), and there was a low mean absolute error of 7.39 μm. A related DL algorithm was also trained to classify fundus photos as either normal or abnormal using the categorical label from the SD-OCT instrument's normative database. The AUC for distinguishing between eyes with and without glaucoma was similar for the DL algorithm and actual RNFL value (AUC = 0.944 and 0.940, respectively; $p = 0.724$). Class activation maps highlighted those regions of the color photograph, mainly the neuroretinal rim and peripapillary RNFL, that were most important in the DL algorithm's prediction (▶ Fig. 14.3). This novel approach offered a distinct advantage by providing SD-OCT as an objective and reproducible reference standard. The reliance on subjective human gradings was thus obviated. Also, since the output of the M2M model is quantitative rather than binary, specificity cut-offs could be established in order to optimize its application in a screening setting. A DL algorithm was also trained to distinguish between normal and abnormal using the classification of the global RNFL by the SD-OCT instrument's normative database. The DL AUC for discriminating eyes with and without glaucoma was 0.944 which was similar to the AUC of 0.940 for the actual RNFL values ($p = 0.724$). Thus, the DL algorithm was able to accurately predict the SD-OCT RNFL value based on its assessment of a color fundus photograph.

In a related study, Thompson et al applied the same approach and labeled color fundus photographs with another summary quantitative SD-OCT parameter of neuroretinal damage, the Bruch's membrane opening–minimum rim width (BMO-MRW) parameter.[22] Studies have suggested

14

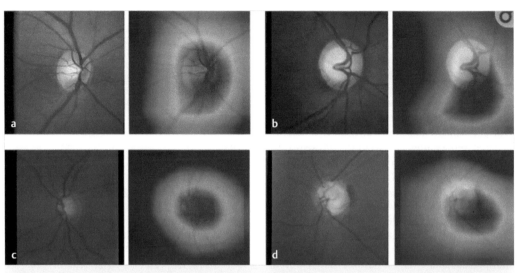

Fig. 14.3 Class activation maps of optic nerve photos. Class activation maps (heat maps) showing the regions of the photograph that had greatest weight in the deep learning algorithm classification. **(a)** Healthy eye. **(b)** Glaucoma suspect. **(c, d)** Glaucomatous eyes. (Reproduced with permission from Elsevier from Medeiros FA,. Jammal AA, Thompson AC. From machine to machine: an OCT-trained deep learning algorithm for objective quantification of glaucomatous damage in fundus photographs. Ophthalmology 2019;126:513–521.)

that BMO-MRW may be more sensitive to early glaucomatous changes,[23] and can be useful for detecting glaucoma when the optic disc is difficult to grade due to high myopia.[24] Similar to the preceding study, there was a high and significant correlation between the DL predictions and the actual SD-OCT BMO-MRW values (Pearson's $r = 0.88$, $p < 0.001$). Also, the DL algorithm performed at least as well as the original BMO-MRW value for distinguishing between glaucoma and healthy eyes (AUC = 0.945 for the DL predictions vs. 0.933 for the actual BMO-MRW; $p = 0.587$). One question raised by these two studies is whether these DL algorithms that have been trained to predict quantitative SD-OCT data from color fundus photographs will perform as well as human graders.

This issue was addressed in a follow-up study by Jammal et al[25] in which the M2M DL algorithm was compared to human graders for the detection of reproducible glaucomatous visual field loss. In this study, the DL algorithm performed at least as well as and sometimes better than human graders. When compared to the probability of glaucomatous optic neuropathy (GON) given by human graders (rho = 0.48), the DL-predicted RNFL thickness had a significantly greater correlation with standard automated perimetry (SAP) mean deviation (rho = 0.54; $p < 0.001$). The partial AUC for the M2M DL algorithm's prediction was also

significantly greater than the probability of GON by human graders (pAUC = 0.529 vs. 0.411, $p = 0.016$). The results of this study suggest that human graders could potentially be replaced by the M2M DL algorithm, thus decreasing the amount of necessary human labor as well as reducing the errors introduced when humans serve as the reference standard. By obviating the reliance on human graders, this and other DL algorithms could potentially improve the feasibility of using color fundus photographs to screen for glaucoma.

14.2.4 Limitations

The field of AI in glaucoma is only in its nascent stages. Although the studies discussed in this chapter have proposed novel ways to train DL algorithms to detect glaucomatous damage either on SD-OCT or on color fundus photographs, the performance of these algorithms has to be interpreted with a modicum of precaution. First, the studies to date have trained algorithms that can discriminate between glaucoma and healthy controls, excluding glaucoma suspects from their training and test samples. However, glaucoma suspects present many of the diagnostic challenges that make the detection of glaucoma so difficult, and glaucoma suspects comprise a substantial proportion of the patients that visit glaucoma specialists. Future algorithms should be trained to distinguish between glaucoma suspects that do not have glaucoma (e.g., physiologic cupping) from those that have true glaucoma (e.g., small optic nerve head with a notch but small cup). Also, the datasets used for training and testing in the studies to date have been free of other comorbid ophthalmic diagnoses. Whether these DL algorithms will perform as well in patients with concurrent diabetic retinopathy or other significant retinal pathology remains to be seen. There is also the concern that the type of machine used to acquire the images heavily influences the performance of the algorithms; in other words, the algorithms will underperform if tested on images acquired by a different camera or SD-OCT machine than the one that obtained the training images. Issues of image quality also need to be addressed since poor quality images can cause algorithms to underperform. DL algorithms could be trained to account for image quality so that the algorithm will differentially weigh information acquired in poor versus high quality images. Finally, these algorithms need to be externally validated in different populations. Patients with high myopia or hyperopia were typically excluded from these studies, and structural differences due to racial variation may also impact the performance of these algorithms. The algorithms also need to be tested in different settings since they are likely to perform better in a clinical setting with a high concentration of glaucoma patients than in screening settings where the prevalence of glaucoma is very low.

14.2.5 Future Directions

Despite the limitations discussed, the early work of AI applied to OCT in glaucoma has been promising. Several groups have demonstrated that DL algorithms can be trained to accurately distinguish between glaucoma and healthy controls on OCT. OCT data can even be used to train DL algorithms that predict quantitative values such as RNFL or BMO-MRW from assessment of color fundus photographs, thus potentially obviating the reliance on human graders. However, the work to date has used cross-sectional datasets and focused on detection of glaucoma, rather than the diagnosis of glaucoma progression. Future studies should investigate whether DL algorithms can detect or predict progression of glaucoma on OCT imaging using large longitudinal datasets. Analysis of OCT angiography data may also provide insights into the impact of blood flow on glaucoma. Acquisition

of electronic healthcare records especially by pooling data across multiple institutions may improve the feasibility of acquiring large datasets for the training and testing of algorithms. Finally, application of these DL algorithms to clinical scenarios and screening settings will be needed to assess whether these algorithms perform well in the real world.

References

[1] Tham YC, Li X, Wong TY, Quigley HA, Aung T, Cheng CY. Global prevalence of glaucoma and projections of glaucoma burden through 2040: a systematic review and meta-analysis. Ophthalmology. 2014; 121(11):2081–2090

[2] Hennis A, Wu SY, Nemesure B, Honkanen R, Leske MC, Barbados Eye Studies Group. Awareness of incident open-angle glaucoma in a population study: the Barbados Eye Studies. Ophthalmology. 2007; 114(10):1816–1821

[3] Ervin AM, Boland MV, Myrowitz EH, et al. AHRQ Comparative Effectiveness Reviews. Screening for Glaucoma: Comparative Effectiveness. Rockville (MD): Agency for Healthcare Research and Quality (US); 2012

[4] Abrams LS, Scott IU, Spaeth GL, Quigley HA, Varma R. Agreement among optometrists, ophthalmologists, and residents in evaluating the optic disc for glaucoma. Ophthalmology. 1994; 101(10):1662–1667

[5] Chan HH, Ong DN, Kong YX, et al. Glaucomatous optic neuropathy evaluation (GONE) project: the effect of monoscopic versus stereoscopic viewing conditions on optic nerve evaluation. Am J Ophthalmol. 2014; 157(5):936–944

[6] Leung CK, Cheung CY, Weinreb RN, et al. Retinal nerve fiber layer imaging with spectral-domain optical coherence tomography: a variability and diagnostic performance study. Ophthalmology. 2009; 116(7):1257–1263, 1263.e1–1263.e2

[7] Chollet F. Deep Learning with Python. Shelter Island, NY: Manning Publications Co.; 2018:386

[8] Weiss K, Khoshgoftaar TM, Wang D. A survey of transfer learning. J Big Data. 2016; 3,:9

[9] Muhammad H, Fuchs TJ, De Cuir N, et al. Hybrid deep learning on single wide-field optical coherence tomography scans accurately classifies glaucoma suspects. J Glaucoma. 2017; 26 (12):1086–1094

[10] Asaoka R, Murata H, Hirasawa K, et al. Using deep learning and transfer learning to accurately diagnose early-onset glaucoma from macular optical coherence tomography images. Am J Ophthalmol. 2019; 198:136–145

[11] Maetschke S, Antony B, Ishikawa H, Wollstein G, Schuman J, Garnavi R. A feature agnostic approach for glaucoma detection in OCT volumes. PLoS One. 2019; 14(7):e0219126

[12] Thompson AC, Jammal AA, Berchuck SI, Mariottoni EB, Medeiros FA. Assessment of a segmentation-free deep learning algorithm for diagnosing glaucoma from optical coherence tomography scans. JAMA Ophthalmol. 2020; 138 (4):333–339

[13] Ting DSW, Cheung CY, Lim G, et al. Development and validation of a deep learning system for diabetic retinopathy and related eye diseases using retinal images from multiethnic populations with diabetes. JAMA. 2017; 318(22):2211–2223

[14] Li Z, He Y, Keel S, Meng W, Chang RT, He M. Efficacy of a deep learning system for detecting glaucomatous optic neuropathy based on color fundus photographs. Ophthalmology. 2018; 125(8):1199–1206

14

[15] Christopher M, Belghith A, Bowd C, et al. Performance of deep learning architectures and transfer learning for detecting glaucomatous optic neuropathy in fundus photographs. Sci Rep. 2018; 8(1):16685

[16] Varma R, Steinmann WC, Scott IU. Expert agreement in evaluating the optic disc for glaucoma. Ophthalmology. 1992; 99 (2):215–221

[17] Jampel HD, Friedman D, Quigley H, et al. Agreement among glaucoma specialists in assessing progressive disc changes from photographs in open-angle glaucoma patients. Am J Ophthalmol. 2009; 147(1):39–44.e1

[18] Kumar S, Giubilato A, Morgan W, et al. Glaucoma screening: analysis of conventional and telemedicine-friendly devices. Clin Exp Ophthalmol. 2007; 35(3):237–243

[19] Lichter PR. Variability of expert observers in evaluating the optic disc. Trans Am Ophthalmol Soc. 1976; 74:532–572

[20] Marcus DM, Brooks SE, Ulrich LD, et al. Telemedicine diagnosis of eye disorders by direct ophthalmoscopy. A pilot study. Ophthalmology. 1998; 105(10):1907–1914

[21] Medeiros FA, Jammal AA, Thompson AC. From machine to machine: an OCT-trained deep learning algorithm for objective quantification of glaucomatous damage in fundus photographs. Ophthalmology. 2019; 126(4):513–521

[22] Thompson AC, Jammal AA, Medeiros FA. A deep learning algorithm to quantify neuroretinal rim loss from optic disc photographs. Am J Ophthalmol. 2019; 201:9–18

[23] Chauhan BC, O'Leary N, AlMobarak FA, et al. Enhanced detection of open-angle glaucoma with an anatomically accurate optical coherence tomography-derived neuroretinal rim parameter. Ophthalmology. 2013; 120(3):535–543

[24] Reznicek L, Burzer S, Laubichler A, et al. Structure-function relationship comparison between retinal nerve fibre layer and Bruch's membrane opening-minimum rim width in glaucoma. Int J Ophthalmol. 2017; 10(10):1534–1538

[25] Jammal AA, Thompson AC, Mariottoni EB, et al. Human versus machine: comparing a deep learning algorithm to human gradings for detecting glaucoma on fundus photographs. Am J Ophthalmol. 2020;211:123 – 131

14

Index

Note: Page numbers set **bold** or *italic* indicate headings or figures, respectively.